Paediatric Audiology 0–5 Years

Third edition

Edited by

BARRY McCORMICK OBE, PhD

W
WHURR PUBLISHERS
LONDON AND PHILADELPHIA

© 2004 Whurr Publishers

First Edition Published 1988
Second Edition Published 1993
Third edition © 2004 Whurr Publishers Ltd
19b Compton Terrace, London N1 2UN, England

British Library Cataloguing in Publication Data
A catalogue record for this book is available from the British Library.

ISBN 186156 217 9

Printed and bound in the UK by Athenaeum Press Limited, Gateshead, Tyne & Wear.

Contents

Contributors

Claire L. Benton MSc, Queen's Medical Centre, University Hospital, Nottingham.

Jacqueline E. Brough MSc, Queen's Medical Centre, University Hospital, Nottingham.

Adrian Davis PhD, MRC Institute of Hearing Research, Nottingham University.

Michelle C. Dodd MSc, Queen's Medical Centre, University Hospital, Nottingham.

Christian J. Durst MSc, MED-EL UK Ltd, Holmfirth.

Philip Evans MSc, Guy's Hospital, London.

Sarah Flynn MSc, University of Southampton.

Kevin Gibbin FRCS, Queen's Medical Centre, University Hospital, Nottingham.

Roger Green PhD, King Edward VII Hospital, Windsor.

Steve Mason PhD, Queen's Medical Centre, University Hospital, Nottingham.

Barry McCormick OBE, PhD, Queen's Medical Centre, University Hospital, Nottingham.

George Mencher PhD, MRC Institute of Hearing Research, Nottingham University.

Jackie Moon MSc, Queen's Medical Centre, University Hospital, Nottingham.

Padma Moorjani PhD, MRC Institute of Hearing Research, Nottingham University.

Paul Shaw MSc, Queen's Medical Centre, University Hospital, Nottingham.

Sally Wood MSc, MRC Institute of Hearing Research, Nottingham University.

Preface

When preparing the first edition of this book in 1988 and the second edition in 1993 it could not have been envisaged that there would be so many new developments to report in this the third edition. Reflecting on nearly 30 years of experience working with deaf children there has never been a more exciting time to be working in the field of paediatric audiology. Developments in neonatal hearing screening, digital hearing aid technology and, of course, cochlear implantation, have influenced the lives of deaf individuals to a degree that could not have been imagined a generation ago. Paediatric audiology is truly a very rewarding and very challenging field in which to work bringing together, as it does, the disciplines of science, technology, medicine and education to enrich the lives of deaf children and their families.

It is hoped that this third edition will appeal to experienced practitioners who wish to keep abreast of the latest developments and also to students who are fortunate enough to be entering the field.

Barry McCormick
August 2003

Chapter 1

An epidemiological perspective on childhood hearing impairment

ADRIAN DAVIS, GEORGE MENCHER, PADMA MOORJANI

Introduction

Hearing impairment is the most prevalent congenital sensory deficit in the human population, with at least one in every 842 babies born in the UK with a permanent hearing loss or deafness detectable at birth (Davis, 1993). Permanent childhood hearing impairment (PCHI) can have a devastating impact on the acquisition of language and development of communication skills, which in turn can lead to poor literacy skills (see, for example, Bench and Bamford, 1979; Conrad, 1979; Levitt et al., 1987; Gallaway et al., 1994; Gregory, 1995). It is also likely that other areas of development will be affected, for example educational achievement (Powers, 1996), mental health (Laurenzi and Monteiro, 1997), self-esteem (Batchava, 1993) and long-term employment opportunities (Gregory et al., 1995) with a high cost to society (Mohr et al., 2000). It is possible that, given adequate support, the effect of these difficulties may be reduced. For example, language development may be enhanced through the use of language-support programmes, residual hearing may be used effectively through adequate amplification (hearing aids or cochlear implants) and family support may be provided through educational services, audiology services and social services. Evidence increasingly shows that such a support programme, used in tandem with early identification procedures, such as universal neonatal hearing screening, is most beneficial the earlier it is embarked upon by the families of hearing impaired children (for example, Yoshinaga-Itano et al., 1998). The assumption that quality-assured services for hearing

1

impaired children are of crucial importance has led to the formulation of a series of quality standards in paediatric audiology (NDCS, 1994, 1995, 1996, 2002). In order to achieve the high levels of continuing care needed by these children in the form of health and educational provision, the services need to be as effective as possible and targeted to groups that will benefit most. Details of the epidemiology of permanent childhood hearing impairment (PCHI) and a current service provision for PCHI informs the public health context in which all these services are provided. To inform priorities concerning prevention, early identification and rehabilitation, an appropriate understanding of the epidemiology is essential.

In this chapter epidemiological data on permanent childhood hearing impairment (PCHI) are presented relating to:

- the prevalence of permanent childhood hearing impairment (PCHI), as a function of severity, onset and demographics;
- the natural history of PCHI;
- the major risk factors for PCHI;
- the differential aetiology of PCHI and the current service indicators, for example the age of referral, confirmation and fitting of hearing aids for PCHI.

Going beyond the epidemiological data, the implications of the data and the changing climate of health service provision such as the provision of family-friendly hearing services and newborn hearing screening will be discussed.

Definitions used in epidemiological studies

Epidemiology is the study of the distribution and determinants of disease frequency in human population. Epidemiological information may be used to 'plan and evaluate strategies to prevent illness and as a guide to the management of patients in whom disease has already developed' (Coggon et al., 1993). Sancho et al. (1988) use the term 'epidemiology' to refer to 'the study of the distribution and determinants of hearing disorders in a population, and the application of the knowledge obtained to the prevention and amelioration of hearing problems.' A *population study* is the primary methodology for gathering information. The word 'population' in this case refers to the whole collection of units from which a sample may be drawn, but is not necessarily limited to a population of people. For example, it may be a collection of hearing aid clinics, schools for the deaf, and so forth. The sample is intended to give results that are representative of the population as a whole. If the population under study is people, the term *cohort* may come into play. A cohort is that component of a population born during a particular period and identified by period of birth, so that its characteristics (for example, prevalence of childhood hearing impairment, age at first hearing aid fitting) can be ascertained as it enters successive time and age periods. If an epidemiological study follows a cohort and studies the group at several different intervals, the project is called a *cohort study*. A cohort study can be a follow-up study, a prospective study, a retrospective or a longitudinal study. A cohort study is essential to understanding change over time and the impact of services.

Another key term associated with epidemiology is *incidence*. This refers to the number of new instances of a specific condition (for example, hearing impairment from meningitis) occurring during a certain period in a specified population. The *incidence rate* is the rate at which this occurs per standard population (for example, 10 new cases per year per 100,000 children). The term *prevalence* is often confused with incidence. However, these are not the same things. Prevalence is the total number of instances within a given population at a specific time in which a specific condition (for example, Pendred syndrome) is present. In the case of hearing loss, prevalence may be described as 'the proportion of individuals with a defined type of hearing impairment in a specified population cohort' (Sancho et al., 1988). Accordingly, *prevalence rate* is the number of individuals who have the condition or attribute divided by the population at risk at a point in time.

When attempting a prevalence study, if there are n children with hearing impairment in the study and the whole population is N, then the prevalence rate is (n*100/N)%. In this case we must be sure that the n hearing impaired children really come from all the birth cohorts of children represented by the population of N and that there is a co-terminosity of n and N, in terms of geographical boundaries. It is quite common to either underestimate n (because not all children with a given condition have been found) or to confuse populations (often because of migration of children into or out of particular districts). A population study is one in which the sample is carefully selected for representativeness of the whole population.

The importance and difficulty of estimating prevalence

One of the most important purposes for the collection of epidemiological information is to use it in planning preventative and rehabilitative services for hearing impaired children. The paucity of data on the prevalence and causes of childhood hearing impairment worldwide is exacerbated by the great difficulty in interpreting the data; perhaps leading to the variability in prevalence rates seen to from study to study. These variations may be due in part to a number of factors; the criteria used to define hearing impairment, adoption of different operational definitions, or use of incompatible methodologies. Agreed definitions for epidemiological studies, such as those outlined in the previous section, can be seen to be of paramount importance. Studies also tend to be cross-sectional and based on retrospective ascertainment rather than longitudinal studies in well-defined geographical areas. The problem of not using a common definition across studies can be seen to hinder estimates of prevalence rates as well as investigating possible risk factors and aetiologies of hearing impairment, this in turn has implications for the planning of service provision. Some commonly used definitions used for the various types of hearing impediment are as given in Appendix 1.

Given the variety of types of hearing impairments presented in Appendix 1, it can easily be understood why there may be some confusion when attempting to define prevalence and/or incidence. The problem is compounded when various generalized categories for the aetiology (cause) of the hearing impairment and the pattern of the hearing loss are taken into consideration. *Temporary hearing impairment* (usually, but not always a conductive hearing loss) can be treated and corrected by medical or surgical intervention. Such an impairment is often short-lived and of a mild nature. On the other hand, *permanent hearing impairment* cannot be treated by surgical or medical intervention and results in a permanent hearing loss greater than 40 dB HL. Both temporary and permanent losses can be *unilateral* (one ear only has either a greater than 20 dB hearing loss through 500, 1,000 and 2,000 kHz or one frequency exceeding 50 dB, with the other ear normal); or *bilateral* (a greater than 20 dB hearing loss through 500, 1,000 and 2,000 kHz or one frequency exceeding 50 dB in both ears).

A unilateral situation is, of course, asymmetrical. However, in studies of hearing, the term *asymmetrical hearing impairment* specifically refers to a greater than 10 dB difference between the ears in at least two frequencies, with the pure-tone average in the better ear exceeding 20 dB HL. Finally, both temporary and permanent losses can be *progressive hearing impairments.* That is, there is a deterioration of greater than or equal to 15 dB in the pure-tone average within a 10-year period.

Historically, the convenient figure of 1 per 1,000 for sensorineural deafness has often been quoted (Fraser, 1976). Further estimates of the prevalence of childhood hearing impairment (worldwide) vary in the literature from 0.5/1,000 to 1.5/1,000 births (for example, Newton, 1985; Das, 1990; Feinmesser et al., 1990; Pabla et al., 1991; Davis and Wood, 1992; Parving, 1993; Fortnum and Davis, 1997).

Note that the terms utilized are 'sensorineural deafness' and 'hearing impairment'. Not only are these different words, but they also represent different things. The term *deaf* is generally associated with the most extreme form of hearing impairment, in which there is no response to auditory stimuli in excess of 120–125 dB at any frequency. This condition is practically never seen and is considered very rare. *Hearing impairment,* on the other hand, primarily refers to a series of descriptive terms that define the decibel level at which an individual responds to sound (see Appendix 2). Hearing impairment is also defined by the frequency range the person can hear. That is, a *low frequency range* is less than 500 kHz; a *mid-frequency range* is 500 kHz to 2,000 kHz; a *high frequency range* is 2,000 to 8,000 kHz; and an *extended high frequency range* is greater than 8,000 kHz. The pattern of the frequencies is also important with some fairly self-explanatory terms such as 'u-shaped', 'low-frequency ascending', 'flat', and 'high-frequency sloping', used as descriptors of the responses plotted on an audiogram.

Prevalence of hearing loss in the UK

General studies

According to published figures, for the general population of the UK prevalence rates are 1–2 per 1,000 for severe/profound sensorineural deafness (see, for example, Newton, 1985; Parving, 1985; Peckham, 1986). Various studies have been carried out in the UK to ascertain accurate prevalence rates;

however, there has been considerable disagreement between the rates established. Such variation may be explained by population differences, for example regional variation, different target age groups, success of ascertainment, degree of hearing loss included in sample; as well as the method used to collect information: for example, ascertainment, prospective, longitudinal, and the reliability and range of the data collected. This can be illustrated best by outlining some of the studies.

Pabla et al. (1991) concluded a prevalence rate of 0.55/1,000 for children born in the Nottingham area from 1981-1985, for children with a bilateral hearing impairment greater than 40 dB. Data included family history, medical examination and audiological testing (distraction test, pure-tone audiometry, electrical response audiometry and tympanometry). However, a further study in the same region (Davis and Wood, 1992) reported a prevalence rate of 1.2/1,000. Their sample included all children born between 1983 and 1986 who had a sensorineural or mixed hearing loss of greater than 50 dB HL. Data from this study included records from a hearing assessment centre, neonatal intensive care unit (NICU) records, records from a targeted screening programme and hearing assessments. Davis et al. (1995) reported a prevalence of hearing impairment of 1.2 per 1,000 live births per annum in Nottingham, Sheffield and Oxford for children born between 1983-8. Hearing loss included bilateral sensorineural or mixed, and at least 40 dB HL. Moderate hearing impairment (40-69 dB HL) accounted for 50% of these, severe (70-94 dB HL) for 23% and profound (greater than 95 dB HL) for 27%. A family history of childhood sensorineural hearing impairment was evident in 25% of the children and 32% had spent time in a NICU. Similar studies have been carried out in the Manchester area (Das, 1990; Newton, 1985; Newton and Rowson, 1988). These studies identified a prevalence rate of between 0.8/1,000 and 1.2/1,000 for bilateral sensorineural hearing loss greater than 25 dB. Audiological, ophthalmic and medical examinations were performed and family history and medical records were also used as sources of information upon which these prevalence rates were based. It is clear from the variability of the prevalence rates obtained in these various studies that care needs to be taken in the definition of hearing impairment for such investigations. Variation in sample populations, hearing levels included in the study, as well as fluctuating numbers of children with hearing impairment are all factors that lead to such variation in prevalence figures.

The Trent Ascertainment Study

Epidemiological studies have largely been based on small populations (Davis and Wood, 1992), often solely using clinic-based lists or registers where information about all levels of severity were not available (for example, Martin et al., 1979; Newton, 1985; Das, 1988; Dias, 1990; Shui et al., 1996; Sutton and Rowe, 1997). However, an extensive study of the epidemiology of permanent childhood hearing impairment (PCHI) has been carried out in the Trent regional health authority (Fortnum et al., 1997). In this study it has been shown there are substantial differences in prevalence over districts in the UK and in the risk profiles of different populations. Prevalence rates of 1.3/1,000 for both acquired and congenital permanent hearing impairment were reported. For congenital hearing impairment alone, the prevalence rate was 1.1/1,000.

All children with a permanent hearing impairment of 40 dB HL or greater in their better ear, averaged over 0.5, 1, 2 and 4 kHz who had been born between 1 January 1985 and 31 December 1993 and were living within the boundary of Trent regional health authority at the time of data collection (June–September 1995) were included in this study. Sources of information included the Education Database, the community audiology and child health database, the neonatal screening database, audiology and medical records, and hearing aid records.

The data collected were divided into two main groups: congenital hearing impairment and acquired hearing impairment. The congenital group were those children presumed to have had a pre-natal or peri-natal hearing impairment. While the acquired group included those whose hearing impairment came later in life due to disease, progressive hearing impairment or late-onset hearing impairment where there was evidence that the child may have been able to hear at an earlier stage. Table 1.1 shows the prevalence rates ascertained for the Trent region divided into the two groups for three severity bands: moderate (40-69 dB HL), severe (70-94 dB HL) and profound (95+ dB HL) hearing loss.

Table 1.1. The prevalence (per 100,000 children) of three broad severity categories of permanent childhood hearing impairment (PCHI) as a function of onset (congenital versus acquired) for the 1985–90 birth cohort in the Trent region

	Severity (dB HL)	Prevalence per 100,000	95% CI
Congenital	40–69	64	56–73
	70–94	23	19–29
	95+	24	20–30
Acquired	40–69	9	7–12
	70–94	5	3–8
	95+	7	5–10

Calculations of prevalence in the UK

Taking the prevalence estimates derived from the Trent region (Fortnum et al., 1997) and data for the number of live births, it is possible to calculate the number of children who may be expected to be hearing impaired for the whole of the UK. As Table 1.2 indicates, we might expect to find approximately 1,000 hearing impaired children in the UK per annual birth cohort with at least a moderate hearing impairment, with just under 84% having a congenital hearing impairment.

Given the estimated number of children born with PCHI in the UK, the need for an early identification programme to reduce the impact of those losses is clear. Undoubtedly this has contributed to a decision by the government of the UK to develop such a programme by the year 2004. Ultimately, a

Table 1.2. The estimated number of children with permanent childhood hearing impairment (PCHI) in the UK per annual birth cohort

Severity of hearing impairment (dB HL)	All PCHI	Congenital PCHI
40	998	840
50	825	675
60	608	480
70	443	353
80	353	278
90	263	210
95	233	180
100	180	135
110	83	68
120	30	23

universal newborn screening programme should enable a more precise appraisal of the prevalence of hearing impairment, provide a more accurate aetiological picture, and provide for earlier audiological and educational intervention programmes to be established.

A more recent questionnaire-based retrospective total ascertainment study to estimate the prevalence of PCHIhas been conducted by Fortnum et al. (1997). This study was designed to overcome the limitation of small sample size (under 700 children) and underascertainment. Children resident in the UK during 1998, born between 1 January 1980 and 31 December 1995 inclusive, with confirmed permanent bilateral hearing impairment exceeding 40 dB HL in the better ear averaged over 0.5, 1, 2 and 4 kHz were ascertained through sources in the health and education sectors by postal questionnaire. Geographical coverage was comprehensive with only two of 122 postcode areas not covered. A total of 26,000 ascertainment forms were received, resulting in 17,160 individual children after eliminating duplicate notifications. The number of cases with date of birth and severity of impairment were converted to prevalences for each annual birth cohort (cases per 1,000 live births) and adjusted for underascertainment using capture-recapture techniques (Cormack, 1999; Bloor et al., 2000).

Results showed that prevalence rose from 0.91 (95% confidence interval 0.85 to 0.98) for children under 3 years old to 1.65 (1.62 to 1.68) for children aged 9–16 years. Adjustment for underascertainment increased estimates to 1.07 (1.03 to 1.12) and 2.05 (2.02 to 2.08).

When the data from this study were compared with those of the Trent ascertainment study, the prevalence increased with age (Figure 1.1).

There are various possible explanations for this. The rise might be due to new cases – that is, acquired hearing losses that were simply not present in the earlier years of life. It may also be that previously 'mild' cases have worsened to such a degree that the hearing impairment now passes the 40 dB HL mark. A similar pattern may happen with unilateral losses: the 'better' ear may also deteriorate and thus increase the prevalence of bilateral losses. Some of the effect might also be due to persistent cases of otitis media with effusion (OME), which can cause long-term hearing loss.

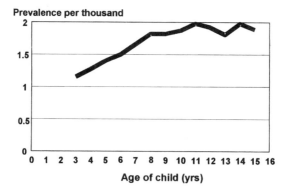

Prevalence per thousand

Age of child (yrs)

Figure 1.1. Prevalence from UK study of support options for deaf and hearing impaired children (hearing loss >40 dB HL, bilateral) as a function of age, N = 18,000.

Risk factors

Sensorineural hearing impairment can lead to problems with communication, academic performance, psychosocial behaviour and emotional development (Bess and McConnell, 1981; Davis et al., 1981; Davis, 1990; Karchmer, 1991; deVilliers, 1992; Holt, 1993). It can also affect the family and society, causing tension and disruption, social isolation and a breakdown in social communication and interaction (Davis, 1988; Maliszewski, 1988; Bess and Paradise, 1994). Early identification and (re)habilitation is essential to try to avoid these various potential complications.

One method of early identification of any pathology involves targeting those considered *at risk* for the problem and applying some sort of screening device to pin-point those individuals who actually have it. *Risk,* in this case refers to the probability that an event will occur – for example, that a child will have a hearing impairment.

Notable risk factors that have been associated with hearing loss include family history of permanent hearing impairment (present since childhood in at least one of the following family members: parent, sibling, grandparent, great-grandparent, aunt, uncle, nephew, niece, cousin), length of stay in NICU, respiratory distress syndrome, neonatal asphyxia, hyper-bilirubinaemia, craniofacial anomalies and retinopathy of prematurity (Kountakis et al., 1997; Mencher, 2000). Borg (1997) has suggested that the total number of risk factors (as indicated by the total length of stay in NICU and the time the baby receives assisted ventilation) are the best predictors of hearing loss of peri-natal origin and that premature babies are more vulnerable than full-term babies. In order to make some sense of the various factors that might be at the root of hearing impairment, and to assist in early identification of the problem, a systematic listing of common aetiological factors has been developed. This list is called the high-risk register for hearing loss.

The best known register for helping to identify hearing impairment is the Joint Committee on Infant Hearing High Risk Register (2000). It consists of a list of indicators by which a neonate or infant can be judged to be 'at risk' for sensorineural and/or conductive hearing loss (Appendix 3). This list should provide the basis for referral for audiological evaluation which should take place between three and six months of age.

There have been a number of studies that test the effectiveness of the high-risk register (Thompson and Folsom, 1981; Stein et al., 1983; Elssman et al., 1987; Halpern et al., 1987; Swigonski et al., 1987; Mauk et al., 1991; Watkin et al., 1991). In general, these studies suggested that between 30% and 50% of children would not be detected using such a register. It should be noted, however, that most of the studies reported here were based upon previous versions of the register and the current version may be a better device than its predecessors. Nevertheless, it is clear from such studies that a high-risk register needs to be supplemented by additional measures. One such measure might be a targeted neonatal hearing screening primarily directed toward children on the register. However, as already indicated, it is likely that a significant number of neonates with congenital hearing impairment are not in the high-risk group, and therefore may be missed by targeted screening. An alternative appears to be to introduce universal neonatal hearing screening – guidelines for good practice that are similar to those of the US Joint Committee on Infant Hearing (JCIH) and those drawn up by the National Deaf Children's Society in the UK (1994, 1996). These set targets for age of identification. The first is to detect 80% of bilateral congenital hearing impairment in excess of 50 dB HL within the first year of life and 40% by the age of six months. A second target is to ensure that by the age of one year all children will have benefited from either a formal screen or a specific surveillance procedure to assess their risk of hearing impairment.

Following the JCIH (1994) report on risk factors, it was noted that the majority of children on the register will actually fall into three larger categories:

- a stay of 48 hours or longer in NICU;
- a family history of permanent childhood hearing impairment; and
- craniofacial anomalies (Davis and Wood, 1992).

In a subsequent study of these elements, Davis and Wood (1992) studied children falling into four categories:

- those with no high-risk factor;
- graduates from the NICU;
- those with a family history of hearing impairment;
- those with a syndrome associated with hearing loss.

These groups were divided into congenital, progressive and acquired. Davis and Wood acknowledged that meningitis-induced profound hearing impairment accounts for a large proportion of children with profound hearing impairment overall. The main conclusions reached from the study were:

- Approximately one child in 900 has a bilateral 50 dB HL hearing impairment or greater.
- Neonatal intensive care unit babies are at least 10 times more likely to have a significant bilateral sensorineural or mixed hearing impairment than non-NICU babies, who have neither family history of hearing impairment, nor a syndrome noticeable at birth.
- The prevalence of substantial other problems in addition to hearing impairment, was approximately 35%. Approximately 70% of the NICU babies had substantial other problems.

In the later Trent study (Fortnum et al., 1997) it was reported that 59% of the congenital PCHI have one or more of the three larger risk factors (history of NICU for 48 hours or longer – 29%; family history of PCHI – 31%; craniofacial abnormality noticeable at birth – 12%). When a stay in the NICU and or a family history have been taken into account for those children with multiple categories, the craniofacial group declines in size to only 3.7%, indicating that the first two categories are the major risk factors for permanent childhood hearing impairment. For children identified in the Trent study who had spent time in the NICU, the proportion of 'acquired' cases was 12%, compared with 10% for those with a family history and 22% for those with no risk factors at all.

In summary then, it has been reported (Davis and Wood, 1992) that children with a history of admission to a neonatal intensive care unit (NICU) have a much increased risk of hearing impairment over children with no risk factors. Other reports also show that there is a high proportion of mild to moderate hearing impairment among children who have attended NICU (Davis et al., 1995). Babies attending NICU suffer many complicating factors and it is often hard to judge, therefore, which of those factors may be causal in the resulting hearing impairment. In general, although there is a specific high-risk register for hearing loss, it does appear as though the items on that list may be reasonably combined into three larger categories which may be used to describe those with an increased risk of hearing impairment. The groupings are considered to be of major importance when planning services for identification of hearing impairments detectable at or around birth. They are:

- admission for 48 hours or longer to a neonatal intensive care unit (NICU);
- a family history of permanent hearing impairment arising in childhood; and
- the presence of craniofacial abnormality (CFA).

These risk factors can also be used when targeting specific groups for neonatal hearing screening. Over half of the babies with detectable hearing impairment might be identified if all those with at least one of the above risk factors was screened within a screening programme that had a sensitive test and high coverage (Davis et al., 1995; Sutton and Rowe, 1997).

Aetiology

Before embarking on a detailed discussion of the various aetiologies of hearing impairment, there are two very important terms that must be defined. All aetiologies fall into one or the other of these two groups:

- *Congenital hearing impairment.* Hearing impairment considered by examination of the case history to be present and detectable using appropriate tests at or very soon after birth.
- *Acquired hearing impairment.* Hearing impairment acquired post-natally, or of late onset, or of progressive nature, which, on the basis of case history, was not considered to be present and detectable using appropriate tests at or very soon after birth.

The frequency of occurrence of some causes of hearing loss has changed over the past 30 years, and further changes will occur with the implementation of new ways of preventing hearing loss. For example, in the US rubella and bacterial meningitis have been greatly reduced though vaccination programmes. In addition, hyperbilirubinaemia, once the major cause of cerebral palsy and approximately 7% to 10% of congenital hearing loss is now nearly a thing of the past with the introduction of photosynthetic lights in the NICU and *in utero* exchange transfusions.

On the other hand, since the 1960s medical advances have ensured that more premature, asphyxic and low birth weight babies now survive, leading to a greater proportion of NICU babies with hearing loss. Thus, hereditary causes, CMV and babies who have attended NICU are now the main causal factors for hearing loss in children. Babies who have attended NICU may typically experience several of the high-risk criteria listed by the Joint Committee on Infant Hearing: low birth weight, low Apgar score, and mechanical ventilation lasting five days or more. Neonatal intensive care unit babies may also experience other identified risk factors such as exposure to ototoxic medications and bacterial meningitis. Children with *in utero* infections such as CMV, rubella, herpes, syphilis and toxoplasmosis; as well as those with craniofacial anomalies or syndromes known to be associated with sensorineural or conductive hearing loss (such as Down syndrome) are frequently admitted to the NICU for associated problems. Roizen (1999) suggests that in the period 1983–92, in the US, the percentage of children with hearing impairment identified by NICU admission increased, with 19% being of low birth weight and 8% having peri-natal factors.

It is clear that since the late 1970s there have been changes in the proportion of children in each broad aetiological group (for example, less rubella, more prematurity, possibly more genetic), but specific determination of the aetiology of any given hearing impairment continues to be difficult. The major aetiological classification system suggested by Davidson et al. (1989) has been used in most recent studies. The categories are:

- genetic;
- pre-natally acquired;
- peri-natally acquired;
- post-natally acquired;
- craniofacial anomalies;
- other; and
- missing.

Unfortunately, however, the major problem with most studies is that children do not always have an ascribed aetiology. There are reports of 30% to 50% of cases of unknown origin (Parving, 1984; Newton, 1985; Davis and Wood, 1992). In the Trent study, 41% of children did not have an identifiable aetiology. Nevertheless, it is possible to impute aetiology from other data such as medical notes. For the Trent study, such a step reduced the percentage who had no aetiological information to approximately 25%.

Table 1.3. Classification of aetiological groups for children with PCHI in the Trent region born between 1985–93 (n = 653), and separated into congenital (n = 556) and acquired (n = 97) hearing impairment

Category (imputed)	Overall %	Congenital %	Acquired %
Genetic	44.7	48.2	24.7
Pre-natal	4.0	4.0	1.0
Peri-natal	16.7	17.6	11.3
Post-natal	6.0	0	41.2
CFA	2.5	2.9	0
Other	2.0	1.0	3.0
Missing	24.6	25.7	18.6

Pre-natal factors

Pre-natal factors often cause sensorineural hearing impairment. They can result from genetic anomalies, infection or maternal drug therapy.

Genetic deafness

Types of genetic hearing losses

At least half of all cases of permanent childhood hearing impairment are known to have a genetic cause (Reardon, 1992). Further, studies have shown that between 30% and 50% of childhood hearing impairment of an unknown aetiology are presumed to be genetically based (Parving, 1984; Newton, 1985; Davis et al., 1995, Parving, 1996). It has been estimated that the common 35delG mutation in the Connexin-26 gene accounts for 20% of all genetic childhood hearing impairment (Kelley et al., 1998). Parker et al. (1999) investigated childhood hearing impairment from a genetic perspective, specifically with reference to Connexin-26 and the 35delG mutation. The families of 526 hearing impaired children (aged four to 13) were sent questionnaires asking about their experience of clinical genetics and they also participated in clinical assessment and molecular sampling. Results pointed toward a definitive relationship between non-syndromal hearing loss and autosomal dominant, autosomal recessive and sporadically based hearing loss. The authors recommend a specific protocol to be used for the investigation of permanent childhood hearing impairment. The protocol contains specific mechanisms to explore the probability of a genetically-based hearing problem. It is clear that recent advances in genetic technology will allow genetic causes to be more readily identified in the future.

Approximately 30% of genetic deafness is syndromal (Bergstrom et al., 1971; Reardon and Pembrey, 1990). There are currently approximately 170 chromosomal disorders and 400 syndromes of single gene or unknown aetiology that have hearing impairment as an associated feature. It has been estimated that 10% of all disease-associated gene mutations can cause some degree of hearing loss (McKusick et al., 1994); indeed, estimates of the proportion of genetically-related hearing impairment have varied from 23% (Das, 1990), to 30 % (Peckham, 1986), to 39.7% (Fortnum and Davis, 1997) up to 50% (Reardon, 1992).

Syndromal hearing impairment can be sensorineural, due to structural anomalies of the auditory system. An association of hearing impairment in children with syndromes should not be overlooked, as it can be important in determining prognosis and intervention measures as well as for estimating the recurrence risks in the family (Mueller, 1996). Chromosomal abnormalities may occur, either during meiosis or mitosis, resulting in too much or too little genetic material. Examples of this, which can result in hearing impairment, include Down syndrome, Patau syndrome, Edward syndrome and Turner syndrome (Northern and Downs, 1991).

The majority of non-syndromal genetic deafness is pre-lingual, inherited in an autosomal recessive way and is extremely heterogeneous. Autosomal recessive deafness is the most common form of genetic deafness, accounting for 40% of profound deafness (Gerkin, 1986). In recessive inheritance, both parents – although not exhibiting the trait – carry a defective gene. There is therefore a 25% chance of the child inheriting both genes and manifesting the genetic disorder, and there is also a 50% chance that the child will become a carrier for that disorder and not manifest the disorder. Such disorders include: Usher syndrome, Cockayne syndrome, Pendred syndrome, Jervell and Lange-Nielson syndrome, Hurler syndrome and Alstrom syndrome (Gibbin, 1988). Numerous non-syndromal recessive hearing impairment genes have been localized. Autosomal recessive inheritance is thought to account for approximately 15% of the cases.

X-linked inheritance accounts for approximately 2% to 3% of the inherited hearing losses (Fraser, 1976; Rose et al., 1977). A more recent review suggests that a constant 5% of congenital male hearing impairment is the result of X-linked recessive inheritance (Bitner-Glindzicz et al., 1994). X-linked deafness, which is sex linked, is probably not present at birth but develops in early infancy. The main characteristic of this type of inheritance is that it affects males only, because they inherit only one X chromosome – if this carries the affected gene deafness will be inherited. Examples of X-linked syndromes include Hunter syndrome, Alport syndrome and Norrie syndrome.

Autosomal dominant non-syndromal hearing impairment usually becomes manifest post-lingually, either because it is congenital and progressive or because it is late-onset, however factors such as infection and noise exposure need to be considered in these cases. Further, hearing impaired children of hearing impaired parents are often identifiable at birth. In dominant inheritance, only one parent need exhibit the trait. When that is the case, there is a 50% chance of the child inheriting the gene and manifesting the genetic disorder, usually as a high frequency bilateral loss. If both parents exhibit the trait, there is a 75% chance of the child manifesting the disorder. Examples of autosomal dominant syndromes include Marshall-Stickler syndrome, Waardenburg syndrome and Treacher Collins syndrome.

Audiological characteristics of genetic hearing losses

There have been various attempts to classify and describe hearing loss. For example, Gorlin (1995) divided genetic sensorineural hearing loss into nine audiometric types. Autosomal dominant could be congenital severe, congenital low-frequency, progressive low-frequency, mid-frequency, high-frequency progressive or unilateral. Autosomal recessive could either be congenital severe to profound or congenital moderate. X-linked stood alone as X-linked congenital and was not sub-divided.

Non-syndromal hearing impairment has also been classified according to audiogram shape (for example, Lui and Xu, 1994; Parving and Newton, 1995). The more established audiogram profiles are sloping (loss greater at high frequencies), ascending (loss greater at low frequencies), U-shaped (loss greater at middle frequencies) and flat (all frequencies falling within a narrow range). It is difficult to distinguish patterns of genetic hearing loss from the confounding effect of age-related hearing loss, which is common in a normal population (Martini et al., 1996). However, this has been attempted by Martini et al. (1996) who have found that dominant inheritance was strongly associated with a sloping audiogram profile, which also equates to the dominant high-frequency progressive type identified by Gorlin. Martini et al. also stated that profound, early-onset hearing impairment is most likely to be recessive. Genetic hearing loss is generally symmetrical (Langenbeck, 1935). Recessive forms are usually profound and present at an early age whereas dominant types are less severe but progressive (Fraser, 1976).

Infections

Infections are considered to be the main cause of pre-natally acquired deafness. In the 1970 and 1980s congenital rubella was the single most common reported cause of sensorineural hearing loss, accounting for 16% to 22% of cases of hearing impairment in babies (Martin et al., 1981, 1982; Parving and

Hauch, 1994). This figure has been reduced dramatically by the introduction of rubella vaccination (Tookey and Peckham, 1999). Lower rates have now been reported at 10% by Newton, (1985) and 5% by Das (1996). If infected during the first month, there is a 50% chance of developing rubella defects. This risk declines throughout pregnancy to approximately 6% chance in the fifth month and beyond. Problems associated with congenital rubella include learning disability, heart disease, cataracts, microcephaly, hepatomegaly, splenomegaly, bone lesions, purpura, glaucoma and hearing impairment (Gerkin, 1984). The hearing impairment is usually severe to profound sensorineural loss, with the mid-frequencies being the most effected (Wilde et al., 1990). Rubella infection may also result in middle-ear anomalies that cause a conductive hearing impairment (Anvar et al., 1984). Hearing loss is the most common permanent manifestation and affects 68% to 93% of children with congenital rubella. Roizen (1999) notes that the SNHL is most frequently profound and bilateral, affects all frequencies equally, and is progressive in some cases.

Other infections such as toxoplasmosis (Gerkin, 1986) and cytomegalovirus (CMV) can also result in sensorineural deafness. These together may account for approximately 15% of children with congenital losses (Davidson et al., 1989). Other studies have suggested that CMV may account for 2.5-3.0% of sensorineural hearing impairment (e.g. Das, 1996; Newton, 1985). Usually hearing impairment is manifest by the age of two in babies who have been infected, although its onset may be later and the hearing impairment may be progressive. Roizen (1999) has observed that cytomegalovirus infection occurs in 2.2% of all newborns, making it the most common intra-uterine infection. Fowler et al. (1997) investigated 307 children with asymptomatic congenital CMV infection and found that 7.2% had sensorineural hearing loss, 3% of which was unilateral and 4% severe to profound loss. Peckham et al. (1987) had previously suggested that children with congenital CMV represented approximately 12% of all children with congenital sensorineural hearing loss.

Maternal drug therapy

Maternal drug therapy during pregnancy can also contribute to congenital deafness. Some substances may permanently injure or destroy the hair cells of the cochlea resulting in a SNHL. For example, alcohol, streptomycin, quinine and chloroquine phosphate may destroy neural elements of the inner ear. Use of Thalidomide can cause damage to structures of the middle and inner ear (Strasnick and Jacobson, 1995). The loss is usually triggered by the ingestion of ototoxic drugs during the first trimester, with damage to the auditory system occurring especially in the sixth and seventh weeks. Conductive loss can result from ototoxicity, primarily as a result of ossicular malformations of the middle ear. Exposure to some drugs causes irreversible SNHL, whereas other drugs cause a loss that can be reversed once the drug is stopped. Of particular note are loop diuretics, aminoglycosides and alcohol (resulting in foetal alcohol syndrome). A hearing impairment due to ototoxicity is usually bilateral and symmetric, but may be of any degree of severity. Such a loss is usually progressive, with the high frequencies affected first.

Peri-natal factors

Peri-natal factors have been associated with approximately 20% of sensorineural hearing impairment in developed countries, generally resulting in elevated high-frequency thresholds (Das, 1996). These include prematurity, anoxia, kernicterus, trauma, apnoea and cyanosis, hyperbilirubinaemia, severe neo-natal sepsis, rhesus incompatibility and low birth weight (Razi and Das, 1994). The incidence of peri-natal factors resulting in hearing impairment has been estimated by various studies. Such estimates range from 2.8% (Das, 1996) and 6.1% (Fortnum and Davis, 1997) as lower estimates, to 9% (Parving and Hauch, 1994), 11.6% (Thiringer, 1984), 13.5% (Newton, 1985) and 14% (Feinmesser et al., 1986) as higher estimates.

Problems associated with prematurity, such as anoxia, hyperbilirubinaemia, increased bacterial and viral infections, treatment with ototoxic drugs and low birth weight are thought to cause hearing impairment (for example, Bradford et al., 1985; Veen et al., 1993). Indeed, Veen concluded that in their study of 890 five-year-olds who had had very low birth weight or had been very premature, the prevalence of sensorineural hearing loss was 15 times higher than the average Dutch population of five-to-seven-year-olds. The incidence of sensorineural hearing loss in infants with a birth weight of 1,500 g or below is estimated to be between 3% and 10% (for example, Newton,1985). In this group of infants it is hard to identify the precise cause of hearing impairment due to the sheer numbers of possible complications such infants may experience. However, it has been suggested that hearing impairment in this group may be caused by bilirubin toxicity, anoxia, exposure to ototoxic drugs, incubator noise, apnoeic spells, pre-natal viral infection or intra-cranial haemorrhage (see, for instance Gibbin, 1988; Gerkin, 1986).

Post-natal factors

It is possible for post-natal causes of hearing impairment to be genetic: such as familial sensorineural deafness or syndromes with delayed-onset of deafness. However, the main post-natal causes are non-genetic, such as meningitis, head injury, measles and ototoxic agents. Otitis media would be included here even though, in and of itself, it is an uncommon cause of permanent hearing impairment, because it may delay the detection of permanent hearing impairment. Parving (1993) reported an incidence of 15% for post-natal causes for hearing impairment. Feinmesser et al. (1986) and Newton (1985) reported lower rates of approximately 4.6%.

Bacterial meningitis is a serious infectious disease both in the neo-natal period and throughout childhood. It is also the most common cause of post-natally acquired hearing impairment. For children who survive meningitis, there are often sequelae, which include learning and speech and language disabilities, hydrocephalus, motor abnormalities, vestibular deficits, psychosis, hyperactivity, visual and sensorineural hearing impairments. Reports have indicated that acquired hearing impairment represents 9.5% of the total childhood hearing impaired population, with 6.5% of these being caused by meningitis (Davis et al., 1995). Meningitis has also been found to be the cause in 16% of children with a profound hearing impairment. Gerber (1990) reported that the most severely deafened children in the study were the product of a meningitis illness and when they studied the most severely deafened children in a local programme for the hearing impaired the children's condition was primarily the product of a meningitis illness. In recent years children who have lost their hearing to meningitis have been considered the best candidates for cochlear implant due to their previous experience with language and their total loss of any auditory neural function.

Fortnum and Davis (1993) reported an average incidence of 16/100,000 with the overall mortality incidence per 100,000 being 1.8. However, Fortnum and Davis (1997) reported considerable variation in the incidence rate with age of onset (see Table 1.4).

Table 1.4. Incidence rate for meningitis in relation to age

Age of onset	Incidence rate (per 100,000)
0–28 days	37.2
1–11 months	115.5
12 months–5 years	28.5
5–16 years	2.8

Meningitis-induced hearing impairment is often bilateral, severe to profound and rapid at onset. Clinical and experimental studies have shown that the loss results from direct damage to the cochlea but it may be exacerbated by additional cochlear damage resulting from any ototoxic drugs used to treat the disease (Francois et al., 1997). The incidence of post-meningitic hearing impairment varies from 6% to 31% depending on the type of meningitis and type of hearing impairment included (see for example Martin, 1982; Fortnum and Hull, 1992; Fortnum and Davis, 1993; Das, 1996).

Evaluation of the aetiology of hearing loss

Every child with hearing loss should be evaluated to determine the cause of the impairment. Medical measures that can be taken include history of pregnancy, labour, delivery, medical history, family history and physical examinations. History of meningitis, NICU attendance, and hearing loss in other family members may also indicate possible causes. If these factors are not present, the most likely cause may be genetic or infection. The identification of a cause can be extremely helpful in determining a successful intervention strategy for the child.

Age of identification

A hearing loss in a child, regardless of the type, can lead to a variety of consequences, not the least of which may be a specific disorder in communication. There can be a significant delay in language development, or a disorder in speech perception and production, or an interference with both receptive and expressive language. Other effects include effects on cognition, educational attainment, social development and family-child interaction. Significant delays in language development and academic achievement, which can be a common consequence of hearing impairment – whether mild-moderate or severe-profound – have led to improvements in hearing aid technology and educational support. However, there is still a long way to go in those areas. Matkin (1988) has indicated that the most successful management of hearing loss in children includes early identification, evaluation and early intervention or treatment. Early intervention for PCHI includes a combination of successful selection of sensory aids (hearing aids, tactile aids, cochlear implants) that reduce the impact of hearing loss and specific treatment that addresses the speech and language delays and disorders that accompany PCHI. Studies have not been entirely definitive in their findings regarding the latest age one can identify a hearing loss in a child and still have a successful intervention with maximum beneficial outcomes.

A constant throughout all the studies of the efficacy of early identification and intervention seems to be the necessity for a high quality of early support given by professionals, which benefits families and children in the enhancement of language development and early educational attainment. For example, Greenberg et al. (1984) suggested that family-focused early intervention enhances family communication skills and reduces the perception of stress. Early intervention in the form of support for parents can be instrumental in developing communication strategies that are less controlling and directive and that enhance joint attention skills, thus modifying their language and interaction strategies.

Until recently there have been few systematic studies that have been able to support the advantages of early identification and intervention. However, there is certainly an increasing amount of evidence supporting the notion that early identification and intervention can lead to considerable benefit for language development. Past studies have focused on 18 months as being an age of early identification and intervention (for example, White and White, 1987; Musselman et al., 1988). From the results of such studies Bess and Paradise (1994) have argued that there is no empirical evidence to support the claim that early identification and intervention leads to better academic outcomes. Such a criticism has prompted further studies (for example, Markides, 1986; Watkins, 1988; Ramkalawan and Davis, 1992; Robinshaw, 1995; Apuzzo and Yoshinaga-Itano, 1995; Moeller, 1996) which have sought to investigate the optimum age at which identification and intervention would enhance language development. These studies clearly show the benefit of early identification and early intervention before six months. For example, Markides (1986) observed better speech intelligibility for children identified and aided less that six months of age. Ramkalawan and Davis (1992) investigated children who were identified at 17 months, whose first referral occurred by approximately 21 months and who were fitted with hearing aids by approximately 29 months. Language measures (MLU, vocabulary size, words per minute, total utterances per minute, proportion of questions, proportion of non-verbal utterances) were found to be significantly correlated with the child's age at intervention. Ramkalawan and Davis concluded that the lower the age of intervention the better the outcome for language development. Robinshaw (1995) showed that children aided between three months and six months, who were severely to profoundly hearing impaired, had similar communicative and linguistic behaviour to that of hearing children of the same age.

In order to address criticisms raised against these studies, a more carefully controlled longitudinal study investigating language development in children with a congenital bilateral hearing loss, has since been carried out by Yoshinaga-Itano et al. (1998). This study has investigated the impact of a relatively intensive, individualized intervention programme on variables including: socio-economic and ethnic group, gender, severity of hearing loss, age at testing, communication mode, cognitive ability and presence of additional disabilities for early- (pre-six months; n = 72) and late-identified (post-six months; n = 78) children. Regardless of severity of hearing loss, language scores, including receptive and expressive scales, from the Minnesota Child Development Inventory (MCDI) were significantly higher for the earlier identified group. Thus, Yoshinaga-Itano (1998) showed clear benefits for early identification and intervention when investigating vocabulary, as well as expressive and receptive language for mild to profoundly hearing impaired children who were identified and entered an intervention programme before the age of six months. Downs (1995) has also shown that children with severe hearing impairment showed the greatest benefit in expressive language (measured by the Minnesota Child Development Inventory) when habilitated early (before three months of age).

In addition to receptive and expressive language and vocabulary, speech perception and personal-social skills have also been shown to be significantly better in children who are identified prior to six months (Moeller, 1998). While early identification has been shown to benefit children at all test ages between 12 months and seven years, a paucity of language development, which continues throughout early childhood, has been shown for children identified between seven and 30 months (Moeller et al., 1998; Stredler-Brown, 1998; Yoshinaga-Itano et al., 1998). Musselman et al. (1988) also showed that the age of intervention (identified between 18 and 23 months) and severity of hearing loss both impacted upon later academic achievement. Another early study by Greenberg (1983) investigated social development of children identified before 24 months, and found that social and communication skills were more advanced for children who had participated in the intervention programme.

Such language delay has been shown to vary depending on severity of hearing loss (Lyders-Gustason, 1998) and other studies (such as Davis and Wood, 1992) have shown that there is considerable variation in the age of identification for children with different levels of hearing impairment. Davis and Wood (1992) noted that the more profound losses were detected earlier and obtained an earlier diagnosis and aiding. For children with a hearing loss between 50 and 79 dB, considerable variation was identified in the age of hearing aid fitting. Reasons for this include surgery, non-attendance at the clinic and other medical complicating factors. Children with losses of less than 50 dB are usually referred and seen at a later age where audiological assessment is more straightforward. Usually, in those cases, the decision to fit a hearing aid is relatively uncomplicated but, nevertheless, due to the timing of the referral to the hearing centre, it usually occurs at a later age for the child. Children with a 50 db HL or greater sensorineural congenital hearing impairment were referred at a median age of 10 months or under. Those children who had a hearing loss of 80 dB or greater were usually fitted with hearing aids by 16 months of age. In a later study (Fortnum and Davis, 1997) there was clear evidence that improvements in terms of lowering both the age of initial prescription and age of actual fitting the hearing aid have occurred (see Table 1.5):

Table 1.5. Mean age in months of hearing aid prescription and fittings as a function of the severity of the hearing impairment from the Trent ascertainment study (Fortnum and Davis, 1997)

Severity of loss	N	Mean age of prescription	N	Mean age of fitting
< 40 dB	223	30.3	336	32.2
40-69 dB	127	40.1	195	42.3
70-94 dB	44	22.4	67	23.5
>95 dB	52	12.8	74	13.9

It has been stressed that the relatively early age at which identification and aiding has been possible is due to a large investment in training of health visitors and the monitoring of health visitor tests and the implementation of a neonatal screening programme. The findings of such studies are clear support for early identification, although success is most likely to be as a result of early intervention and emphasis must therefore be placed on the nature of such intervention – especially in preparation for universal neonatal hearing screening. Indeed, in the UK there has been a considerable effort to reduce the age of identification from a median age of three years in the 1970s (Martin et al., 1981), to a present age of approximately 20 months (Davis et al., 1997; Fortnum and Davis, 1997). The most significant steps in that direction have evolved as the result of the development of infant hearing screening programmes.

Hearing screening in the UK

As far back as the 1930s hearing screening was being implemented at school entry, although no standardized procedure was being used. Ewing (1957) recommended that all children should undergo a school entry screen using a pure-tone 'sweep' test. This is still used in the UK and is seen as a beneficial measure to identify any children who may not already have been identified. However, it has long been argued that identification of hearing impairment at the age of school entry is far too late (Ewing and Ewing, 1944). As early as the 1950s it was demonstrated that testing could be adequately carried out on babies as young as nine months. This led to the introduction of universal hearing screening using the Health Visitor Distraction Test. It is currently used with infants of seven to eight months of age and consists of localization responses to low-level sounds presented to the child by a tester while the attention of the child is suitably manipulated by a second tester. However, this test has been criticized for its low yield, low sensitivity and poor credibility with parents (NDCS, 1983). Nevertheless, it remains in use as a screening tool despite the ongoing concerns about its focus, performance, coverage, yield and cost-effectiveness (NCDS, 1994; NHS HTA programme commissioning document, 1994).

In addition to doubts about the poor identification rate of the HVDT, concern was also expressed about the importance of the age of identification for language and communicative development; the HVDT would be performed at seven to eight months, which was thought to be less than optimal, as evidence presented by Markides (1986) showed that early identification and intervention was beneficial to the development of the hearing impaired child. Other screening devices have therefore been developed. In the UK, the Auditory Response Cradle (Bennett and Lawrence, 1980) was developed as a behavioural test of hearing that could be used with neonates. The use of such devices at such an early age have enabled research to identify at-risk populations and prevalence rated (for example, Newton, 1985; Davis and Wood, 1992). For instance, it has been found that newborn babies in need of special care in NICU for more than 48 hours are an at-risk group, a finding that has led to the increasing implementation of targeted neonatal hearing screening for this population.

Advances in technology have also aided the development of suitable screening tools for use with neonates. Automated auditory brainstem response (ABR) testing has proved to be a powerful diagnostic tool. Since the discovery of otoacoustic emissions (OAEs) (Kemp, 1978) they have also been used in the screening of neonates (Kemp and Ryan, 1995).

Targets for the identification of all children with permanent childhood hearing impairment in the UK have been set by NDCS (1994) in the guidelines drawn up for quality standards, such that 40% of children with moderate or greater permanent childhood hearing impairment should be identified by the age of six months and 80% by 12 months.

The quality standards document led directly to a critical review of the role of neonatal screening in the detection of congenital hearing impairment, commissioned by the Health Technology Assessment (HTA). This review was commissioned because of the increasing doubt about the ability of screening programmes – mainly the health visitor distraction test (HVDT) at seven to eight months – to identify children with congenital hearing impairment, and technological advances which have made neonatal hearing screening an alternative option. The commissioning brief noted that there is a need to consider 'whether available evidence is sufficient to justify a reassessment of policy and practice in particular, to identify the review the evidence for the effectiveness and cost-effectiveness of neonatal and target screening for the early detection of hearing loss in young children'. For a more detailed review the reader is referred to the Davis and Bamford et al. (1997) report to the Department of Health under the Health and Technology Assessment programme.

Implications for health service provision

Given the general nature of the evidence to support the benefits of early identification and intervention of hearing impaired children, and the general improvement in technology that permits earlier and earlier identification, in June 2000 Britain's health minister announced the introduction of universal neonatal hearing screening in England with an initial pilot programme with a hospital or clinic based protocol in 17 areas and a community protocol in three areas. The key to the whole programme is the provision of a 'family-friendly hearing service' (FFHS). A FFHS is based on the rationale that any success the child achieves will be through family intervention, and therefore, the family must be an equal partner in the hearing management team. Furthermore, if family intervention determines outcome, then ultimately the outcomes for any child with hearing loss significantly depend on the support and care that each individual and child's family receives and the extent to which family concerns and anxieties are taken into consideration (Davis et al., 1997; Luterman and Kurtzer-White, 1999; Moeller, 1996; Roush and McWilliam, 1944). Such an approach is congruent with recent UK Government initiatives on 'Supporting Families' (1999), and other health initiatives to become 'family-centred' (for example, Maxton 1997). The following elements indicate the underlying culture of family-friendly hearing services:

1. Service provision by all professional sectors in a positive family-friendly culture that encourages
   - collaboration that is 'seamless';
   - responsiveness that meets families' real needs; and
   - provision of appropriate information between all agencies and for parents that enables families to make informed choices about services for their children;
2. paediatric audiology that exceeds a minimum standard in terms of quality and accessibility;
3. a culture of service evaluation, including peer review with an element of feedback from parents and their hearing impaired children.

These three elements of family-friendly hearing services represent a culture shift in the provision of services and rely on the realignment of current resources. The success of a FFHS is predicted on the understanding of certain principles (Appendix 4). From these principles, four main elements of what families want and what constitutes a family-friendly service can be identified:

- collaboration;
- responsiveness;
- optimal provision of information;
- continuous evaluation of services.

Bamford et al. (1998) looked at what parents want and do not always get from services supporting hearing impaired children. They identified parents' right to knowledge of factors affecting their child's development, and parents' right to expect services to offer a standard of care that reflects current evidence-based knowledge. SCOPE (1994) identified what parents want and what is good practice in regard to how parents are told that their child has a disability. Good practice is rooted in the valuing of the child and the respect for both children and parents. Effective two-way communication, being 'in tune' with the parents, and following their lead in responding to them are critical to parents remaining in control. Their role is active not passive and more progress is likely when respect is demonstrated for parents. Often parents are put into a position of 'reactive advocacy' (DesGeorges,1998) where they have to attempt to change the system to meet the needs of their child in an already-established programme. Involving parents in the strategic management of services helps build services based not only on professional training and expertise, but also on family-friendly principles making the programme work for real families in real life settings.

Bamford et al. (1998) also noted that parents have a very strong preference for identification at birth but this is dependent upon the existence of good and sensitive information and assessment. They want early identification of hearing loss, better information, a more holistic view of the child and family, better co-ordinated services, less delay in hearing aid fitting and better support after identification. In the US, Gallaudet researchers Meadow-Orlans et al., in a communication on work carrying on from their 1997 national survey of support services for parents and their children who are deaf and hard of hearing have indicated that parents want involvement in the decision-making process and for information not to be withheld by professionals. Parents want information about support in the areas of social development and behavioural guidelines for children with hearing loss. In terms of education, they found that deaf parents were concerned that their children's educational programmes were not challenging enough and that they were not receiving what parents would consider age-appropriate programmes and experiences. Deaf parents felt that professionals do not have high enough expectations for deaf children. They want their children to have deaf friends and deaf adults in early intervention and pre-school programmes for their children to look to as role models, and they want their children to have the same access to outside-of-school experiences as other children.

Summary and conclusions

Since the early 1980s our understanding of the epidemiology of permanent childhood hearing impairment in the UK and in other 'developed' countries has increased substantially. There is a realization that there are at least 1.1 per 1,000 children born with a such a condition that is bilateral and that the organization of services for these children needs to be based on evidence of (1) what parents and children need and want (2) what services are associated with better outcomes. For these children, early identification may be the key to better outcomes and there is substantial service development based around newborn hearing screening and the impetus it has given to service development in health, education and social services.

In addition to the children with bilateral moderate severe or profound deafness, there is a growing awareness that the children with mild bilateral or any sort of unilateral deafness are an important group (there are probably 0.6 per 1,000 unilateral and 0.4 per 1,000 mild we can currently detect). Whether these children should become a priority for newborn screening and what sort of services these children need should be the subject of research activity in the next five years or so.

However, there is a substantial need to make sure the screening programmes are audited systematically, to audit the process beyond screening and to analyse the outcomes for children and their families.

The children who acquire, develop or have a late-onset deafness or hearing impairment are also an important group but there has been no systematic work looking at the impact on these children at different ages, with the exception of those children with meningitis.

The NDCS quality standards for the children with meningitis indicate that best practice is for all such children to have a formal audiological assessment. Parental and professional concern should also be associated with a referral for such an assessment. There is a continued need to screen hearing at school entry. Such screening should not be implemented unless there is an agreed written protocol for testing and referral, and data collected for annual audit. It is not appropriate to screen without audit!

Future years should see the improvement of health and education services in part due to the introduction of newborn hearing screening but also in response to guidelines for intervention after early identification of potential childhood conditions (such as deafness). The challenge is there for the professions to develop the services to meet the needs of children and their families.

Appendix 1: definitions of the various types of hearing impairment

- Sensorineural: related to disease/deformity of the inner ear/cochlear nerve with an air-bone gap less than 15 dB averaged over 0.5, 1 and 2 kHz.
- Conductive: related to disease or deformity of the outer/middle ears. Audiometrically there are normal bone conduction thresholds (less than 20 dB) and an air-bone gap greater than 15 dB averaged over 0.5, 1 and 2 kHz.
- Mixed: related to combined involvement of the outer/middle ears and the inner ear/cochlear nerve. Audiometrically greater than 20 dB HL in the bone conduction threshold together with greater than or equal to 15 dB air-bone gap averaged over 0.5 kHz, 1 kHz and 2 kHz.
- Sensory: a subdivision of sensorineural related to disease or deformity in the cochlea.
- Neural: a subdivision of sensorineural related to a disease or deformity in the cochlear nerve.
- Central: sensorineural hearing loss related to a disease or deformity in the central nervous system rostral to the cochlear nerve.

Appendix 2: definitions of hearing impairment in dB levels

- *Average hearing level:* the level of the thresholds (in dB HL) measured in the better hearing ear at 0.5, 1, 2, 4 kHz.
- *Mild:* average hearing level 20–39 dB HL.
- *Moderate:* average hearing level 40–69 dB HL.
- *Severe:* average hearing level 70–94 dB.
- *Profound:* average hearing level greater than 95 dB HL.

Appendix 3: Joint Committee on Infant Hearing High Risk Register for Identification of Hearing Impairment (1994)

For use with infants (birth – 28 days)

1. Family history of hereditary childhood sensorineural hearing impairment.
2. *In utero* infection (such as CMV, rubella, syphilis, herpes, toxoplasmosis).

3. Craniofacial anomalies.
4. Birth weight less than 1,500 g.
5. Hyperbilirubinaemia at a serum level requiring exchange transfusion.
6. Ototoxic medications.
7. Bacterial meningitis.
8. Apgar score of 0–4 at one minute and 0–6 at five minutes.
9. Mechanical ventilation lasting five days or more.
10. Stigmata associated with a syndrome known to include sensorineural and/or conductive hearing loss.

For use with infants 29 days – two years when health conditions develop that require rescreening

1. Parental concern regarding hearing, speech, language and/or developmental delay.
2. Bacterial meningitis and other infections associated with sensorineural hearing loss.
3. Head trauma associated with loss of consciousness or skull fracture.
4. Stigmata associated with a syndrome known to include sensorineural and/or conductive hearing loss.
5. Ototoxic medications.
6. Recurrent or persistent otitis media with effusion for at least three months.

For use with infants (aged 29 days – three years) who require periodic monitoring of hearing

1. Family history of hereditary childhood hearing loss.
2. *In utero* infection.
3. Neurofibromastosis type II and neurodegenerative disorders.

Indicators associated with conductive hearing loss include:

1. Recurrent or persistent otitis media with effusion.
2. Anatomic deformities and other disorders that effect Eustachian tube function.
3. Neurodegenerative disorders.

Appendix 4: Essential elements of understanding in a family-friendly hearing service (FFHS; Baguley, Davis and Bamford, 2000)

- Families are all different.

- Families and professionals should work in partnership.
- There needs to be an ongoing partnership between agencies.
- Families have a right to accurate, up-to-date and comprehensive information.
- Families deserve continuity of care.
- The attitudes of professionals should be characterized by listening.
- The family-professional dialogue should be undertaken in the appropriate language.
- The FFHS should be responsive.
- When a family cannot go to the FFHS, the FFHS should go to the family.
- Family representative should be involved in the strategic management of the FFHS.
- The physical environment of the services should be family friendly.
- Meeting the needs of the family is more important than adhering to targets and standards.

References

Anvar B, Mencher GT, Keet SJ (1984) Hearing loss and congenital rubella in Atlantic Canada. Ear and Hearing 5(6): 340–5.

Apuzzo ML, Yoshinaga-Itano C (1995) Early identification of infants with significant hearing loss and the Minnesota Child Development Inventory. Semin Hear 16: 124–37.

Baguley DM, Davis AC, Bamford JM (2000) Principles of Family-Friendly Hearing Services for Children.

Batchava Y (1993) Antecedents of self-esteem in deaf people: a meta-analytic review. Rehabil Psychol 38: 221–34.

Bench R, Bamford J (1979) The spoken language of hearing impaired children. London: London Academic Press.

Bennett MJ, Lawrence R (1980) Trials with the auditory response cradle II. British Journal of Audiology 14: 1–6.

Bergstrom L, Hemenway WG, Downs MP (1971) A high risk registry to find congenital deafness. Otolaryngologic Clinics of North America 4(2): 369–99.

Bess F, Dodd-Murphy J, Parker R (1998) Children with minimal sensorineural hearing loss: prevalence, educational performance and functional status. Ear and Hear 19(6): 339–54.

Bess FH, McConnell FE (eds) (1981) Audiology, Education and the Hearing Impaired Child. St.Louis MO: CV Mosby.

Bess FH, Paradise JL (1994) Universal screening for infant hearing impairment: not simple, not risk-free, not necessarily beneficial, and not presently justified. Pediatrics 93(2): 330–4.

Bess FH, Tharpe AM (1984) Unilateral hearing impairment in children. Pediatrics. 74: 206–16.

Bitner-Glindzicz M, de Kok Y, Summers D, Huber I, Cremers FP, Ropers HH, Reardon W, Pembrey ME, Malcolm S (1994) Close linkage of a gene for X linked deafness to three microsatellite repeats at Xq21 in radiologically normal and abnormal families. Journal of Medical Genetics 31(12): 916–21.

Bloor M, Wood F, Palmer S (2000) Use of mark-recapture techniques to estimate the size of hard-to-reach populations. J Health Serv Res Policy 5: 89–95.

Borg E (1997) Perinatal asphyxia, hypoxia, ischemia and hearing loss. An overview. Scandinavian Audiology, 26(2): 77–91.

Bradford BC, Baudin J, Conway MJ, Hazell JWP, Stewart AL, Reynolds EOR (1985) Identification of sensory neural hearing loss in very preterm infants by brainstem auditory evoked potentials. Archives of Disease in Childhood 60: 105–9.

Coggon D, Rose G, Barker D (1993) Epidemiology for the Uninitiated. London: British Medical Journal.

Conrad R (1979) The Deaf School Child. London: Harper & Row.

Cormack RM (1999) Problems with using capture-recapture in epidemiology: an example of a measles epidemic. J Clin Epidemiol 52: 909–14.

Das V (1988) Aetiology of bilateral sensorineural deafness in children. Scand Audiol Suppl 30: 8107-593.

Das V (1990) Prevalence of otitis media with effusion in children with bilateral sensory hearing loss. Archives of Disease in Childhood 65: 757–9.

Das V (1996) Aetiology of bilateral sensorineural hearing impairment in children: a 10 year study. Archives of Disease in Childhood 74: 8–12.

Davidson J, Hyde ML, Alberti PW (1989) Epidemiologic patterns in childhood hearing loss: a review. International Journal of Pediatric Otorhinolaryngology 17(3): 239–66.

Davis A (1988) Response times as an indicator of access to frequency-resolved information. British Journal of Audiology 22: 305–8.

Davis A (1990) What are the prerequisites for identifying priorities in social science research and deafness? Paper presented at RNID Seminar.

Davis A (1993) The prevalence of deafness. In Ballantyne J, Martin A, Martin M (eds) Deafness. London: Whurr, pp. 1–11.

Davis A, Wood S (1992) The epidemiology of childhood hearing impairment: factors relevant to planning services. British Journal of Audiology 26: 77–90.

Davis AC, Bamford J, Wilson I, Ramkalawan T, Forshaw M, Wright S (1997) A critical review of the role of neo-natal screening in the detection of congenital hearing impairment. Health Technology Assessment 1(10).

Davis A, Sancho J (1988) Screening for hearing impairment in children: a review of current practice in the UK with special reference to the screening of babies from special baby units for severe/profound impairments. In Gerber SE, Mencher GT (eds) International Perspectives on Communication Disorders. Washington: Gallaudet University Press, pp. 237–75.

Davis A, Wood S, Healy R, Webb H, Rowe S (1995) Risk factors for hearing disorders: epidemiological evidence of change over time in the UK. J Am Acad Audiol 6: 365–70.

DeVilliers PA (1992) Educational implications of deafness – language and literacy. In Eavey RD, Klein JO (eds) 102nd Ross Conference on Pediatric Research – Hearing Loss in Childhood: a Primer. March 24–27, 1991. Ross Laboratories.

DFES 'Together from the start' www.dfes.gov.uk

Downs MP (1995) Universal newborn hearing screening – the Colorado story. Int J Pediatr Otorhinolaryngol 32: 257–9.

Elssman SF, Matkin ND, Sabo MP (1987) Early identification of congenital sensorineural hearing impairment. The Hearing Journal 40(9): 13-17.

Ewing I (1957) Screening tests and guidance clinics for babies and young children. In Ewing A (ed.) Educational Guidance and the Deaf Child. Manchester: Manchester University Press.

Ewing IR, Ewing AC (1944) The ascertainment of deafness in infancy and early childhood. The Journal of Laryngology and Otology (September): 309-33.

Feinmesser M, Tell L, Levi H (1986) Etiology of childhood deafness with reference to the group of unknown cause. Audiology 25: 65-9.

Feinmesser M, Tell L, Levi H (1990) Decline in the prevalence of childhood deafness in the Jewish population of Jerusalem: ethnic and genetic aspects. The Journal of Laryngology and Otology 104: 675-7.

Fortnum H, Davis A (1993) Hearing impairment of children after bacterial meningitis; incidence and resource implications. British Journal of Audiology 27: 43-52.

Fortnum H, Davis A (1997) Epidemiolgy of permanent childhood hearing impairment in Trent region, 1985-1993. British Journal of Audiology. 31: 409-46.

Fortnum H, Hull D (1992) Is hearing assessed after bacterial meningitis? Archives of Disease in Childhood. 67: 1111-12.

Fowler KB, McCollister FP, Dahle AJ, et al. (1997) Progressive and fluctuating sensorineural hearing loss in children with asymptomatic congenital cytomegalovirus infection. J Pediatr 130: 624.

Francois M, Laccourreye L, Huy ETB, Narcy P (1997) Hearing impairment in infants after meningitis: detection by transient evoked otoacoustic emissions. Journal of Pediatrics 130(5): 712-17.

Fraser G (1976) The Causes of Profound Deafness in Children. Baltimore: John Hopkins University Press.

Gallaway C, Nunes A, Johnston M (1994) Spoken Language Development in Hearing Impaired Children: A Bibliography Covering Research from 1996-Present. Manchester: CAEDSP, University of Manchester.

Gerkin KP (1984) The high risk register for deafness. ASHA 26(3): 17-23.

Gerkin KP (1986) The development and outcome of the High Risk Register. In ET Swigart (ed.) Neonatal Hearing Screening. Philadelphia: Taylor & Francis, pp. 31-46.

Gibbin KP (1988) Otological considerations in the first five years of life. In B McCormick (ed.) Paediatric Audiology, 0-5 years. London: Taylor & Francis, pp. 1-33.

Gorlin RJ (1995) Genetic hearing loss asssociated with endocrine and metabolic disorders. In Gorlin RJ, Toriello HV, Cohen MM (eds) Hereditary Hearing Loss and its Syndromes. Oxford: Oxford University Press, pp. 318-54.

Greenberg MT (1983) Family stress and child competence: the effects of early intervention for families with deaf infants. American Annals of the Deaf 128: 407-17.

Greenberg MT, Calderon R, Kusche C (1984) Early intervention using simultaneous communication with deaf infants: the effect on communication development. Child Development 55(2): 607-16.

Gregory S (1995) Deaf Children and their Families. Cambridge: Cambridge University Press.

Gregory S, Bishop J, Sheldon L (1995) Deaf Young People and Their Families. Cambridge: Cambridge University Press.

Haggard M, Gatehouse S, Davis A (1981) The high prevalence of hearing disorders and its implications for services in the UK. British Journal of Audiology 15: 241-51.

Halpern J, Hosford-Dunn H, Malachowski N (1987) Four factors that accurately predict hearing loss in 'high risk' neonates. Ear and Hearing 8(1): 21-5.

Holt JA (1993) Stanford Achievement Test - 8th edition: reading comprehension subgroup results. Am Ann Deaf Ref Iss 138: 172-5.

Joint Committee on Infant Hearing High Risk Register for Identification of Hearing Impairment (2000). Principles and Guidelines for Early Intervention Programs: Year 2000 Position Statement. See www.audiology.org and/or www.asha.org.

Karchmer MA (1991) Causal factors and concomitant impairment. In Matz GJ (ed.) Early Identification of Hearing Impairment in Infants and Young Children: NIH Consensus Development Conference. Bethesda, Maryland: National Institute of Hearing.

Kelley PM, Harris DJ, Corner BC, Askew JW, Fowler T, Smith SD, Kimberling WJ (1998) Novel mutations in the connexin 26 gene (GJB2) that cause autosomal recessive (DFNB1) hearing loss. American Journal of Human Genetics 62(4): 792-9.

Kemp D (1978) Stimulated acoustic emissions from within the human auditory system. J Acoust Soc Am 64: 1386.

Kemp D, Ryan S (1995) The use of transient evoked otoacoustic emissions in neonatal hearing screening programs. Semin Hear 14: 30-45.

Kountakis SE, Psifidis A, Chang CJ, Stiernberg CM (1997) Risk factors associated with hearing loss in neonates. American Journal of Otolaryngology 18(2): 90-3.

Langenbeck B (1935) Das symmetriegesetz der erblichen taubheit. Zeitschrift fur Ohrenheilkunde 223: 261.

Laurenzi C, Monteiro B (1997) Mental health and deafness - the forgotten specialism. ENT News 6: 22-4.

Levitt H, McGarr N, Geffner D (1987) Development of language and communication in hearing impaired children. ASHA: Monogr 26: 9-24.

Lui X, Xu L (1994) Nonsyndromic hearing loss: an analysis of audiograms. Annals of Otology, Rhinology and Laryngology 103(6): 428-33.

Lyders-Gustason R (1998) The effect of degree of hearing loss on language ability of early and late identified deaf and hard of hearing children. Unpublished masters thesis, May 1998.

Maliszewski SJ (1988) The impact of a child's hearing impairment on the family: a parent's perspective. In Bess FH (ed.) Hearing Impairment in Children. Parkton MD: York Press.

Markides A (1986) Age at fitting of hearing aids and speech intelligibility. British Journal of Audiology 20: 165-7.

Martin J (1982) Aetiological factors relating to childhood deafness in the European Community. Audiology 21: 149-58.

Martin J, Bentzen O, Colley J, Hennebert D, Holm C, Iurato S, de Jonge G, McCullen O, Meyer M, Moore W, Morgan A (1981) Childhood deafness in the European Community. Scandinavian Audiology 10: 165-74.

Martin J, Hennebert D, Bentzen O, et al. (1979) Childhood Deafness in the European Community. Brussels: Commission of the European Communities.

Martini A, Prosser A, Mazzoli M, Rosignoli M (1996) Contribution of age-related factors to the progression of non-syndromic hereditary hearing impairment. Journal of Audiological Medicine 5: 141-56.

Matkin ND (1984) Early recognition and referral of hearing impaired children. Pediatrics in Review 6: 151-6.

Matkin ND (1988) Re-evaluating our approach to evaluation: demographics are changing - are we? In Bess F (ed.) Hearing Impairment in Children. Parkton MD: York Press.

Mauk GW, White KR, Mortenson LB, Behrens TR (1991) The effectiveness of screening programs based on high-risk characteristics in early identification of hearing impairment. Ear and Hearing 12: 312-18.

McKusick VA, Francomano CA, Antonorakis SE, Pearson P (1994) Mendelian Inheritance in Man: A Catalog of Human Genes and Genetic Disorders. Baltimore: John Hopkins University Press.

Mencher GT (2000) Challenge of epidemiological research in the developing world: overview. Audiology 39: 178-83.

Mencher LS, Mencher GT (000?) Neonatal asphyxia, definitive markers and hearing loss. Audiology 38(6): 291-5.

Moeller M (1996) Family matters: making sense of complex choices. In Proceedings of the 4th International Symposium on Childhood Deafness, Kiawah Island, South Carolina.

Mohr PE, Feldman JJ, Dunbar JL, McConkey-Robbins A, Niparko JK, Rittenhouse RK, et al. (2000) The societal costs of severe to profound hearing loss in United States. Int J Technol Assess 16: 112-35.

Mueller RF (1996) Genetic counselling for hearing impairment. In Martini A, Read A, Stephens D (eds) Genetics and Hearing Impairment. London: Whurr, pp. 255-64.

Musselman CR, Wilson AK, Lindsay PH (1988) Effects of early intervention on hearing impaired children. Except Child 55: 222-8.

NDCS (1983) Discovering Deafness. A report for National Deaf Children's Week. London: National Deaf Children's Society.

NDCS (1994) Quality Standards in Paediatric Audiology Vol I: Guidelines for the Early Identification of Hearing Impairment. London: National Deaf Children's Society.

NDCS (1996) Quality Standards in Paediatric Audiology Vol II: the Audiological Management of the Child with Permanent Hearing Loss. London: National Deaf Children's Society.

NDCS (2002) Quality Standards in the Early years: Guidelines on Working with Deaf Children under Two Years Old and their Families. London: National Deaf Society.

NHS (1994) Health Technology Assessment Programme Commissioning Document. London: NHS Executive.

NIH (1993) Early Identification of Hearing Impairment in Infants and Young Children. Bethesda, Maryland: National Institutes of Health.

Newton V (1985) Aetiology of bilateral sensori-neural hearing loss in young children. The Journal of Laryngology and Otology suppl 10: 1-57.

Newton V, Rowson V (1988) Progressive sensorineural hearing loss in childhood. British Journal of Audiology 22: 287-95.

Niskar AS, Kieszak SM, Holmes A, Esteban E, Rubin C, Brody DJ (1998) Prevalence of hearing loss among children 6 to 19 years of age. JAMA 279: 1071-5.

Northern J, Downs M (1991) Hearing in Children. Baltimore: Williams & Wilkins.

Pabla H, McCormick B, Gibbin K (1991) Retrospective study of the prevalence of bilateral sensorineural deafness in childhood. International Journal of Pediatric Otorhinolarygology 22: 161-5.

Parker MJ, Fortnum H, Young ID, Davis AC (1999) Variations in genetic assessment and recurrence risks quoted for childhood deafness: a survey of clinical geneticists. Journal of Medical Genetics 36(2): 126–30.

Parving A (1984) Early detection and identification of congenital early acquired hearing disability – who takes the initative? Int J Pediatric Ontorhinolaryngology 7: 107–17.

Parving A (1985) Hearing disorders in childhood, some precedures for detection, identification and diagnostic evaluation. International Journal of Pediatric Otorhinolaryngology 9(1): 31–57.

Parving A (1993) Epidemiology of hearing loss and aetiological diagnosis of hearing impairment in childhood. International Journal of Pediatric Otorhinolaryngology 5: 151–65.

Parving A (1996) Study group in the epidemiology of genetic hearing impairment. HEAR Info Letter 2 (November): 18–22.

Parving A, Hauch A (1994) The causes of profound hearing impairment in schools for the deaf – a longitudinal study. British Journal of Audiology 28: 63–9.

Parving A, Newton V (1995) Editorial: guidelines for description on inherited hearing loss. Journal of Audiological Medicine 4: ii-v.

Peckham C (1986) Hearing impairment in childhood. Br Med Bull 42: 145–9.

Peckham C, Stark O, Dudgeon JA, Hawkins G (1987) Congenital cytomegalovims infection: a cause of sensorineural hearing loss. Archives of Disease in Childhood 62(12): 1233–7.

Powers S (1996) Deaf pupils' achievements in ordinary subjects. J Br Assoc Teachers Deaf 20: 111–23.

Ramkalawan TW, Davis AC (1992) The effects of hearing loss and age intervention on some language metrics in young hearing impaired children. British Journal of Audiology 26: 97–107.

Razi MS, Das VK (1994) Effects of adverse perinatal events on hearing. International Journal of Pediatric Otorhinolaryngology 30: 29–40.

Reardon W (1992) Genetics of deafness: clinical aspects. British Journal of Hospital Medicine 47: 507–11.

Reardon W, Pembrey M (1990) The genetics of deafness. Archives of Disease in Childhood 65: 1196–7.

Robinshaw HM (1995) Early intervention for hearing impairment: differences in the timing of communicative and linguistic development. British Journal of Audiology 29: 315–34.

Roizen NJ (1999) Etiology of hearing loss in children: nongenetic causes. Pediatric Clinics of North America 46(1): 49–64.

Rose SP, Conneally PM, Nance WE (1977) Genetic analysis of childhood deafness. In Bess FH (ed.) Childhood Deafness. New York: Grune & Stratton, pp. 19–36.

Sancho J, Hughes E, Davis A, Haggard M (1988) Epidemiological basis for screening Hearing. In B McCormick (ed.) Paediatric Audiology, 0–5 years. London: Taylor & Francis, pp. 1–33.

SCOPE Working Group (1994) Right From the Start Strategy – The Template. SCOPE Publications.

Shui J, Purvis M, Sutton G (1996) Detection of Childhood Hearing Impairment in the Oxford Region. Report of the Regional Audit Project. Oxford: Oxfordshire RHA.

Stein LK, Clark S, Kraus N (1983) The hearing-impaired infant: patterns of identification and habilitation. Ear and Hearing 4(5): 232–6.

Strasnick B, Jacobson JT (1995) Teratogenic hearing loss. Journal of the American Academy of Audiology 6(1): 28–38.

Stredler-Brown A (1998) The development of pre-school-aged deaf and hard of hearing children in Colorado. Report to the Colorado Department of Education.

Sutton G, Rowe S (1997) Risk factors for childhood deafness in the Oxford region. Br J Audiology 31: 39–54.

Swigonski N, Shallop J, Bull MJ, Lemons JA (1987) Hearing screening of high risk newborns. Ear and Hearing 8(1): 26–30.

Thiringer K, Kankkunen A, Liden G, Niklasson A (1984) Perinatal risk factors in the etiology of hearing loss in preschool children. Developmental Medicine and Child Neurology 26: 799–907.

Thompson G, Folsom R (1981) Hearing assessment of at-risk infants: current status of audiometry in young infants. Clinical Pediatrics 20(1): 257–61.

Tookey PA, Peckham CS (1999) Surveillence of congenital rubella in Great Britain, 1971–96. British Medical Journal 318(7186): 769–70.

Veen S, Sassen ML, Schreuder AM, Ens-Dokkum MH, Verloove-Vanhorick SP, Brand R, Grote JJ, Ruys JH (1993) Hearing loss in very preterm and very low birthweight infants at the age of five years in a nationwide cohort. International Journal of Pediatric Otorhinolaryngology 26: 11–28.

Watkin PM, Baldwin M, McEnery G (1991) Neonatal at risk screening and the identification of deafness. Archives of Disease in Childhood 66: 1130–5.

Watkins S (1988) Long-term effects of home intervention with hearing impaired children. American Annals of the Deaf 132: 267–71.

White SJ, White REC (1987) The effects of hearing status of the family and age of intervention on receptive and expressive oral and language skills in hearing impaired infants. In Levitt H, McGarr NS, Geffner D (eds) Development of Language and Communication Skills in Hearing Impaired Children. ASHA Audiology Superconference. ASHA 21: 38–47.

Wild NJ, Sheppard S, Smithells RW, Holzel H, Jones G (1990) Delayed detection of congenital hearing loss in high risk infants. British Medical Journal 301: 903–4.

Yoshinaga-Itano C, Sedley A, Coulter D, Mehl A (1998) Language of early- and later-identified children with hearing loss. Pediatrics 102(5): 1161–71.

Chapter 2
Otological considerations in the first five years

KEVIN GIBBIN

Introduction

Paediatric otology covers a wide spectrum of disease and requires understanding of basic embryological development of the ear, post-natal anatomical development, otophysiology and otopathology. It also requires an understanding of some aspects of developmental paediatrics.

Most aspects of paediatric otology mirror adult practice although there are differences including some anatomical differences, for example the course of the facial nerve in early life, and differences in spectrum of disease. Middle-ear mucosal disease, both acute and chronic, is particularly prevalent in childhood.

The paediatric otologist carries responsibility for all aspects of managing children with deafness including diagnosing the causes of the loss as well as its treatment. In addition to the management of hearing loss the paediatric otologist is also concerned with other aspects of ear disease including ear infections, dizziness, facial nerve problems and cosmetic deformities of the outer ear.

Embryology

The human ear develops from three separate sources. The inner ear is a neuro-ectodermal derivative developing from the otic placode to form the primitive auditory vesicle or otocyst, which then develops into the membranous labyrinth. The semicircular canals are well developed by the sixth week; the cochlea begins to form at this stage and at four months is almost in its adult

41

form. The primitive otocyst carries with it a layer of mesoderm that subsequently differentiates into the otic capsule, initially cartilaginous but ultimately bony.

The middle-ear cleft, comprising the Eustachian tube, middle ear, mastoid antrum and related air cell system, develops from the tubotympanic recess, an outpouching of the first pharyngeal pouch. By the end of the second foetal month the Eustachian tube may be identified; by this stage the ossicles are appearing, developing from the first and second branchial arch mesoderm.

The mastoid antrum is present by the seventh month but the mastoid air cells do not appear until the end of foetal life.

The inner ear is fully developed at birth. The middle ear is almost at its full development at birth although growth of the tympanic annulus is not complete until the first year of life, developing in parallel with the mastoid process. During the first five years there is further development of the skull, some growth occurring in the mastoid area.

Management of deafness

All aspects of managing deafness must be considered including its diagnosis and treatment. The logistics of managing children with deafness depend on many factors including the age of the child at presentation or suspicion of the hearing loss, the degree of the deafness, the likely nature of the cause or aetiology of the loss, social and developmental background and whether there is any other concomitant or related pathology. The management of a baby with a profound congenital hearing loss, for example, will differ considerably from the management of an older child with deafness due to otitis media with effusion. The role of the parents or carers is, of course, crucial in the management of the deaf child and how the otologist approaches the parents with the diagnosis of their child's deafness may influence subsequent dealings; it is important to present a positive view of the child's hearing loss stressing what the child *can* hear.

Irrespective of age of child or degree or nature of the deafness some basic principles apply – a careful history is taken including, where relevant, family and pregnancy history, history of any peri-natal events, neonatal history and history of early life. Fortnum and Davis (1997) have shown that three factors carry a major increased risk of hearing impairment: admission to a neonatal unit for 48 hours or longer, a family history of permanent hearing impairment since childhood and the presence of a craniofacial anomaly. Sutton and Rowe (1997) demonstrated a number of risk factors including low birth weight. Birth weight below 2,500 g gave a significantly increased risk with an odds ratio of 4.5, rising to 9.6 for weight below 1,500g. It should be noted also that low birth weight is also associated with other disability (Power and Li, 2000).

Details of inoculations given should be sought.

Parents should be questioned about their child's responses to sounds and other stimuli and an account of the child's speech development should be obtained. It is essential to obtain a general developmental history for the child, particularly in relation to cognitive development in view of the interaction of any developmental delay in acquisition of communication skills; delay in speech development may arise purely from hearing loss but may also be influenced by many other factors.

The next element of the management involves a careful examination of the child with particular reference to examination of the ears although careful note should be made of any craniofacial dysmorphic features. It is also important to note the child's ability to communicate. A full otolaryngological examination is required, especially in the case of older children with possible upper respiratory tract disease. In many children, particularly those with non-syndromic sensorineural deafness, there may be no demonstrable clinical abnormality.

Audiometry, either behavioural or objective, will then demonstrate the degree and possibly the nature of the underlying hearing loss although as discussed elsewhere in this book, age of the child and any other factors such as developmental delay may preclude a detailed evaluation.

Investigation of children with deafness will depend on the nature of the underlying hearing loss and may include various blood tests, specialized radiological investigation including magnetic resonance image scanning (MRI) or computerized tomographic scans (CT).

Often other specialist opinion is required and in some cases may be an essential part of the 'work-up' of these children – developmental paediatric opinion in the case of children with any form of developmental delay. A clinical geneticist should always be included in the investigative team where an otherwise unexplained sensorineural deafness is demonstrated and similarly in those cases where there is a clear family history of deafness. Clinical genetics input may also prove invaluable in children with a syndromic cause for the deafness (Reardon, 1992).

In a small number of children there may be other general medical problems and liaison with a paediatric physician will be essential.

Classification of deafness

There are many ways to classify the cause, nature and degree of deafness. The simplest approach is to consider the locus of the pathology causing the loss and therefore the nature of the deafness. Deafness may be caused by pathology in the outer, middle or inner ear or more centrally within the central auditory pathways from the cochlea to the auditory cortex. Lesions of the outer or middle ear cause a conductive loss, those of the inner ear or neural pathways a sensorineural deafness, loosely and colloquially called a 'nerve' deafness; most cases of sensorineural deafness are, in fact, cochlear or sensory losses. However sensorineural deafness in childhood is much less common than conductive deafness. Davis et al. (1995) have shown the prevalence of all bilateral sensorineural hearing impairment of at least 40 dB HL to be about 1.2 children per 1,000 live births per annum. A recent study (Fortnum et al., 2001) published in the *British Medical Journal* has shown that this may be an underestimate with a prevalence rising to 1.65 for children aged between nine and 16 years.

The commonest cause of deafness in children is a conductive loss due to otitis media with effusion (OME) with prevalence peaking at age two years (20%) and again at about five years (17%) (Zeilhuis et al., 1990). It should be noted that a sensorineural hearing loss may coexist with deafness due to OME; the modal loss due to OME with a fluid filled ear is 30 dB (Fria et al., 1985) ranging typically up to 50 dB although theoretically a conductive loss of up to 60 dB may be observed. Any child who presents with OME and a hearing loss of greater than 50 dB should therefore be investigated for a possible underlying sensorineural hearing impairment in addition to the effects of the OME.

Deafness in childhood may also be classified according to the timing of its onset in relation to birth – pre-natal, peri-natal and post-natal.

Pre-natal causes

- Genetic causes.
- Intra-uterine infections:
  - cytomegalovirus;
  - toxoplasmosis;
  - rubella.
- Intra-uterine exposure to ototoxic agents:
  - thalidomide.
- Other developmental anomalies.

Peri-natal causes

- Prematurity.
- Low birth weight.
- Hypoxia.
- Jaundice.

Post-natal causes

Post-natal acquired causes of deafness are many and varied and may cause either sensorineural deafness or conductive losses or both and include:

- infections – most commonly middle ear – acute and chronic otitis media, although bacterial meningitis is the commonest cause of acquired severe to profound sensorineural deafness (Martin, 1982; Davis and Wood, 1992; Fortnum and Davis, 1997);
- viral labyrinthitis including measles and mumps;
- complications of otitis media.
- immunization;
- chronic non-infective middle ear disease – OME;
- chronic suppurative otitis media;
- genetic causes. Examples of acquired sensorineural deafness in association with genetic abnormalities include Pendred syndrome, which may be associated with large vestibular aqueduct syndrome (LVAS) (Jackler and De La Cruz, 1989; Cremers et al., 1998) and branchio-oto-renal syndrome (Chen et al., 1995). Large vestibular aqueduct syndrome may be associated with either a sudden loss of hearing often after even a minor head injury or with a progressive, often fluctuating sensorineural loss.

Genetics and deafness

At least half of all cases of permanent childhood hearing impairment have a genetic cause of which approximately 30% is syndromal (Reardon, 1992). Parker et al. (2000) state that the majority of genetic hearing impairment is inherited in an autosomal recessive manner.

Genetic transmission of deafness may be:

- autosomal dominant;
- autosomal recessive;
- X-linked;
- mitochondrial.

Deafness of genetic origin may be syndromic or non-syndromic. Between 1995 and 2002, 32 autosomal and 30 autosomal dominant loci were mapped and between 2000 and 2002 seven autosomal recessive and 10 autosomal dominant genes have been cloned (Mueller RF, personal communication). The Connexin-26 35delG mutation has been associated with approximately 10% of non-syndromal hearing impairment (Parker et al., 2000) and has been associated with hearing impairment of all degrees of severity (Mueller et al., 1999).

Some genes can be involved with different types of deafness such as both dominant and recessive, syndromic and non-syndromic (Steel, 2000). One particular genetic mutation is known to predispose carriers to deafness induced by aminoglycoside antibiotics (Steel, 2000).

Editorials in the *British Medical Journal* in successive years have shown the advances made in genetics, Richards in 1999 noting that there is uncertainty in what genomic medicine will deliver and Cardon and Watkin (2000) predicted that the identification of novel pathways and mechanisms of disease may be a realistic and important goal. Kaprio (2000) predicted that greatest progress will be made in understanding the genetic contribution to the intermediate phenotypes linking genes and disease. However gene transfer techniques have already been used to regenerate inner ear hair cells in rats (Berger, 2000). In other human developments gene therapy has been reported as saving children born with human immunodeficiency disorder (Cavazzana-Calvo et al., 2000) indicating the potential for this type of treatment.

Genetics is already a major contributor to our understanding of sensorineural deafness (Lalwani and Castelein, 1999). Steel (2000) predicted that within five to 10 years cheap diagnostic tools based on DNA chips would become available to allow rapid detection of the commonest gene mutations associated with deafness but that it would be some 10 to 20 years before gene therapy becomes available to halt or reverse progression of hearing loss. Lalwani (personal communication) has noted that safe and long-term gene transfer has been demonstrated in cochlear and vestibular tissues and that safe stable and therapeutic gene transfer is feasible in the cochlea. Molecular biology including gene therapy, coupled with intra-uterine diagnosis will, it is hoped, prevent most if not all genetically determined deafness in the longer term.

The reader is referred to a useful Web site for keeping abreast of developments in the field of genetic deafness – http://dnalab-www.uia.acbe/dnalab/hhh.

Syndromic deafness

Grundfast (1996) has tabulated physical abnormalities and their associated syndromes related to hearing loss. Sakashita et al. (1996) provide a detailed account of the various congenital anomalies of the outer and middle ear, many of which have a genetic cause although other aetiological factors exist. For more detailed accounts the reader is referred to one of the major texts such as Gorlin and Pindborg (1964).

Conductive deafness

Classification of conductive deafness

Disorders of the outer ear

- Congenital.
- Atresia and aplasia of the pinna and external auditory canal.
- Wax – rarely causes more than a minor conductive loss.
- Foreign bodies – rarely cause any significant hearing loss.
- Infections of the ear canal – acute and chronic otitis externa – these are very uncommon in this age group.
- Acquired stenosis of the external auditory canal – this is very uncommon in this age group and may arise as a result of either infection or trauma.

Disorders of the middle ear

- Congenital:
  - atresia and aplasia of middle-ear structures (Sakashita et al., 1996).
- Acquired:
  - infections;
  - acute suppurative otitis media;
  - chronic suppurative otitis media – tubotympanic and attico-antral disease;
  - non-infective otitis media, including OME;
  - trauma to the middle ear.

It should be noted that this list is not exhaustive but refers to the commonest causes of deafness under the various sub-headings.

Disorders of the external auditory canal

Apart from the presence of wax in the ear canal which in itself rarely causes any significant degree of deafness congenital anomalies of the ear canal probably represent one of the larger groups of conditions causing a conductive loss due to ear canal disease. Wax may, however, be of importance as a result of it obstructing the ear canal and preventing a view of the tympanic membrane; it may also require removal, for example, when fitting a hearing aid.

Anomalies of the external ear may represent either an isolated lesion, often unilateral, or may form part of a congenital syndrome associated with either unilateral or bilateral anomalies. All degrees of hypoplasia of the external auditory canal are seen including total aplasia, the latter associated with a conductive loss of up to 60 dB. Congenital anomalies of the ear canal may be associated with middle-ear anomalies in view of their closely related intra-uterine development. In view of the different periods of foetal development during which the ear canal and inner ear are formed it is extremely uncommon for ear-canal anomalies to be associated with sensorineural deafness.

Clinical examination and diagnosis of a child with aplasia/hypoplasia of the external auditory canal is usually straightforward; if a syndromic condition is considered it is wise to involve a clinical geneticist in the diagnostic team.

Infective/inflammatory disorders of the ear canal are very uncommon in childhood but may sometimes be seen as a secondary feature of chronic suppurative otitis media (CSOM) as a result of an eczematous reaction to the presence of purulent discharge from the middle-ear in the ear canal. Such a condition should always be suspected in the case of children with otitis externa.

Middle-ear pathology and conductive deafness

As already discussed, otitis media with effusion, the commonest form of middle-ear disease in children, accounts for the great majority of cases of deafness in children, far exceeding the numbers of cases of severe to profound sensorineural hearing loss. However there are other causes of conductive deafness in children and the diagnosis of these other conditions must be considered if a child presents with a conductive loss and evidence of OME can be excluded. Examples of other middle-ear pathology include other infective conditions of the ear and their sequelae, congenital anomalies of the middle ear that, as already discussed, may be part of a syndrome such as Treacher Collins or may be isolated developmental anomalies. The diagnosis of many of these anomalies rests with a surgical exploratory procedure on the middle ear, an exploratory tympanotomy, in itself only indicated if it is the intention to attempt surgical reconstruction of any abnormality found.

Classification of inflammatory/infective disorders of the middle ear

Infections

* Acute suppurative otitis media (ASOM).
* Chronic suppurative otitis media (CSOM):
  - tubotympanic disease;
  - attico-antral disease.
* Non-suppurative otitis media.
* Otitis media with effusion.
* Adhesive otitis media.
* Atelectasis.
* Tympanosclerosis.

It should be noted that the above conditions are often inter-related and form, in effect, a spectrum or continuum of disease.

Acute suppurative otitis media (ASOM)

This is rarely seen in hospital practice in the UK unless either it fails to resolve or it results in a complication such as acute mastoiditis, the infection having spread into the mastoid air cell system. Referral may also be made in cases of recurrent acute suppurative otitis media. Acute suppurative otitis media presents a considerable workload in general practice with an overall episode rate of 27.6 per 1,000 (Royal College of General Practitioners, 1986). The highest incidence is at six months to 12 months of age with a second peak at about the time of entry into school (Brook and Burke, 1992). The majority of children have experienced an episode of ASOM at some stage during their early years (Brownlee et al., 1969).

Acute suppurative otitis media typically occurs behind an intact tympanic membrane but can recur in children with a persistent perforation of the eardrum. The condition is characterized by an acute febrile illness with severe ear pain often followed by a discharge from the ear as the tympanic membrane ruptures.

Although ASOM usually presents with a typical clinical picture of pain, pyrexia and then discharge, in infants the presentation may be much more non-specific with a history of an unwell child with pyrexia and vomiting.

Acute suppurative otitis media causes deafness but this is usually only temporary, the deafness being of secondary importance. However some children suffer recurrent episodes of ASOM; in a number of these there may be an underlying cause such as persistent otitis media with effusion or a persistent perforation. In these instances then there may be an associated hearing loss. It should be recognized that effusions might persist for many weeks after an episode of ASOM.

Debate has occurred as to whether any treatment should be offered at all in the majority of these cases with the issue remaining largely unresolved (Del Mar et al., 1997; Harkness et al., 1998; Cates, 1999; O'Neill, 1999; Damoiseaux et al., 2000; Little et al., 2001). Some authors have suggested that the use of antibiotics in ASOM may predispose to the development of chronic middle-ear effusions. A useful reference article on the subject of acute otitis media is by Klein (1994).

Chronic suppurative otitis media

Chronic suppurative otitis media is usefully considered under two broad headings, tubotympanic disease and attico-antral disease. In both conditions there is chronic infection in the middle-ear cleft but its nature and significance differ in the two groups.

Tubotympanic disease

This condition is characterized by a chronic infection of the mucosal lining of the middle ear, a mucositis, the infection initially developing as a result of spread up the Eustachian tube from upper respiratory tract sepsis and may be the long term outcome of unresolved ASOM. Symptoms of tubotympanic disease may consist only of a persistent discharge from the ear or may include the symptom of deafness; the discharge itself is usually thick and mucoid or muco-purulent. Pain is an uncommon presenting feature.

In addition to the presence of a discharge the main clinical finding is of a perforation in the pars tensa of the tympanic membrane; this may be of any size from a minute pinhead appearance to a sub-total defect of the pars tensa. Although less common than in attico-antral disease defects in the ossicular chain may occur; such abnormalities may not be visible on clinical otoscopy unless there is a large posterior perforation.

Examination of the upper respiratory tract may demonstrate evidence of infective rhinitis, sinusitis or adenoiditis; tonsillitis is not considered to be a cause of acute or chronic suppurative otitis media.

Attico-antral disease

Attico-antral disease is associated with an attic defect, a perforation or pocket in the pars flaccida, the upper or attic part of the tympanic membrane. In many cases the defect may be difficult to visualize and initial otoscopy may show only a small crust in the attic region.

It is usually associated with a scanty but offensive discharge from the ear, from which can be cultured coliform bacteria and other Gram-negative organisms such as Proteus and Pseudomonas species. Attico-antral disease is typically considered as a less safe or unsafe form of CSOM in view of the risk of more severe complications developing if left untreated, complications such as facial palsy, labyrinthitis and intra-cranial infection such as meningitis and temporal lobe abscess.

Often microscopic examination of the ear is required both to define the nature of the underlying pathology but also to allow suction toilet of the ear as part of the initial treatment; in young children this will usually need to be carried out under a short general anaesthetic.

Attico-antral disease is typically associated with cholesteatoma, the collection of epidermal debris – keratin – in the middle ear. Cholesteatoma may cause erosive changes to the structures of the middle ear and may erode into the inner ear producing a labyrinthine or cochlear fistula, a pathological communication between the fluid compartments of the inner ear and the normally air containing space of the middle ear. Cholesteatoma in young children is often more extensive than in adults, extending into a well pneumatized mastoid air cell system; in adults cholesteatoma tends to occur in a sclerotic petrous temporal bone. It is uncommon for cholesteatoma to occur bilaterally. In a study in Finland Karma et al. (1989) showed the risk of a child under the age of 16 years developing cholesteatoma to be 1:1,400.

Both tubotympanic and attico-antral infections may cause a conductive deafness dependent on the nature of the pathology in the individual case; the presence of a perforation does not necessarily cause any degree of deafness at all, for example in the presence of a small anterior perforation or even in the case of the attic defect. Even a large cholesteatoma may be associated with normal or nearly normal hearing if, for example, the disease extends purely postero-superiorly into the attic and mastoid antrum without eroding the ossicular chain; alternatively hearing may be occurring by transmission of sound through a mass of cholesteatoma.

The whole question of chronic suppurative otitis media and its management is beyond the scope of a text such as this and the reader is referred to one of the larger textbooks of otolaryngology such as *Scott-Brown's Otolaryngology.*

Non-suppurative otitis media

Chronic middle-ear inflammatory disease represents a spectrum of related conditions including tubotympanic infections at one end of the spectrum through such conditions as otitis media with effusion to adhesive otitis and atelectasis – collapse – of the middle ear structures with gross retraction of the pars tensa of the tympanic membrane (see Proctor, 1989). All of these conditions may be seen in childhood although, as noted previously, OME is the commonest cause of deafness in childhood and indeed the commonest otological condition in the paediatric age group.

Estimates of the prevalence of OME vary widely with age and with the method of diagnosis. Tos et al. (1986) carried out a study on three cohorts of Danish children using tympanometry as the basis of initial assessment. In their first cohort 60% of 150 children tested at 12 months showed abnormal tympanograms, 13% with flat, type B traces (Jerger, 1972). At ages two and three years prevalence varied from 7% to 19% and at four and five years from 11% to 18%. They also demonstrated a seasonal variation. Giebink et al. (1982) showed mucoid otitis media to be most prevalent in the below one-year age group. Birch and Elbrond (1984) showed that in a group of children age nine months to seven years in day care centres the maximum proportion of Type B tympanograms was found in one-year-olds. Van Cauwenburge (1986) has shown that 16% of apparently healthy pre-school children aged from 2;6 to six years had effusions, the highest percentage being at age two to three years. Similar findings were demonstrated by Rach et al. (1986) who also noted a marked seasonal effect.

Although OME has been recognized since the early nineteenth century, Black (1984) has been unable to find details of incidence or prevalence of the condition and Fiellau-Nikolajsen et al. (1979) have questioned whether there has been a genuine increase in its prevalence. Haggard et al. (1992) showed that improved screening yields a large increase in the numbers failing the early screening; they showed that as a result the number of children in the first year of life requiring referral for an otological opinion corresponded to about 1.5% of the age cohort.

Aetiology and pathogenesis of OME

Many factors contribute to the development of OME in children and some groups of children are at particular risk, notably those with Down syndrome and those with cleft palate. The high, almost endemic, incidence of OME in this latter group of children (Paradise et al., 1969) suggests one of the factors involved in the aetiology to be abnormal Eustachian function; further evidence for this is provided by the occurrence of OME in adults with nasopharyngeal carcinoma where tumour may directly obstruct the Eustachian opening. Bluestone and Beery (1976) felt that such obstruction could be either mechanical or functional and that nasal obstruction may also be involved in the pathogenesis of OME.

The role of the adenoids in the pathogenesis is poorly understood. Hibbert and Stell (1982) quoted 26 authors who blamed large adenoids for the presence of OME but they found no difference between the size of the adenoids in a group of children with OME and a control group supporting the views of Fiellau-Nikolajsen et al. (1980), Sade (1979) and Widemar et al. (1985). Maw (1983), however, showed that adenoidectomy (but not tonsillectomy) confers benefit in the management of children with OME. Nieto et al (1983) came to a similar conclusion. Tuohima and Palva (1987) supported the view that the adenoids are a risk factor for OME. Linder et al. (1997) carried out a bacteriological study on the adenoids removed from children with OME and showed an elevated count of pathogens in these children compared with a control group. The role of the adenoids was further discussed by Haggard (personal communication, 2001) in his lecture at the Royal Society of Medicine when he reported that the strength of indicator as professed by ORLs (Otolaryngologists in the UK surveyed by Professor Haggard) and the strength of interaction term in the original data justified indicator status. There is thus evidence that the adenoids have a role in the aetiology of OME and also that there is an evidence base for the practice of adenoidectomy in OME.

Studies of risk factors for OME may also help understand the pathogenesis; evidence is provided by Strachan et al. (1989) and Maw et al. (1992) that parental smoking may be a factor; Kraemer et al. (1983) showed a fourfold incidence of OME in children of parents who smoked. The role of smoking was questioned by Pukander et al. (1985) who found a slight but not significant increase in risk for *acute* otitis media attributable to smoking; Barr and Coatesworth (1991) felt that smoking was unlikely to be a risk factor but may have an association with OME.

In the UK, the 'Trial of Alternative Regimens in Glue Ear Treatment' (TARGET), a large multi-centre study of OME, has been undertaken, organized by the Medical Research Council Institute of Hearing Research. A cohort of 639 children aged between 3.25 and 6.75 years with OME was recruited. After a period of 'watchful waiting' of 12 weeks, a spontaneous resolution rate of between 26% and 65%, depending on the audiometric cutoff by which a persisting condition was defined, was seen (MRC Multi-centre Study Group, 2001). In this age group three significant risk factors were identified – time of year when first seen, hearing level ($\geq$ 30 dB HL in the better ear) and route of referral that included audiometry prior to the hospital appointment. These three risk factors in combination can increase the odds ratio of persistence more than sixfold.

This study has researched a wide range of factors including predictive and risk factors as well as looking at outcomes from a three-arm trial of treatment, the arms being

- non-surgical or medical treatment;
- insertion of grommets;
- insertion of grommets plus adenoidectomy.

The results are being published under the joint authorship of the MRC Multi-centre Study Group.

A variety of other risk factors for OME has been proposed – see Gibbin (1993) for a review of various risk factors.

Effects and clinical presentation of OME

Otitis media with effusion has effects in two main domains:

- hearing;
- otopathological sequelae.

Sade (1979) has termed OME the 'silent syndrome' due to its effect on the hearing and its often insidious presentation. The hearing loss in OME averages 28 dB but varies from normal to about 50 dB HL (Cohen and Sade, 1982).

Deafness may present in these children in a number of ways including by detection of a mild to moderate loss of hearing on routine screening tests. Haggard et al. (1992) have shown that the hearing loss due to OME in children being referred for further hearing assessment following the six to nine month health visitor screen results in a significant otological workload equating to 1.3% of the age cohort. Bamford and Saunders

(1985) have discussed reasons why children may pass the health visitor screen despite the presence of middle ear effusions; it should be noted that the hearing in OME may fluctuate. It is clear that OME is a disease also of infancy and may have significant impact on the child's development particularly of communication skills. Delay in the acquisition of spoken language may be a sequel of OME and children with such difficulties should have their hearing tested as an initial step in their management. Downs (1977) has noted a possible secondary effect of fluctuating conductive loss on the development of auditory strategies for speech perception and that this effect may be irreversible.

Hall and Hill (1986) have postulated five variables that must be considered in the assessment of why OME can have such a variable impact on children:

* the age at which the disorder occurs;
* the duration of the episodes;
* the severity of the loss;
* intrinsic qualities in the child;
* the child's environment.

The hearing loss may present in many other ways and this may depend *inter alia* on the age of the child and its environment; such secondary effects of the deafness may include behaviour difficulties in children of all ages, especially in the case of younger children who are less able to articulate their frustrations.

Otological/otopathological sequelae include:

* Frequent/ recurrent attacks of acute suppurative otitis media.
* Earache – often mild – a common problem in OME, not necessarily indicating that a child has infection; these bouts should be distinguished from the more severe pain of ASOM.
* Vertigo in children is well recognized by otologists and has been reported by Blayney and Colman (1984). Jones et al. (1990) have shown a significant effect of OME on balance in young children, the balance restoring to normal on ventilation of the ears.
* Other chronic non-suppurative otitis media such as atelectasis, a collapse of the pars tensa of the tympanic membrane as a result of loss of the supportive middle layer of

the membrane due to the effects of chronic inflammation of the ear coupled with chronic Eustachian insufficiency. Adhesive otitis media results when intra-tympanic adhesions occur as a result of previous inflammation. Tympanosclerosis is a hyaline degeneration in the sub-mucosa of the ear, most commonly and typically seen in the ear drum itself but may occur in other parts of the middle ear. Cholesterol granuloma is an inflammatory condition of the middle ear, often associated with OME; clinically the ear drum may appear dark blue – the so-called idiopathic haemotympanum. Histologically cholesterol crystals may be seen in the sub-mucosa surrounded by a foreign body giant cell reaction.

- Cholesteatoma may be rarely seen following OME and may be related to the same underlying pathology of Eustachian dysfunction (Deguine, 1986).

Examination of the child with suspected OME

As with any child with a suspected hearing loss a full otological examination should be undertaken and this will also include examination of the child's nose, pharynx and, where possible, the nasopharynx. Otoscopy may be performed using either a head mirror or headlight and speculum or by means of an electric otoscope; pneumatic otoscopy should also be performed if feasible. It is essential to be able to visualize the whole tympanic membrane inspection of the membrane being carried out methodically.

In cases of OME the appearance of the tympanic membrane may vary widely from an almost normal appearance to distinct abnormality. The effusion itself may manifest as a dull appearance to the drum or a colour varying from yellow to blue; a typical appearance is of a pinkish membrane. Air bubbles and fluid levels may be seen but more rarely than supposed. If otopathological sequelae are present then evidence of these may be visible.

Management of children with OME

The management of OME in children has perhaps been more widely discussed and debated than almost any other condition in otology; Mills (1996) reviewed the management and noted that there is no medical treatment available which has been shown to influence the natural history of OME. See also Maw (2001). Autoinflation has been proposed as a non-surgical treatment and was the subject of a systematic review in 1999 by Reidpath et al. (1999) who concluded that the evidence for its use was conflicting and of poor quality; they could not recommend its use. Mills (1996) discussed the role of surgery and concluded that the only treatment that has been shown to promote resolution of OME is adenoidectomy, citing three studies carried out in the UK. The benefits of ventilating tubes are currently being evaluated from analysis of the TARGET data, early results of outcomes suggesting that there is almost certainly benefit to be gained in the short term from the use of grommets and possibly also in the longer term. The Effective Health Care Bulletin (Leeds University, 1992) raised awareness of the condition of glue ear in children and resulted in a reduction in the numbers of children undergoing this particular line of treatment (Mason, Freemantle and Browning, 2001).

There is now almost universal agreement that there should be a period of 'watchful waiting' of about three months in managing these children and obviously this needs to be accompanied by careful advice to the parents and carers of the children to ensure that appropriate support is provided. From the TARGET trial it was noted that in approximately half the children seen initially the effusions had resolved at the three-month visit (MRC Multi-centre Otitis Media Study Group, 2001). Browning (2001) has noted that in the UK where there are long waits for even the minor surgery associated with OME a policy of OME review clinics would reduce the numbers both waiting for and requiring surgery for OME and also reduce the waiting time for such surgery.

Management of the children with persistent effusions should depend on the degree of disability manifested by the child. In some children a policy of continued observation may be the most appropriate method. It is hoped that TARGET will produce evidence to help determine practice in children requiring surgery for their disability. There is little doubt that insertion of grommets produces significant improvement in hearing but that the effect is limited to the period during which the grommets are *in situ* and patent, typically between six and nine months in the case of the Shephard type grommet (Gibb and Mackenzie, 1985), slightly longer if larger tubes are used. From the evidence to date there is longer term benefit from performing adenoidectomy.

Finally, in considering the management of children with middle-ear effusion there are two groups of children especially susceptible to its development – those with a cleft palate and those with Down syndrome. Both groups demonstrate craniofacial dysmorphism but in addition the Down syndrome group may have other predisposing causes such as tendency to infection. It is the practice of this author to ventilate the ears of the child with a cleft palate using a long-term vent, typically a Per Lee grommet. Down syndrome children present other problems including often extremely narrow external auditory canals and in these children it is often preferable to provide hearing aids for aural rehabilitation.

Summary

Children with hearing loss present many potential otological problems. Sensorineural deafness is less common than conductive hearing loss but its effects may be more severe. In the longer term, development of understanding of the genetics of this group of conditions looks likely to provide the basis for management of the problem and hopefully even prevention. Considerable efforts continue to be made in the understanding and management of otitis media with effusion; the hearing loss in these children is often easier to manage than the otopathological sequelae.

Appendix: syndromes associated with deafness

Association with skeletal/craniofacial abnormalities

Apert

Acrocephalosyndactyly; craniofacial synostosis, brachycephaly, hypertelorism, proptosis, saddle nose and spina bifida.

Crouzon

Autosomal dominant; mixed deafness; fused skull sutures with central prominence of the forehead. Often many middle-ear anomalies.

Cleft palate

Palatal defects and associated Eustachian tube dysfunction cause otitis media with effusion.

Goldenhars

Oculo-auriculo-vertebral dysplasia; conductive deafness due to microtia/atresia of the external auditory canal; unilateral facial hypoplasia.

Klippel-Feil

Cervico-oculo-acoustic dysplasia; fusion of cervical vertebrae; both inner and middle-ear anomalies may be present. Recurrent meningitis has been described with this syndrome (Richards and Gibbin, 1977).

Moebius

Bilateral facial palsy; recessive sensorineural or conductive deafness.

Osteogenesis imperfecta

Autosomal dominant; otosclerosis-like changes in the stapes footplate causing a conductive deafness; 'brittle bone disease', labelled Van der Hoeve syndrome when associated with deafness.

Pierre Robin

Now more correctly known as the Robin sequence; mandibular hypoplasia and cleft palate with OME.

Treacher Collins

Autosomal dominant. Hypoplastic malae, anti-mongoloid palpebral fissure, notching of the lower eyelids, low-set pinnae and outer and middle-ear anomalies including total aplasia.

Association with neurological disorders

Cerebral palsy

Sensorineural deafness; spasticity, abnormal limb movements; mental handicap may be associated.

Association with ectodermal or pigmentary anomalies

Ectodermal dysplasia

Autosomal dominant; progressive sensorineural or conductive deafness; lobster claw hand and foot deformity; cleft lip and palate; sometimes microcephaly.

Pili torti

Severe sensorineural deafness and dry, brittle, twisted hair.

Waardenburg

Autosomal dominant; mild to severe sensorineural deafness; white forelock, eyebrows, eyelashes; heterochromia iridis.

Association with ophthalmological disorders

Duane syndrome

A recessive sensorineural and/or conductive loss associated with the typical bilateral sixth cranial nerve (abducens) palsy. Other ear anomalies have been described.

Laurence-Moon-Biedl syndrome

This is a recessive progressive sensorineural loss associated with retinitis pigmentosa, mental handicap, hypogonadism and spastic paraplegia.

Refsum syndrome

Recessive sensorineural deafness with delayed onset blindness, ataxia, obesity, ichthyosis and polyneuritis.

Usher syndrome

Recessive. Moderate to severe sensorineural loss. Blindness of delayed onset due to retinitis pigmentosa. There may be mental handicap, vertigo and epilepsy.

Chromosomal abnormalities

Down syndrome (trisomy 21)

This is the most common of the chromosomal abnormalities causing deafness. Typical facial features with hyponasality and frequent or persistent upper respiratory tract disorders. Mental handicap is present but may appear worse than it is because of the associated hearing loss. Typical otological features include a very high incidence of otitis media with effusion, narrow hairy ear canals with dry scaling skin.

Long-arm 18 deletion syndrome

This condition involves growth and mental impairment, microcephaly, malformation of pinnae and ear canals. It is typically associated with a conductive loss.

Trisomy 13-15

Microphthalmia, cleft lip and palate, often with mental handicap. Microcephaly and seizures are associated with this condition. Both conductive and sensorineural loss may be found with abnormalities of ear canals, ossicles and inner ear.

Trisomy 18

This condition involves microcephaly and mental handicap. Deformities of the ear may be present. Typically the hearing loss is profound.

Turner syndrome

Turner syndrome is associated with a sensorineural or conductive loss. The readily recognizable defects include webbed neck, webbing of digits, high arched palate, micrognathia.

Deafness associated with metabolic/endocrine/renal disorders

Alport syndrome

An autosomal dominant condition, affecting men more severely than women. Progressive hereditary nephritis associated with progressive sensorineural deafness, starting in pre-adolescence.

Nephrosis and urinary tract malformations

Sex-linked or recessive disorder comprising renal anomalies and conductive deafness.

Pendred syndrome

A recessive profound deafness associated with goitre, which in some cases may be noted at birth. May be associated with large vestibular aqueduct syndrome.

Renal genital syndrome

Recessive. Renal and genital abnormalities, low set ears, aplastic external auditory canals and conductive deafness.

Miscellaneous

CHARGE syndrome

Congenital, non-hereditary defects – syndrome comprising *C*oloboma, *H*eart disease, *A*tretic nasal choanae, *R*etarded development, *G*enital hypoplasia and (external) *E*ar anomalies. Usually associated with sensorineural deafness.

Jervell and Lange-Nielson syndrome

Recessive. Profound sensorineural deafness associated with electrocardiographic abnormalities. Death usually occurs in childhood.

Pre-auricular abnormalities

Dominant. Conductive loss with pre-auricular pits, tags and sinuses.

References

Bamford J, Saunders E (1985) Hearing Impairment, Auditory Perception and Language Disability. London: Edward Arnold.

Barr GS, Coatesworth AP (1991) Passive smoking and otitis media with effusion. British Medical Journal 303: 1032–3.

Berger A (2000) Cochlear hair cells regenerated in mammals after birth. British Medical Journal 320: 1360.

Black NA (1984) Is glue ear a modern phenomenon? A historical review of the medical literature. Clinical Otolaryngology 9: 155–64.

Blayney AW, Colman BH (1984) Dizziness in childhood. Clinical Otolaryngology 9: 77–86.

Bluestone CD, Beery QC (1976) Concepts on the pathogenesis of middle ear effusions. Annals of Otology, Rhinology and Laryngology 85: (suppl. 25).

Browning GG (2001) Watchful waiting in childhood otitis media with effusion. Clinical Otolaryngology 26: 263–4.

Brownlee RD, de Loach WR, Jackson HP (1969) Otitis media in children. Incidence, treatment and prognosis in pediatric practice. Journal of Pediatrics 76: 636–42.

Cardon LR, Watkin H (2000) Waiting for the working draft from the human genome project. British Medical Journal 320: 1223–4.

Cates C (1999) An evidence-based approach to reducing antibiotic use in children with acute otitis media: controlled before and after study. British Medical Journal 318: 715–6.

Cavazzana-Calvo M, Hacein-Bey S, De Saint Basile G, Gross F, Yvon E, Nusbaum P, Selz F, Hue C, Certain S, Casanova J-L, Bousso P, Le Deist F, Fischer A (2000) Gene therapy of human severe combined immunodeficiency (SCID)-X1. Disease Science 288: 669–72.

Chen A, Francis M, Ni L, Cremmers CW, Kimberling WJ, Sato Y, Phelps PD, Bellman SC, Wagner MJ, Pembrey M (1995) Phenotypic manifestations of branchio-oto-renal syndrome. American Journal of Medical Genetics 58(4): 365-70.

Cohen D, Sade J (1982) Hearing in secretory otitis media. Canadian Journal of Otolaryngology 11: 27-9.

Cremers CWRJ, Bolder C, Admiraal RJC, Everett LA, Jooston FBM, van Hauwe P, Green ED, Otten BJ (1998) Progressive sensorineural hearing loss and a widened vestibular aqueduct in Pendred syndrome. Archives of Otolaryngology – Head and Neck Surgery 124(5): 501-5.

Damoiseaux RAMJ, van Balen FAM, Hoes AW, Verheij TJM, de Melker RA (2000) Primary care based randomised, double blind trial of amoxicillin versus placebo for acute otitis media in children aged under two years. British Medical Journal 320: 350-4.

Davis A, Wood S (1992) The epidemiology of childhood hearing impairment: factors relevant to planning of services. British Journal of Audiology 26: 77-90.

Davis A, Wood S, Healy R, Webb H, Rowe S (1995) Risk factors for hearing disorders: epidemiological evidence of change over time in the UK. Journal of the American Academy of Audiology 6: 365-70.

Deguine C (1986) The relationship between secretory otitis and cholesteatoma. In Sade J (ed.) Acute and Secretory Otitis Media. Amsterdam. Kugler, pp. 11-16.

Downs MP (1977) The expanding imperatives of early identification. In Bess F (ed.) Childhood Deafness: Causation, Assessment and Management. New York: Grune & Stratton.

Fiellau-Nikolajsen M, Lous J, Vang-Pedersen S, Schousboe HH (1979) Tympanometry in three year old children. Archives of Otolaryngology 105: 461-6.

Fiellau-Nikolajsen M, Falbe-Hansen J, Knudstrup P (1980) Adenoidectomy for middle ear disorders: a randomised controlled trial. Clinical Otolaryngology 5: 323-7.

Fortnum H, Davis A (1997) Epidemiology of permanent childhood hearing impairment in Trent Region, 1985 -1993. British Journal of Audiology 31: 409-46.

Fortnum MH, Summerfield AQ, Marshall DH, Davis AC, Bamford J (2001) Prevalence of permanent childhood hearing impairment in the United Kingdom and implications for universal neonatal hearing screening: questionnaire based ascertainment study. British Medical Journal 323: 536-40.

Fria JJ, Cantekin EI, Eichler JA (1985) Hearing acuity of children with otitis media with effusion. Archives of Otolaryngology 111: 10-16.

Gibb AG, Mackenzie IJ (1985) The extrusion rate of grommets. Archives of Otolaryngology, Head and Neck Surgery 93: 695-9.

Gibbin K (1993) Otological considerations in the first five years. In B McCormick (ed.) Paediatric Audiology 0-5 Years. London: Whurr Publishers.

Giebink GS, Le CT, Paparella MM (1982) Epidemiology of otitis media with effusion in children. Archives of Otolaryngology 108: 563-6.

Gorlin RJ, Pindborg JJ (1964) Syndromes of the Head and Neck. New York. McGraw-Hill.

Grundfast KM (1996) Hearing Loss in Pediatric Otolaryngology. 3 edn (eds Bluestone CD, Stool SE, Kenna MA). Philadelphia: WB Saunders.

Haggard MP, McCormick B, Gannon MM, Spencer H (1992) The paediatric otological case load resulting from improved screening in the first year of life. Clinical Otolaryngology 17: 34-43.

Hall DMB, Hill P (1986) When does secretory otitis media affect language development? Archives of Disease in Childhood 61: 42-7.

Harkness MJ, Melhus A, Hermansson A, Rosenfeld RM, Paradise JL, Froom J, Culpepper L (1998) Controversies: treatment of acute otitis media. Journal of the American Medical Association 279: 1783-5.

Hibbert J, Stell PM (1982) The role of enlarged adenoids in the aetiology of secretory otitis media. Clinical Otolaryngology 7: 253-6.

Jackler RK, De La Cruz A (1989) The large vestibular aqueduct syndrome. Laryngoscope 99: 1238-42.

Jerger J (1972) Studies in impedance audiometry. Acta Oto-laryngologica 96: 513-23.

Jones NS, Radomskij P, Prichard JN, Snashall SE (1990) Imbalance and chronic secretory otitis media in children; effect of myringotomy and insertion of ventilation tubes on body sway. Annals of Otology, Rhinology and Laryngology 99: 477-81.

Kaprio J (2000) Genetic epidemiology. British Medical Journal 320: 1257-9.

Karma PH, Sipila MM, Pukander JS, Perala ME (1989) Occurrence of cholesteatoma and secretory otitis media in children. In Tos M, Thomsen J, Peitersen E (eds) Cholesteatoma and Mastoid Surgery. Proceedings of the Third International Conference on Cholesteatoma and Mastoid Surgery. Amsterdam: Kugler & Ghedini Publications.

Kraemer MJ, Richardson MA, Weiss NS, Furukawa CT, Shaapiro GG, Pierson WE, Bierman CW (1983) Risk factors for persistent middle ear effusions. Otitis media, catarrh, cigarette smoke exposure and atopy. Journal of the American Medical Association 249: 1022-5.

Lalwani A, Castelein CM (1999) Cracking the auditory genetic code: nonsyndromic hereditary hearing impairment. American Journal of Otology 20: 115-32.

Leeds University (1992) The treatment of persistent glue ear in children. Effective Health Care Bulletin 1992. Number 4.

Little P, Gould C, Williamson I, Moore M, Warner G, Dunleavey J (2001) Pragmatic randomised controlled trial of two prescribing strategies for childhood acute otitis media. British Medical Journal 322: 336-42.

Martin JAM (1982) Aetiological factors relating to childhood deafness in the European Community. Audiology 21: 149-58.

Mason J, Freemantle N, Browning G (2001) Impact of Effective Health Care bulletin on treatment of persistent glue ear in children: time series analysis. British Medical Journal 323: 1096-7.

Maw AR (1983) Chronic otitis media with effusion (glue ear) and adenotonsillectomy: prospective randomised controlled study. British Medical Journal 287: 1586-8.

Maw AR (2001) http://www.orl-baohns.org/members/clineffe.htm.

Maw AR, Parker AJ, Lance GN, Dilkes MG (1992) The effect of parental smoking on outcome after treatment for glue ear in children. Clinical Otolaryngology 17: 411-14.

Mills R (1996) The management of childhood otitis media with effusion. Journal of the Royal Society of Medicine 89: 132-4.

MRC Multi-centre Study Group (2001) Risk factors for persistence of bilateral otitis media with effusion. Clinical Otolaryngology 26: 147-56.

Mueller RF, Nehammer A, Middleton A, Houseman M, Taylor GR, Bitner-Glindzciz M, Van Camp G, Parker M, Young ID, Davis A, Newton VE, Lench NJ (1999) Congenital non-syndromal sensorineural hearing impairment due to Connexin-26 gene mutations – molecular and audiological findings. International Journal of Pediatric Otorhinolaryngology 50(1): 3-13.

Nieto CS, Calvo RM, Garcia PB (1983) Aetiological factors in chronic secretory otitis in relation to age. Clinical Otolaryngology 8: 171-4.

Northern JL, Downs MP (1978) Hearing in Children. Baltimore: Williams & Wilkins.

O'Neill P (1999) Acute otitis media. British Medical Journal 319: 833–5.

Paradise JL, Bluestone CD, Felder H (1969) The universality of otitis media in 50 infants with cleft palate. Pediatrics 44: 35–42.

Parker M J, Fortnum H J, Young I D, Davis AC, Mueller RF (2000) Population-based genetic study of childhood hearing impairment in the Trent region of the United Kingdom. Audiology 39: 226–31.

Power C, Li L (2000) Cohort study of birthweight, mortality, and disability. British Medical Journal 320: 840–1.

Proctor B (1989) Surgical Anatomy of the Ear and Temporal Bone. New York: Thieme Medical Publishers.

Pukander J, Luoptonen J, Timonen M, Karma P (1985) Risk factors affecting the occurrence of acute otitis media among 2–3 year old urban children. Acta Oto-laryngologica 100: 260–5.

Rach GH, Zielhuis GA, Van den Broek P (1986) The prevalence of otitis media with effusion in the two year old children in the Netherlands. In Sade J (ed.) Acute and Secretory Otitis Media. Amsterdam: Kugler, pp. 135–7.

Reardon W (1992) Genetic deafness. Journal of Medical Genetics 29: 521–6.

Reidpath DD, Glasziou PP, Del Mar C (1999) Systematic review of autoinflation for treatment of glue ear in children. British Medical Journal 318: 1177.

Richards SH, Gibbin KP (1977) Recurrent meningitis due to a congenital fistula of stapedial footplate. Journal of Laryngology and Otology 91: 1063–71.

Richards T (1999) The genomic challenge. British Medical Journal 318: 3410–12.

Royal College of General Practitioners (1986) Morbidity Statistics from General Practice: Third National Study 1981–82. London:.HMSO.

Sade J (1979) Secretory Otitis Media and its Sequelae. New York: Churchill Livingstone.

Sakashita T, Sando I, Kamerer DB (1996) Congenital anomalies of the external and middle ears. In Bluestone CD, Stool SE, Kenna MA (eds) Pediatric Otolaryngology. Philadelphia: WB Saunders.

Steel KP (2000) New interventions in hearing impairment. British Medical Journal 320: 622–5.

Strachan DP, Jarvis MJ, Feyerabend C (1989) Passive smoking, salivary cotinine concentration and middle ear effusions in seven year old children. British Medical Journal 298: 1549–52

Sutton GJ, Rowe SJ (1997) Risk factors for childhood sensorineural hearing loss in the Oxford region. British Journal of Audiology 31: 39–54.

Tos M, Stangerup SE, Hvid G, Andreassen UK, Thomsen J (1986) Epidemiology and natural history of secretory otitis. In Sade J (ed.) Acute and Secretory Otitis. Amsterdam: Kugler, pp. 95–106.

Tuohima P, Palva T (1987) The effect of tonsillectomy and adenoidectomy on intratympanic pressure. Journal of Laryngology and Otology 101: 892–6.

Van Cauwenburge PB (1986) The character of acute and secretory otitis media. In Sade J (ed.) Acute and Secretory Otitis. Amsterdam: Kugler, pp. 95–106.

Widemar L, Svenson C, Rynnel-Dagoo B, Schiratzki H (1985) The effect of adenoidectomy on secretory otitis media; a two-year controlled prospective study. Clinical Otolaryngology 10: 345–50.

Zeilhuis G, Rach GH, Van den Bosch A, Van den Broek P (1990) The prevalence of otitis media with effusion. A critical review of the literature. Clinical Otolaryngology 15: 283–8.

Chapter 3

Behavioural hearing tests for infants in the first years of life

Barry McCormick

Introduction

Behavioural hearing tests are used more widely than any other techniques in paediatric audiology. This situation will probably prevail despite increasing availability of the objective test techniques, described in other chapters of this book. Behavioural tests can assess the integrity of the entire hearing pathway and sample functional auditory behaviour. Objective tests provide limited information about isolated areas of the hearing pathway:

- otoadmittance measurements assess middle-ear function;
- acoustic reflex measurements extend information to the brainstem and to the central pathway;
- otoacoustic emissions assess cochlear function;
- tympanic membrane displacement measurements can indicate abnormal pressures in the cochlea;
- electric response audiometry can be used to measure responses from the hearing pathway up to the cortex.

In contrast with these tests speech audiometric testing extends our investigations into the important domain of disability. Faced with the limitations of information from objective tests there will always be the need for good behavioural tests to demonstrate a child's functional hearing ability. For the mature child, behavioural test results provide the gold standards for hearing measurements against which objective test results can be calibrated and evaluated. Not only do behavioural tests provide more extensive information about the child's auditory behaviour but they are normally quicker to administer than , say, auditory brainstem tests, and they are less demanding on equipment and on other resources thus making them very cost-effective for service providers. With the expansion of neonatal hearing screening programmes and the increasing trend to fit hearing aids within the first months of life (and cochlear implants within the first or second year) there is clearly a need for good and reliable tests to measure a child's performance prior to and during the fitting of hearing aids or cochlear implants, and then following their provision. The criteria for paediatric cochlear implantation are based on findings from behavioural test techniques (McCormick, 2002) and behavioural test techniques are needed to justify findings from objective measurement techniques such as neural response telemetry.

In practice a range of tests with a mixture of behavioural and objective techniques will normally be available to the clinician but the more expensive objective tests should be reserved for the very young or for complex cases for whom there may be doubts about the reliability of clinical findings. To give some sort of perspective here, a survey was undertaken in the author's paediatric audiology service, which, at that time, served a population of one million (12,000 births per year) and had a well-recognized reputation as a model service with an open access referral system (McCormick et al., 1984). It was found that auditory brainstem testing was needed to back up the audiological investigations in 3% of cases (Mason, McCormick and Wood, 1988). The introduction of neonatal hearing screening will, of course, increase the need for objective test applications in the first weeks of life at a time when behavioural tests have limited application.

Most practitioners use behavioural techniques based on those described initially by Ewing and Ewing (1944) and by Suzuki and Ogiba (1961). Visual reinforcement audiometry (VRA) is given detailed coverage in Paul Shaw's chapter in this volume. The current chapter includes detailed descriptions of the author's modifications to the Ewings' tests, which have been progressively improved over a period of three decades of clinical practice. It places particular emphasis on the practical application of the techniques because, by their very nature, behavioural techniques require high levels of tester skill to administer successfully. They represent an interesting blend of art and science within a clinical service context. To the casual observer the tests may appear to be very straightforward and easy to administer as, indeed, they can be on occasions. To be successful and to establish an appropriate level of rapport with the many non-straightforward/difficult-to-assess children requires a particular level of expertise that can only be acquired through practice and experience.

Tips and guidelines are provided in this chapter but the practitioner must practise the techniques under the guidance of an experienced tester. This will help to consolidate the learning and enable a repertoire of alternative conditioning strategies to be acquired to suit individual children. Skilled application of test technique will be needed to secure the child's interest in the activity and to maintain co-operation for the successful completion of the test. Some of the teaching points presented in this chapter may appear to be very trivial and obvious but the incorporation of these finer points of detail in a test situation can make all the difference between success and failure with the test application. Before discussing the tests in detail it is useful to consider auditory development and the emergence of auditory responsiveness in the first months of life.

The development of auditory responsiveness

Neonates (birth to one month)

Studies have revealed a consistent finding that newborns are more responsive to low-frequency sounds than to high-frequency sounds (Hutt et al., 1968; Eisele, Berry and Shriner, 1975; Weir 1976) and Weir (1976) concluded that they are actually more sensitive to low-frequency sounds and not just more responsive. Various workers have attempted to estimate hearing thresholds for neonates (Olsho et al., 1987; Werner and Gillenwater, 1990; Werner and Mancl, 1993) and despite obvious methodological problems the general conclusion is that at one month of age infants' thresholds are 35 dB to 45 dB higher than adults' with smaller differences for frequencies below 500 Hz.

Behavioural responses, including head turns and startle and other reflex responses, can be elicited in response to intense sounds within hours of birth and have been used with varying degrees of success in hearing screening procedures. The auditory response cradle was developed as a neonatal hearing screening procedure in the UK and has received widely differing

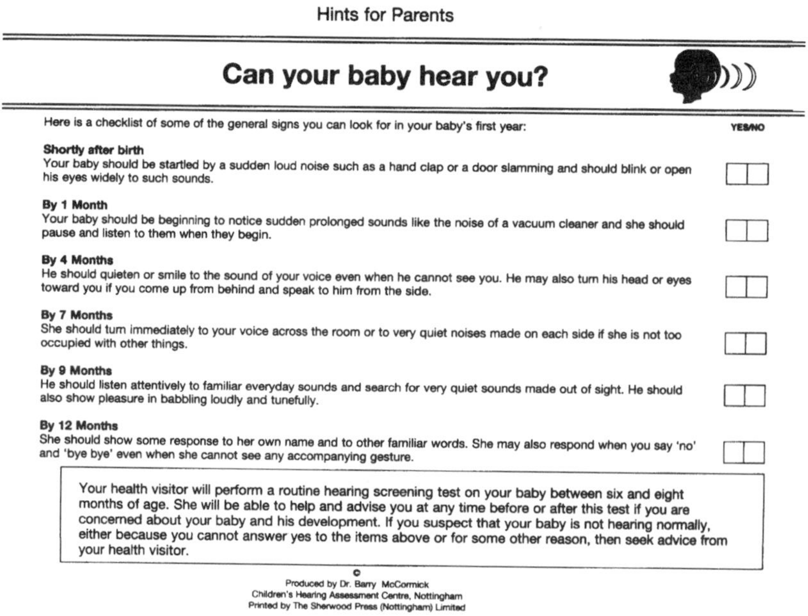

Hints for Parents

Can your baby hear you? 　)))

Here is a checklist of some of the general signs you can look for in your baby's first year: YES/NO

Shortly after birth
Your baby should be startled by a sudden loud noise such as a hand clap or a door slamming and should blink or open his eyes widely to such sounds.

By 1 Month
Your baby should be beginning to notice sudden prolonged sounds like the noise of a vacuum cleaner and she should pause and listen to them when they begin.

By 4 Months
He should quieten or smile to the sound of your voice even when he cannot see you. He may also turn his head or eyes toward you if you come up from behind and speak to him from the side.

By 7 Months
She should turn immediately to your voice across the room or to very quiet noises made on each side if she is not too occupied with other things.

By 9 Months
He should listen attentively to familiar everyday sounds and search for very quiet sounds made out of sight. He should also show pleasure in babbling loudly and tunefully.

By 12 Months
She should show some response to her own name and to other familiar words. She may also respond when you say 'no' and 'bye bye' even when she cannot see any accompanying gesture.

> Your health visitor will perform a routine hearing screening test on your baby between six and eight months of age. She will be able to help and advise you at any time before or after this test if you are concerned about your baby and his development. If you suspect that your baby is not hearing normally, either because you cannot answer yes to the items above or for some other reason, then seek advice from your health visitor.

©
Produced by Dr. Barry McCormick
Children's Hearing Assessment Centre, Nottingham
Printed by The Sherwood Press (Nottingham) Limited

Figure 3.1. The 'can your baby hear you' form for parents.

reviews (Bennett, 1975; Bennett, 1979; Bennett and Lawrence, 1980; Bhattacharya, Bennett and Tucker, 1984; Davis, 1984; McCormick, Curnock and Spavins, 1984). This cradle attempted to objectify the recording of behavioural responses to intense sounds by using transducers to record head turn responses, startle responses, breathing changes and general body activity. Although admirable in its intentions to record behavioural responses, which are associated with meaningful use of hearing, the reliability with which such responses could be recorded in neonates (particularly those in special care) has been questioned. It is interesting that the recording of otoacoustic emissions and auditory brainstem responses have proved to be more popular in neonatal hearing screening programmes and these responses can be elicited to sounds of moderate levels.

First year of life

Olsho et al. (1988) reviewed the studies that had reported hearing threshold levels for babies in the first year of life and they undertook their own investigation. They investigated hearing threshold development for three- to 12-month-old infants and compared the findings with those for adults. They found that by three months the infant's thresholds were 20 dB to 25 dB higher than those for adults between 250 Hz and 4 kHz but 30 dB higher for 8 kHz. For six- to 12-month-olds the thresholds in the 250 Hz to 1 kHz region were 15 dB to 20 dB higher than those of adults but at 2 kHz and above their thresholds were within 10 dB of the adults'. The findings were broadly in line with other published papers (Berg and Smith, 1983; Nozza and Wilson, 1984; Nozza and Henson, 1999; Sinnott, Pisoni and Aslin, 1983; Trehub et al., 1980) and they concluded that the typical six-month-old child should have hearing thresholds within 10 dB to 20 dB of adult thresholds. Nozza and Henson (1999) estimated six- to nine-month-old infants' normal thresholds to be 20 dB HL at 500 Hz, 15 dB HL at 1 kHz and 10 dB HL at 2 kHz.

It is interesting to note that although the newborn shows poorer responsiveness to high-frequency sounds within a few months of birth the responsiveness to high frequencies approaches adult thresholds before that of the low frequencies. The differential rates of maturation must depend upon a complex combination of factors including changes in the middle ear and external auditory meatus (Gerber, 1977; Keefe et al., 1993; Roush et al., 1995), changes in the primary auditory nervous system, and the development of selective attention to sound. A detailed review of these factors is given by Werner and Marean (1996). Nozza and Henson (1999) attempted to separate the sensory from non-sensory contributions to infant-adult differences in behavioural hearing thresholds and they concluded that the greater difference between infant and adults at 500 Hz relative to 2 kHz was not a result of non-sensory factors alone but was largely due to differences in sensory processing. Only about 4 dB of the difference between six- and nine-month-old infants and adults in the unmasked threshold could be attributed to non-sensory factors and the effect is not frequency specific. Suggestions that the frequency-related changes in infant-adult differences are due to frequency-specific non-sensory influences, such as frequency-specific differences in ability to attend to signals or in the amount of training required to reach optimum performance for different frequencies, were not supported by their data. Clearly there is still much to learn about infants' responses.

Having discussed the development of hearing sensitivity within the first year of life it is interesting now to consider aspects of auditory behaviour that can be observed during this period. It is particularly important to obtain a careful history from parents and to ask parents about their child's responses to sound and about the emergence of vocalizations. Care must be taken when trying to interpret the significance of reported vocalizations in the first months of life because deaf and hearing babies produce almost identical sounds up to six months of age (Stoel-Gammon and Otomo, 1986) and it is not until about eight months that clear differences can be detected (Kent et al., 1987).

Figure 3.1 shows a form developed by the author, which has found widespread use within child health surveillance settings in the UK. The form was designed to be used by parents to monitor their child's responses to sounds knowing that parents are often the first to notice signs of deafness. Any parental suspicion about lack of their baby's responsiveness to sound should be taken seriously and it should be assumed that deafness may be present until it can be proved otherwise (Latham and Haggard, 1980; Watkin, Baldwin and Laoide, 1990). Not all parents of deaf children do detect the signs of deafness, however, and Watkin et al. (1990) and McCormick (1991) found that only about one family in five detected the signs of permanent childhood deafness even when prompted with the use of a questionnaire form. Maw and Tiwari (1998), Hammond et al. (1997) and Rosenfield, Goldsmith and Madell (1998) all concluded that parental awareness was not a reliable indicator of the presence of conductive hearing loss. Thus although a parent handout approach may help to identify deafness in some cases this technique should not be used in isolation without the full backup of hearing screening programmes. All parents, including those who are suspicious of deafness, need careful and sensitive conveyance of test results. If deafness had been suspected and is confirmed the parents might not be totally surprised at the news but they will, nevertheless, face the natural shock when the permanency of the condition is confirmed. The needs of parents and of professional workers at this sensitive time has been discussed by the author elsewhere (McCormick, 1975) and although the article was written over 25 years ago the needs of parents are just the same now as they were then, the main difference is that the deafness is generally confirmed much earlier. The needs will not be covered here but all workers who have to convey unexpected and unwelcome news to parents should be aware of the variety and sequence of reactions that may be experienced and that may include denial, defence, grieving for the normal child they thought they had, retreat, fantasy searching for rescue solutions, possible anger and apportioning blame and, of course, there will often be tears of sadness.

Behavioural observation audiometry

This rather grand term embraces a very basic and mostly subjective method of clinical assessment. A review of the literature on this method is given by Wilson and Thompson (1984). The baby is observed in a normal (quiet) state and also during the presentation of sound to see if there is any change of behaviour in the form of a startle, eye movement, eye widening or blinking (auropalpebral response), arousal from sleep, distress, crying-cessation, stilling, sucking (cessation or initiation), head turn or any other response. However crude the method may seem it does have its place in a clinical context, particularly when testing the very young, when testing infants with multiple problems and when assessing hearing aid fitting and cochlear implant speech processor fittings. At best all that can be stated from this form of testing is that the baby shows awareness or responsiveness (in the form observed) to particular sounds at measured levels. A variety of sounds can be used and the hand-held noisemakers are now available with digitally stored waveforms of a variety of everyday sounds including vowel and consonant sounds, animal sounds and bells, all of which can be presented at calibrated levels at a set distance. This test method serves as a last resort if the child cannot be tested with any of the other behavioural methods outlined in this book. Clearly it will be necessary to arrange for objective tests to be undertaken in these circumstances.

Testing babies from six months to 18 months

The two main behavioural tests applicable to babies within this age range are the distraction test and visual reinforcement audiometry. The only well-controlled study to have attempted a direct comparison between the two methods was that performed by Gliddon, Martin and Green (1999). This interesting study, however, included very small numbers of infants (N = 20) with age ranges from 12 months to 25 months (mean 18 months) and the results must, therefore, be interpreted with caution. The distraction test is designed primarily for babies in the first year of life and it is well accepted that VRA is more appropriate for babies above the age of one year. Their study showed that there was no significant difference in the performance of the two tests with the younger babies in the age group tested but the distraction test became less sensitive than VRA with the older age group.

It must be accepted that both tests do have their particular merits and shortcomings. Visual reinforcement audiometry is increasingly the test of choice for most clinicians but distraction tests should not be disregarded for certain cases and they have valuable application either as a useful adjunct to, or replacement for, VRA when the child will not co-operate or condition for the latter. Visual reinforcement audiometry is viewed with sufficient importance to justify a chapter devoted solely to its application in this book and the focus of attention here will, therefore, be on the distraction test and how to perform this to best effect in the circumstances in which it is needed.

The distraction test is based on the general principles first described by Ewing and Ewing (1944). They termed the test the 'distracting test' and it has been progressively modified and improved over the years, the greatest changes having been made by the present author working within the Nottingham paediatric audiology service where the test has been evaluated extensively (McCormick, 1983; McCormick, 1986; McCormick, 1990; Haggard et al., 1992; Wood, Davis, McCormick, 1997). There are many potential pitfalls that can influence the reliability of the distraction test and it is unfortunate that the finer points of details that need to be taken into account to administer the test correctly have not been given sufficient attention by some workers. This historical problem applies particularly to the application of the test when used by health visitors in a community hearing screening context. The reasons for poor standards of success with the health visitor distraction test and suggestions for improvement have been detailed by the author elsewhere (McCormick, 1988; McCormick, 2000). The main shortcomings arose because of lack of adherence to well-defined standards and poor local support with training. With tight control over such factors the distraction test has been shown to work extremely well in the screening context using a simplified version of the test described in detail in this chapter and a screening sensitivity of 88% was sustained over many years in the author's service (Davis and Wood, 1992) and 93% in another service (Watkin, Baldwin and Laoide, 1990). The reader is advised to refer to McCormick (1988) to complement this chapter by extending the distraction test to the screening context for those areas that do not have the facility of universal neonatal hearing screening.

The distraction test

This test is based on the principle that the normal response observed when sound is presented to a baby is a turn to locate the source of the sound. The response is most likely to occur with the very young baby if the sound is presented in the horizontal plane of the ear. In the developmental hierarchy babies respond to sounds at and below ear level before they respond to sounds located in planes above ear level and they have particular difficulty locating sounds above and behind the ear.

Test arrangement

Two testers are required to undertake the test (Figure 3.2) one remains out of the baby's attention and presents sound stimuli at the appropriate time rewarding any responses. The second tester has the more skilful task of controlling the baby's attention in the forward direction so that the sound stimuli can be presented when the baby is in an appropriate attention state without competing auditory, visual and tactile stimulation.

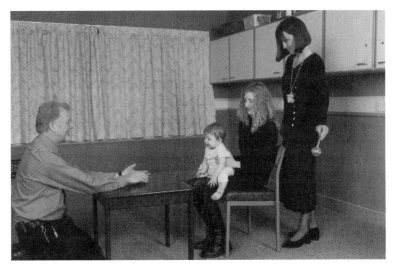

Figure 3.2. Test arrangement for the distraction test.

To perform the test in its normal form the baby must have matured to the stage of being able to sit erect on a parent's knee and be able to perform stable head turn responses. These requirements are usually met at six months of age but in some cases the test can be applied, in a modified form, with babies of three or four months of age if given sufficient head and back support in a reclining seat or by letting the baby's head rest against the parent's chest. There is no strict upper age range for the test application but it becomes much more difficult to apply in the normally developing baby beyond the first year of life because by then the child is socially attuned to the surroundings and is much more likely to be aware of the presence of the second tester. Tips on how to modify the test for application beyond the first year of life will be given later.

The test is undertaken with the baby seated on a parent's knee facing forward and sitting erect. Parents must be instructed not to react in any way when the sound stimulus is presented, for even the slightest movement on their part could initiate a response from the baby and invalidate the test. It is the role of the tester at the front to capture and then control the baby's attention to just the right degree in preparation for the insertion of the sound stimulus. This is best done by attracting the baby's attention down to a table surface situated between the tester and the baby. A useful technique to achieve this is to spin a small brightly coloured object on the table to captivate the baby's attention to a peak (Figure 3.3) and then to cover the spinner with the hands to phase the interest (Figure 3.4). The sound stimulus should be presented as soon as the spinner is covered and the sound should be maintained for a duration of up to 10 seconds or until the baby turns to locate the sound (Figure 3.5). It is undesirable for the baby to look at the tester but the tester must watch the baby's eyes and facial expressions carefully to ensure that the attention is being maintained appropriately and to observe the nature of any responses. If the baby does not turn quickly to the sound but starts to look up to the distractor's face the distracter should move his or her fingers gently on the table to maintain the attention on the table surface. If the baby looks up quickly the tester's fingers should be moved into the baby's field of vision and then be brought down onto the table surface again to bring the baby's eye gaze down to the table (Figure 3.6). If the sound stimulus is presented continuously during this activity, and if it is audible to the baby, a response in the form of a glance down to the table and then an immediate turn to the sound stimulus will often be seen. The objective is to keep the baby's attention on the table surface rather than on the tester.

The second tester's role is to remain out of the baby's attention and the seating and lighting arrangements must be checked very carefully to ensure that there are no unwanted

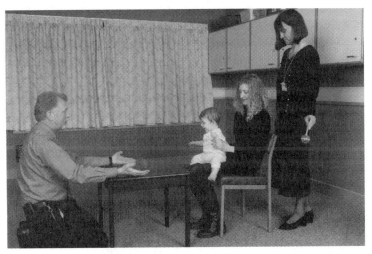

Figure 3.3. Using a spinning toy to capture a baby's attention in the distraction test.

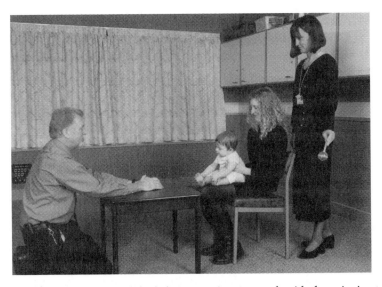

Figure 3.4. Having captured the baby's attention to a peak with the spinning toy the item is then covered to reduce (phase) the attention in preparation for the sound stimulus.

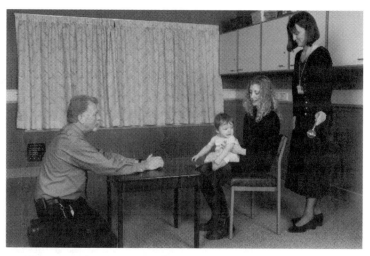

Figure 3.5. A localizing response in the distraction test.

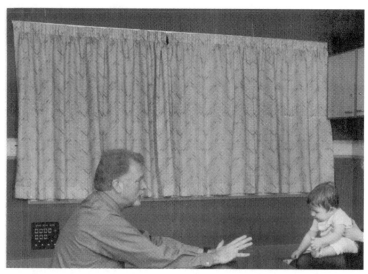

Figure 3.6. The tester applying a fine degree of control over the baby's attention by gently moving his fingers.

reflections or shadows to give away the presence of the tester. The test can be invalidated by rustling clothes, squeaking shoes, creaking floorboards, perfumes or after-shaves, and any movements or shadows within the baby's peripheral vision (assumed to extend to at least 90 degrees to either side). The sound should be presented in the horizontal plane of the baby's ear at an angle set back from the ear of at least 30 degrees but no more than 45 degrees. Nothing must be allowed to enter the baby's peripheral vision including the tester's hair or shoes and so forth. Inadvertent visual cueing is probably the most common invalidator of the distraction test. It is vital, of course, that the distractor should not glance at, or gesture to, the second tester because the baby will be alerted to his or her presence.

Noisemakers with outputs calibrated at set distances should be used for diagnostic clinic application. It is desirable to present the sounds 50 cm or less from the ear to make maximum use of head shadow and thus to increase the chance of stimulating each ear separately. Correct application of a distraction test should enable unilateral hearing loss or asymmetrical hearing loss to be detected if stimuli are presented very close to the ear, within a few centimetres, to make maximum possible use of head shadow effects. Some noisemakers are calibrated for use at 15 cm in which case the dial readings can be taken at that distance or, alternatively, they can be used at any distance as long as the same distance is reproduced when measuring the level on a sound level meter after the response has been recorded. The errors will be small and tolerable (well within 5 dB) with careful matching of distance. As a rule of thumb, when measuring sounds within one metre from the source each halving of distance will increase the level by 6 dB. With skilled testing differences of 10 dB or so between the hearing thresholds for each ear should be measurable.

Response requirements

The normal response expected from the baby in the distraction test is a full head turn in the direction of the sound. There may be reasons, not relating to hearing, which prevent the child from responding in this way. The child might not be developmentally ready for the test because of mental or physical disabilities or might simply not be in an appropriate attention state. A quick check of the baby's physical maturation and readiness for the test can be made by bringing a bright object into the child's central vision and then moving it smoothly through a 90-degree arc on each side to see if the baby can track it visually and can perform the head turn response. If the baby can do this but still fails to respond to sounds then responses to other modalities of touch and vision should be checked by touching the ear or head from the side and by deliberately moving into peripheral vision. If quick responses are observed to touch and vision but not to sound then there are clear indications of hearing difficulties and the hearing thresholds should be chased with very intense sounds containing vibrotactile components if necessary. Boothroyd and Cawkwell (1970) reported that vibrotactile responses can be expected at air conduction levels of 80–110 dB HL for a 250 Hz tone and 100–120 dB HL for a 500 Hz tone (the corresponding levels for bone conduction are 20–40 dB HL for 250 Hz and 55–70 dB HL for 500 Hz). If lack of response is recorded to all modalities then the child is either not in a good state for the test on the day or is developmentally not ready for the test. Objective test techniques will need to be employed in these cases or in any cases where the reliability of the test is in question.

Consideration of the number of trials to administer for each stimulus may be influenced by drifts in the baby's attention but the objective is to find the minimum level at which the baby responds on two out of three occasions when the attention state is judged to be ideal.

Response reinforcement

When the baby has turned to a sound the tester should reward the response by simple means such as a smile or a tickle on the arm. She should then stay in position until the attention has been regained in the forward direction by the distractor and only then should she move back and into position for the next stimulus. The sounds should be presented in an unpredictable sequence from the left or right sometimes presenting twice on the same side so that the baby cannot anticipate where the next stimulus will appear. Response reinforcement is important and is often not performed well. Some warble tone instruments now incorporate light reinforcement systems to supplement human reinforcement. If a baby shows apparently no response to a particular sound it may be that the hearing sensitivity is reduced but it is also possible that the baby has simply lost interest in that particular sound. Above the age of 10 months babies may turn only once to each sound to satisfy their curiosity and then not turn again if the same sound is presented even at louder levels. It is wise to vary the sequence of sound presentations to heighten the novelty factor. Another useful technique to adopt with the more mature baby is to play with the noisemaker at the front and then, when this is hidden, the baby is mystified to hear it again from the side and will often turn out of curiosity.

No-sound trials

The child's checking or searching behaviour must be assessed during the test and this is best done by including 'control' trials or 'no-sound' trials during the test. The baby's attention should be captured, controlled and phased in the normal way and the tester should move into position as if to present a stimulus but without actually including a sound. The baby's general responsiveness should be observed noting particularly if there is a tendency to turn to one side or the other rather than stay in the mid-line. If a localizing response is observed the nature and speed of response should be judged relative to those when sounds are present to see if there are differences. Normally differences will be apparent and the observation of these will help to improve the interpretation of responses. If a child is checking repeatedly to one side during the no-sound trials the hearing thresholds for the contra-lateral ear should be chased for a while until the checking behaviour has ceased. These no-sound trials must form a necessary part of every test and they should be included at frequent intervals throughout the test to assess the child's general checking and searching behaviour. With some babies it will be necessary to include as many no-sound trials as sound trials.

An additional tip for increasing the number of response possibilities when testing mature infant is to say 'Where's the noise?' when the sound stimulus appears (assuming, of course, that the baby has been shown to have sufficient hearing to hear the request). This will often trigger a response from a child who has lost interest in the sounds but care must be taken to include control (no-sound) trials in which the same request is made but without there being any sound. If the child looks puzzled when there is no sound present but turns quickly and accurately to the sounds it can be assumed that the responses are to the stimulus and not to a general search.

Recording the results

The distraction test results may be measured in dB SPL or dB(A). It is common clinical practice to use a sound level meter with an A weighting characteristic and to measure each sound after each response by duplicating the same distance and angle of presentation using the microphone of the meter to replace the child's ear. There will inevitably be some errors bearing in mind that the sound field cannot be duplicated exactly because of factors such as body mass, location and orientation, but in practice these errors are small and tolerable within upper limits of only 2 or 3 dB. Attempts to use probe microphones close to the location of the baby's ear have proved to be unworkable in practice and they cannot be placed at the exact position of the ear without disturbing the child and thereby occupying their attention and interfering with the test. When levels are recorded in dB (A) it will be necessary to apply conversion factors if the results are to be plotted on a conventional audiogram in dB HL units.

It is debatable whether conversion factors should be adopted given that the signals are not pure tones and they are of varying bandwidths. Moreover, the normal concept of hearing threshold may not apply in the first year or so of life. Nevertheless, on occasions, it might be of interest to plot the results on an audiogram style chart using best estimate conversion factors to achieve hearing level values (dB HL). The steps needed to achieve such conversions have been discussed by Nolan (1978, 1987) and by Lutman and McCormick (1987) and the general topic has been discussed by Haggard et al. (1992) and by Beynon and Munro (1993). The conversion factors from Lutman and McCormick are given in Table 3.1. The last column in Table 3.1 gives the composite conversion factor derived according to the assumptions made above. Since the publication of the original article by Lutman and McCormick in 1987 the original ISO 226 standard has been replaced by BS EN ISO 389-7 (1998) and this alters the conversion factors slightly to the values shown in brackets in Table 3.1.

Until more is known about true threshold values for babies and the relationship between pure-tone and complex-tone hearing thresholds is more fully understood, it is probably more convenient simply to quote the measured dB (A) values if the sounds are measured live with sound level meters.

The influence of the types of test stimuli

It has been shown that sound field and earphone testing can give equally reliable and repeatable results (Byrne and Dillon, 1981; Arlinger and Jerlvall, 1987). Pure tones cannot be used with any degree of reliability in a sound field situation because of the potential risk of standing wave effects (interaction between direct and reflected waves according to the phase relationships on arrival at the ear: if they arrive 180 degrees out

Table 3.1. Conversion factors from dB (A) to HL equivalent

Frequency (Hz)	Conversion dB (A) to dB SPL	Minimal audible field (Bin) dB SPL from ISO 226	True conversion values dB (A) to dB HL equivalent (ISO 389-7 update in brackets)	
250	+9	+12	-3	(-2)
500	+3	+6	-3	(0)
1000	0	+4	-4	(0)
2000	-1	+1	-2	(+1)
4000	-1	-4	+3	(+4)

From Lutman and McCormick (1987)

of phase there will be a cancelling effect which will significantly reduce the level of sound received by the child). When performing sound field testing it is desirable to use warble tones or narrow band noises to avoid unwanted interactions between the direct and reflected signals. A great deal has been written about babies' responsiveness to test sounds of different nature – for example, Ewing and Ewing (1944), Mendel (1968), Hoversten and Moncur (1969), Moore, Wilson, Thompson (1977), Samples and Franklin (1978), Thompson and Folsom (1985) and McCormick (1986). The consensus finding has been that infants are more responsive to sounds of wider bandwidth and there is good responsiveness to warble tones and narrow band noises. In a study by Orchik and Rintelmann (1978) on children from 3.5–6.5 years of age, warble tones gave 5 dB better thresholds than narrow band noises and 1 dB to 2 dB better thresholds than for pure tones across all ages. It was assumed that this was because of attention/ interest factors but the bandwidth of the sounds could have had a bearing on the findings. The same authors reported progressive improvements in the thresholds with age with those for six-year-old children being 5 dB better than those for the three-year-old children.

Test techniques 18 to 30 months

By the age of 18 months a hearing child should be able to understand simple verbal instructions. This broadens the horizon for testing hearing beyond the confines of auditory detection into the area of auditory recognition and discrimination. This age group is, however, by far the most difficult and challenging to test because of the emergence of the negative phase of development often termed the 'terrible twos' stage. The typical 18-month-old child may cry a lot and often want to do the opposite of what adults desire or request. The child's natural negativism and short variable attention span may challenge the skills of the tester to the full. The tests described here are based on play methods, one of which was described by Ewing and Ewing (1947) as the 'co-operative test'.

Testing auditory recognition and discrimination of speech

For children above the age of three years it is possible to undertake speech audiometry using simplified adult-type testing and plotting performance/intensity function scores. This type of task is, however, too demanding for the younger child and it is necessary to simplify both the task and the method of scoring to suit the child's vocabulary level and to accommodate the short concentration span of the child. The simplest and most widely accepted approach is to find the quietest listening level at which the child can discriminate between simple familiar instructions or requests. For speech presented in the live mode the quietest level at which the child will respond correctly with an accuracy of 80% (four correct responses out of five requests) is a reasonable target to aim for and the child with normal hearing should be able to achieve this score at a listening level of 40 dB (A). It is not possible to define more precise target scores at this age because of the practical difficulty of presenting live material at levels below 40 dB (A) and because of the constraints imposed by the child's vocabulary, development, concentration, attention and co-operation. Children's spoken and receptive vocabulary will vary widely between 18 and 30 months.

The Four-toy Eyepointing Test (McCormick, 1988)

This test, described by the author in 1988, is probably the simplest available for this age group and it requires a minimum degree of co-operation from the child. Two pairs of items from the McCormick Toy Discrimination Test (described in full detail later) are used , namely cup/duck and spoon/shoe, these being the ones known to the typical 18-month-old child. The test is undertaken with the child seated on a parent's knee (for added security) and facing the tester. The four toy items are placed in a semicircular arc on a table with a spacing of at least 20 centimetres so that the tester can see at which toy the child is looking (Figure 3.7). The child is conditioned to look at each item in response to the requests such as 'where is the duck?' or 'look at the cup'. It is, of course, necessary to check that the child understands the names of the items and this is best done by asking the parent to confirm this as each item is introduced to the child at the start of the test. The tester should use a loud conversational level of voice initially and sign language and lipreading clues can be given at this stage of the conditioning. Once the child has responded by looking at the correct item on request, lipreading and signing cues should be removed and the voice level should be progressively reduced to determine the quietest level at which the child obtains an 80% score. With only four items in the display there is a 25% probability of a chance response, or of a learning effect, if the toys are requested in a set sequence. To minimize problems it will be necessary to avoid any set sequence and sometimes request the same item twice in succession. If the child's attention drifts it may be helpful to swap the position of the toys to recapture the interest for a few more responses.

It will be appreciated that this test is very simple in principle, as indeed it has to be for young children of this age. There are, however, certain pitfalls that must be avoided when using

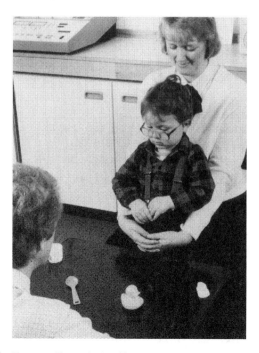

Figure 3.7. The Four-toy Eyepointing Test.

eyepointing techniques – the chief one being the avoidance of premature praise as the child's eyes sweep across the toys. The response should be judged only when the child's eyes have settled clearly on one item. The more mature child might co-operate by fingerpointing in which case the test can be performed on each side in an attempt to assess each ear separately. It is sometimes possible to measure a difference of 10 dB or more between the ears but the possibility of cross hearing cannot be excluded in any sound field test when the stimulus is presented at more than a few centimetres from the ear. By being at 90 degrees to the side and at very close proximity to the ear, the head shadow effect can be used to the full in an attempt to record separate thresholds for each ear. If performed from the front using eyepointing no claims can be made as to which ear is being tested and the objective is to determine if the child can discriminate speech in at least one ear either at normal levels (≤40 dB A), in which case the child is not at risk in terms of developing spoken language, or at raised levels, in which case the degree of disability can be assessed. An example of the reporting of the findings might be: 'He could not identify simple instructions below a listening level of 60 dB (A) without signing or lipreading cues.'

The test can, of course, be used with signing and/or lipreading to assess the child's total communication capabilities. If signs are used the parent should be asked which signs the child is familiar with because there are considerable regional variations.

The Co-operative Test

This is the technique suggested by Ewing and Ewing (1944) and the child is conditioned to perform a 'giving' game. In some cases it offers a useful alternative to the Four-toy Eyepointing Test but it does require a higher degree of co-operation from the child and it takes longer to administer. It can be an appropriate test technique for the more mature very active child. The objective is to develop an activity with the child giving a brick (or other toy item) to a teddy, baby or mummy on request. The items are chosen to sound alike and it will be noticed that they have the same number of syllables. The aim is to record the quietest listening level at which the child will respond to the instructions when listening without lipreading or signing cues. The first stage of the test is to determine if the child understands the names of the items and then the game is established by demonstrating the giving activity in response to instructions presented at a loud level and with signing and lipreading cues if necessary. After a few demonstrations at the loud level the child should be invited to take part and it may be helpful to place the giving item in the child's hand, restrain the hand until the request has been given, and then guide the child's hand to the appropriate response item. This introduces discipline for the test but some children will insist on giving the toy to the item of their choice and may push the tester's hand away to achieve this. The child might be encouraged to co-operate better if the game is demonstrated with the parent, and the tester, giving the items initially and then gradually coercing the child to take part giving clear praise for each correct response. Once a pattern of conditioning has been achieved, lipreading and signing cues should be removed leaving only the listening task and lowering the voice level to establish the quietest level at which an 80% score is obtained.

Test techniques two to three years

Between the ages of two years and 2.5 years infants will normally become more compliant and more able to restrain their impulses. The opportunity is now afforded to establish games that can be fun for the child and that can be used to measure hearing thresholds and auditory discrimination ability in greater depth.

The Performance Test (play audiometry)

By 2.5 years of age children can sometimes be conditioned to wait for a sound and then to respond with some play activity (Figure 3.8). This establishes the ground for a very useful test known as the Performance Test (play audiometry), which really marks a transitional stage to performing conventional audiometry. The inclusion of a play activity such as placing a man in a boat, a ball on a stick or knocking a skittle off a table, helps to motivate the child and attract interest for long enough to record hearing thresholds for a few frequencies on each side. A particular merit of this test is that the child can be conditioned to perform the task by pure demonstration without verbal instruction and this is useful when testing children who may not have developed functional spoken language skills, perhaps

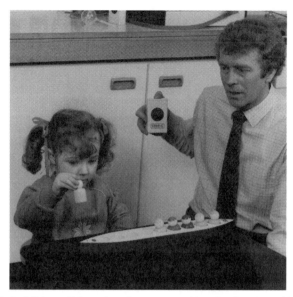

Figure 3.8. A child conditioned ready to respond in a Performance Test.

because they are deaf, or because they do not understand spoken English for other reasons.

Children should be seated on a low chair adjacent to the parent, or on the parent's knee for reassurance if they are nervous or clingy. The test material, for example the boat, is placed on a low table bringing out only one response item (man) at a time so that the child does not become distracted with an array of materials. The remaining items and other reserve toys should be kept out sight. It might be useful to demonstrate the play activity using vibrotactile and visual stimulus clues if profound deafness is suspected. Conditioning will not be possible without some clearly perceived stimulus.

The conditioning sequence starts with a demonstration in which the tester holds the response item poised ready to respond and then promptly inserts the man in the boat (for example) when the stimulus (for example a warble tone of at least one second duration) is presented. After a few demonstrations of this nature using visual and vibratory clues if necessary, the child should be offered the man and the tester should guide a few responses reminding the child to wait for the noise. Natural gestures with a cupped hand at the ear for the sound and a stop sign with the palm of the hand or an authoritative finger for the wait command should be used. The responses should be rewarded with a hand-clap gesture and vocal praise with a smile and approving facial expression. If, after a few demonstrations, the child shows no clear signs of conditioning or constraint the stimulus level should be increased to vibrotactile levels if necessary and more use should be made of visual prompting with head nods to signal the need to respond. As many as 20 guided responses may be needed to condition the very young child and if no pattern of restraint can be detected after this number of demonstrations then it is unlikely that performance technique will be successful. In these circumstances the time can be better spent using other methods (distraction testing or VRA). Even with the mature child it might be wise to cross-check the findings using different methods to compile an audiological profile.

If and when the conditioning has been established, the hearing thresholds can be determined after removing all visual or other clues leaving just the sound stimulus. The sound presentation intervals should be varied in an unpredictable sequence sometimes waiting just a second or so and on other occasions waiting for up to 10 seconds. A common mistake observed with newcomers to this technique is the adoption of a pattern of quick presentations of the sounds without checking to see if the child is demonstrating anticipatory or random response behaviour. Long pauses between sound stimuli will help the tester to assess the reliability of the conditioning. A very mature child might be conditioned with only four or five demonstrations but other children may require many more guided responses.

If portable sound field noise generators are used they should be held out of the child's visual field and there should be no visual cues such as a movement of the tester's eyes, arm or finger when the interrupter switch is operated and, of course, the switch must be operated silently. Whenever the stimulus frequency is changed the tester should be prepared to re-condition the child to the new stimulus. If there is uncertainty about the reliability of the response or if the child's attention is drifting it might be useful to perform a few quick guided responses at high stimulus levels just to remind the child about the response requirement. Four or five responses of this nature will help to keep the child's attention on the task.

It might be necessary to change the activity fairly frequently if the child becomes bored and a range of reserve toys should be available (out of sight, behind closed cupboard doors). A good activity to use with a lively child is that of knocking a plastic skittle off the table perhaps aiming it at a doll or teddy on the floor. Another activity often used with success to motivate an otherwise uninterested child is that of nudging one of the 'men-in-a-boat' toy men off the table into a box on the floor, sometimes hitting the box and sometimes missing the box to keep the child guessing. The tester will need to exercise ingenuity to determine the most suitable activity for each child and this is where the tester's experience really does determine success or otherwise when difficult children are being tested.

If a child accepts the test situation and shows a good level of maturity it might be possible to introduce the bone conduction vibrator and later insert phones or headphones to obtain pure-tone audiometric thresholds for a few frequencies. The golden rule, however, is to obtain sound field thresholds for two or three frequencies first because the point at which the child might lose interest can be quite unpredictable. The introduction of insert phones or headphones might be offputting for some children during the early conditioning stage. If a few sound field air conduction thresholds have been established and no obvious difference can be detected in the response levels for each ear it will be wise to try to obtain a few bone conduction thresholds next rather than use the headphones for further air conduction measurements. It will be wise to work on the principle that the next response might be the last before the child loses interest in the task. With this in mind the intention should be to obtain as much diagnostic information as possible within a limited time frame.

The term 'threshold' has been used in this section in a rather loose sense. The objective is to attempt to apply a standard threshold tracing method using the Hughson and Weslake ascending threshold chasing technique (described by Carhart and Jerger, 1959), using step sizes of 5 dB. It will be appreciated that this might not always be possible and it might be necessary to use larger increments or decrements to home in on the threshold region fairly quickly. A useful variation of technique to adopt with hand-held noisemakers is to sweep the instrument in smoothly from 1 m to within 10 cm or so from the child's ear (remaining out of sight) knowing that each halving of distance increases the sound level by 6 dB. The response level recorded for the child can then be deduced either from a pre-determined calculation or it can be measured directly with a sound level meter simply by reproducing the same distance. An experienced tester can easily gauge distances and reproduce sound levels within limits of 2 dB or 3 dB. It is, of course, preferable to work in a calibrated sound field setup using speakers at a set distance, as for VRA, but this will not always be possible in every clinic environment where these tests are undertaken. The objective should be to use insert phones or headphones as soon as possible and the tester's role becomes much more straightforward once this can be achieved. There is, however, an intermediate stage when some children will not accept the imposition of such equipment and when VRA techniques do not always work sufficiently well for a variety of reasons. It is in such cases that the performance test in the hands of a skilled tester can often help to complete the audiological profile by providing information about the child's hearing sensitivity for frequency-specific sounds. With mature children above the age of three years it might be possible to progress to full audiometry. With some children, however, it will be appropriate to continue to use the performance technique up to the age of five years.

In an interesting study of a cohort of 15,17 children between the ages of 3.25 and 6.75 years included in a multi-centre otitis media study (MRC, 2000) the influence of age, type of audiometry and child's concentration on hearing threshold recordings was assessed with stringent statistical analysis techniques. It was concluded that play audiometry (performance testing) should be employed in the three- to five-year-old age group if conventional audiometry is not feasible. Furthermore, the magnitude of the effect of poor concentration rated 'fair/poor' versus 'good' was slightly greater on play as opposed to conventional audiometry (+5 dB versus + 3 dB). It is rather difficult to disentangle the effects of age, ability of the child to perform a particular task, the skill of the tester, and the child's attention, motivation and concentration levels, in an attempt to determine whether there is a genuine improvement in hearing sensitivity with age. This had been debated by Wightman and Allen (1992) and the MRC (2000) study did not provide conclusive guidance despite the rigorous statistical control. The MRC study did, however, indicate no effect of gender on hearing thresholds in the three- to six-year-old age groups and an improvement of 0.1 dB for bone conduction thresholds for each month of increase in age during this period of growth. The conclusion can be drawn that by the age of three years it should be possible to record hearing thresholds very close to adult values if the child is conditioned appropriately.

Speech discrimination tests

Although children between two and three years of age have usually developed a wide receptive and expressive vocabulary it is not usually possible to undertake conventional speech audiometric measures, using a series of word lists, simply because of the child's relatively short attention span. Consequently it is necessary to simplify the task. The writer's Toy Discrimination Test (McCormick, 1977), shown in Figure 3.9, was developed for use as a simple hearing screening test but it is now widely used in diagnostic audiology clinics, having been adopted by manufacturers for various computerized implementations. These will be described later. Other techniques have been described by Boothroyd (1991, 1984), Boothroyd, Hanin and Eran (1996) and Dawson et al. (1998), but the tests described by these authors have been used in research investigations rather than in routine clinical contexts in the UK. Boothroyd developed a technique known as the Imitative Test of the Perception of Speech Pattern Contrasts (IMSPAC), which assesses a child's auditory capacity for discriminating the minimal acoustic differences which signal a change in the meaning of a word. The child is asked to imitate a nonsense syllable using auditory-visual clues (and written clues if appropriate) and then using auditory information alone. The responses are recorded and later evaluated by a group of listeners who judge if there is accurate representation of vowel place and final consonant voicing of syllables such as /uk/, /ug/, /ik/, /ig/. Although children as young as three years have performed the test Boothroyd (1984) emphasizes that the test is not suitable for pre-lingually deaf children with poor speech production skills.

Dawson et al. (1998) reviewed the speech perception measures that had been developed mostly in America and then developed a technique based on a modification of play audiometry to assess speech discrimination ability in severe-profoundly deaf two- to four-year-old children. The aim was to develop an assessment procedure that was independent of language and speech production ability to test speech feature discrimination in deaf children. The child's task was to respond to a change in speech stimulus in a play audiometry situation when exposed to a speech stimulus that was presented continuously through a speaker. The change occurred at random intervals. Half of the two-year-old children and 82% of three- and four-year-old children tested were able to condition and complete testing of eight speech contrasts in three 20-minute sessions. This test and the IMSPAC test may have research application for the future but they are too time-consuming for normal clinical application.

A novel computer based implementation of the Iowa Matrix Test (Tyler and Holstad, 1987), which measures word identification and cognitive skills, has been described by Nakisa et al. (2001). A matrix of six pictures forming three columns and two rows appears on a VDU screen and the child is required to point to a sequence of words represented on the screen (for example, 'small blue bikes', 'two girls laugh'). This test has been used in a research context with good success for deaf and hearing children between the ages of three years and six years. It is likely that interactive computerized tests of this nature will appear in the field for more routine clinical applications. The following test is already being used in a wide variety of clinic applications both in community and diagnostic clinic settings.

The McCormick Toy Discrimination Test

This test is designed for quick hearing screening and clinical application. It consists of a series of carefully selected toys. There are 14 toys in total, divided into seven near 'minimal' pairs, which sound similar when heard at very quiet listening levels. The author selected the items following field trials with a wide range of alternatives and the final list was chosen according to the following criteria:

- the words, and their toy representations, should be known to a normal child with a mental age of two years;
- paired items of monosyllabic words are used;
- the words within each pair have a maximum degree of acoustic similarity within the vocabulary constraints of the two-year-old child.

The full display is shown in Figure 3.9.

The test is administered by setting out a display containing only the paired items known to the child and the child is

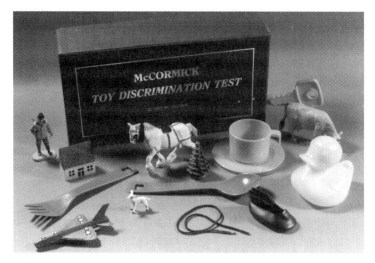

Figure 3.9. The McCormick Toy Discrimination Test.

requested to point to each toy on request. Children with normal hearing can identify the items with 80% accuracy at a quiet listening level of 40 dB(A) for live spoken voice. The objective is to determine the quietest listening level at which a child can obtain an 80% score (four correct out of five requests) and to measure any deviations from the 40 dB level.

Practical details of the test administration will now be discussed and it is worth emphasizing that a very young child's co-operation might be maintained only for a brief spell and it will be necessary for the tester to develop skills in timing and in child handling to maximize the amount of information that can be obtained.

It is recommended that the child be seated in a low chair adjacent to a parent or on a parent's lap if shy or withdrawn. With the tester kneeling, or seated at a low table, and facing the child each toy item should be brought out individually to see if the child recognizes the toy and can name it. The presence and quality of the child's articulation can be assessed taking special note of the clarity of high frequency consonants. If the child will not name the toys the parent should be asked which ones they would expect the child to know. The final display should contain only those pairs of items that the child knows well and the tester can then demonstrate to the child that they should point to the toy when they hear the word using the phrases 'Point to the cup' , 'Where is the spoon?' or 'Show me the cow' and so forth. A loud level of voice should be used initially and the child should be permitted to watch the tester's face for visual clues. If the child responds to the items the tester should then cover the child's face to obliterate any lipreading clues and the voice level should be lowered to determine the quietest level at which the 80% score can be achieved. If the child's attention drifts a quick re-arranging of the toys on the table might re-captivate attention sufficiently for a few additional responses. If a child tries to manipulate the toys the use of a pointing stick held by the child with both hands (such as a drum stick) should help to stop the manipulations. Another technique is to have the pointing stick in one hand and the child to keep the other hand on a 'magic' box (the empty Toy Test box) positioned on the table adjacent to the toys. They often enjoy discipline of this nature at this age and a game can be made out of the instruction 'Keep your hand on the box and do not let it move.' This technique helps to occupy fiddly fingers.

In the case of the very shy or withdrawn child or child with motor difficulties, the eyepointing technique can be used with a limited range of toys spaced out well apart on the table. If a child is known to have a hearing problem and uses a combined mode of communication the signs for each toy can be used to establish the conditioning and then the signs and lipreading clues can be removed to see if the child is able to respond to auditory information alone and if so at what level. The reporting of success with and without visual, signing and auditory clues can give a very useful information about the child's communication strategies.

One advantage of a sound field speech discrimination test is that the parents can witness the nature of their child's hearing abilities. Parents are impressed if the hearing levels are normal and they witness at first hand the child's difficulties when deafness is present. The difference between sound detection and speech discrimination can be demonstrated and the observation of word confusions at quiet listening levels (for the child) will be apparent. Children with mild or moderate degrees of hearing loss will often say 'what?' or 'pardon?' at the quiet listening levels and children with more severe losses will often attempt to watch the speaker's face for lipreading clues. These signs offer useful indications and verifications of the child's difficulties and they should be discussed with the parents.

The validity of the test when used in community settings by health visitors with varying experience has been assessed by Harries and Williamson (2000). In an interesting study they compared the results of the McCormick Toy Discrimination Test, administered by health visitors, in typical non-ideal community settings, with gold standard audiometry, clinical examination and tympanometry undertaken by experienced clinicians. They found that the health visitor application of the Toy Test was capable of identifying conductive hearing loss in three-year-old children with 100% sensitivity, 94% specificity and with a positive predictive value of 82%. It even identified children with mild unilateral hearing loss and some children with normal hearing were able to perform the Toy Test for health visitors but had difficulty with the audiometry. It was concluded that the Toy Test may have advantages for difficult-to-test children in these circumstances. Its value increases both for diagnostic audiology clinical application and for community clinic application if one of the automated versions of the test discussed below is used.

The Automated Institute of Hearing Research /McCormick Toy Discrimination Test

There are advantages and limitations in the live presentation of speech test material to very young children.

Advantages

- The material is presented in a very natural communication situation;
- visual lipreading and signing clues can be used;
- the test is non-intrusive requiring minimum equipment and without the potentially disturbing or distracting effect of headphones or other accessories.

Limitations

- Inter- and intra-subject variability in voice level and intelligibility can influence the results;
- the accurate monitoring of voice level can be problematic;
- it may be difficult to score responses accurately while maintaining close rapport with the child;
- there are practical constraints on the minimal level of voice that can be used.

The Automated IHR/McCormick Toy Discrimination Test (Ousey et al., 1989; Palmer, Sheppard and Marshall, 1991; Summerfield et al., 1994) provides an innovative solution to many of the problems and offers an accurate method for obtaining stable, reliable, and repeatable audiometric speech test results from very young children above the age of two years. The original version of this test is no longer available commercially but alternative versions have been and will be appearing in the field and they all work on similar principles to those described here. A more simplified version is known as the Parrot (Figure 3.10). The latter version uses digitally recorded words but does not incorporate an automated scoring facility.

It is worthwhile providing a detailed description of the principles of the Automated IHR/McCormick test because its novel departure from current speech test methods makes it accessible for application with the very young.

The test uses a speaker presentation of digitally stored speech waveforms of the 14 words in the Toy Discrimination Test and incorporates an adaptive scoring algorithm under microprocessor control. The advantage of digitally stored speech materials is that the words can be presented in any order and in any combination to suit the child's vocabulary. Words not known to the child can be excluded from the test, together with the matching pair, and then the test randomly cycles through the remaining items.

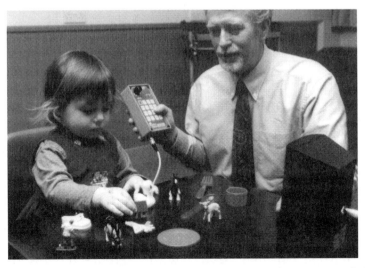

Figure 3.10. Another digitized implementation of the McCormick Toy Discrimination Test - The 'Parrot'.

The components of the test include a keypad handset linked to a control unit housed in a speaker stand. The tester programmes the test by means of the handset control which includes a display for the tester indicating the output word for the current trial and the running estimate of the threshold.

The automated test takes approximately two or three minutes to administer to the typical two- to five-year-old child and shows an excellent test/retest correlation of 0.93 for such children (Ousey et al., 1989). For children in this age group the normal score in quiet (typical ambient noise level less than 30 dB A) for the 71% correct score for six adaptive reversals is 30–35 dB(A). For adults in the same environment the 71% score is obtained at 20 dB (A). A useful feature of the test is that there is no floor or ceiling effect even for adults. Testing starts with a word presented at 72 dB (A) and consists of a running-in phrase 'Point to the . . .' followed by the stimulus word. Initially the level is reduced by 12 dB following each correct response until the child makes an error and then the level is increased by 12 dB. After the next correct response an adaptive procedure is used to control the stimulus level and to estimate the level giving the 71% correct response. The level is reduced by 6 dB following two correct responses and increased by 6 dB following an error. The transition from increasing to decreasing level, or vice versa, constitutes a reversal. The threshold is then estimated as the mean of the stimulus levels at six reversals at which time the test automatically stops.

The correlation between the speech-in-quiet score and the average pure-tone threshold for 500 Hz, 1 kHz and 4 kHz is high with a 95% confidence interval of 11 dB (Palmer, Sheppard and Marshall, 1991). The word discrimination threshold (WDT) in dB (A) measured by this test has been shown to relate to the average better-ear hearing level at 0.5, 1 and 4 kHz (AT in dB HL) according to the formula AT = 0.877 × WDT −9.28 (Palmer et al., 1991). This link between hearing threshold and speech discrimination ability is very interesting. Furthermore it has been shown that there is a strong relationship between the IHR-McCormick word discrimination threshold and wider measures of speech perception which sample aspects of everyday auditory communication skill. A correlation of 0.71 has been reported (McCormick, 2002) with a connected discourse tracking test (de Filippo and Scott, 1978) and 0.59 with the Iowa Matrix Test (Tyler and Holstad, 1987) (both correlations being significant p < 0.50). Use of the speech-in-noise test facility offered in the automated version of the test affords the possibility of investigating aspects of hearing disability in more depth and the full potential of the test has yet to be fully explored in a clinical context. The IHR-McCormick Automated Toy Discrimination Test has already found application in assessing relative performance of hearing aid and cochlear implant users and in helping to determine audiological selection criteria for cochlear implantation (McCormick, 2002; Nakisa et al., 2001).

Assessing hearing in infants with physical and learning difficulties

A very useful review of this subject has been presented by Coninx and Lancioni (1995) and space here only permits a brief account of the author's contribution to this work (McCormick, 1995). This is an important topic because one third of children with severe/profound deafness will have additional problems and audiology services have the responsibility to assess all children with multiple problems to exclude the possibility of deafness. At the time of the audiological assessment it is possible that other conditions may not have been confirmed, or even suspected, and the audiologist will need to determine the child's capabilities including the level of responsiveness and ability to condition for the tests. If the child cannot be conditioned for a performance test it might be possible to undertake a co-operative test and if this does not work a distraction test or VRA might be appropriate. Failing this behavioural response audiometry will be needed together with a range of objective test techniques. Exactly the same sequence of logical progression should be used when testing children of any age with multiple problems.

The following represent just a few examples of how tests might have to be modified to suit children with different difficulties. For children with cerebral palsy the child's physical response capabilities must be assessed and checked with the parents/caregivers. It might, for example, be possible to condition a child to nudge a skittle off a stand with a simple head movement if the child does not have the physical capability to manipulate a toy. The test situation for VRA might have to be rearranged by bringing the visual reward closer to the child or more directly into vision to accept eye glance responses if the child cannot perform clear head turn responses. Some children with learning difficulties may be disinterested in, or be frightened by, the visual rewards used for VRA but can be conditioned to respond in a distraction test with human reward such as a smile or tickle on the arm or cheek. Children with visual problems can be conditioned to reach out for a tactile reward when a sound is presented on the same side (see later discussion). The assessment of responsiveness to touch and visual stimulation in the distraction test situation is particularly useful when testing children with complex combination of problems.

The auropalpebral (eye blink) reflex (APR) is quick and simple to observe and its appearance can indicate the presence of a considerable amount of hearing although not necessarily normal hearing. If it can be elicited to stimuli presented at 80/90 dB and behavioural responses can also be observed at 40/50 dB it can be concluded that the child must have reasonably normal hearing at some frequencies and this can be a good strategy to apply during the early stage of a clinical assessment. The auropalpebral reflex has been used in studies of reflex modulation (Reiter, 1981). This refers to a general class of phenomena in which a weak but supra-threshold auditory, visual or tactile pre-stimulus can alter (by facilitation or inhibition) the normal or control magnitude of an elicited reflex. If the presentation of a pure tone is shown to inhibit the magnitude of the blink reflex then that tone can be said to have been perceived. Reiter (1981) found that pure tones as low as 10 dB to 15 dB sensation could inhibit the eyeblink reflex to an air puff. The auropalpebral response has also been used in conventional forms of classical conditioning (Lancioni et al., 1985; Lancioni et al.,1990). The role of this approach for hearing assessment has been reviewed by Lancioni and Coninx (1995) and the reader is referred to the original work for further details.

Further tips and suggestion for testing special categories of children

Blind infants

Infants with some degree of vision will often turn to locate the source of a sound but totally blind infants can usually be conditioned to reach out for the sound and the response can be rewarded by letting the child handle the noisemaker when a correct response is obtained. Fraiberg (1977) observed such behaviour in babies beyond a mental age of eight months when object permanency is developing. She noted that the five- to eight-month-old blind child did not reach out for a toy removed from grasp even when the toy was a noisemaker. Sonksen (1979) noted that once the visually handicapped baby started to locate sounds there was a marked difference in the reactions to familiar and unfamiliar sounds to the degree not witnessed in sighted children. Yarnall (1983) assessed the benefits of using various reinforcers, including food, sounds and vibrations in an operant conditioning audiometry task with deaf-blind infants and concluded that the results were comparable with those obtained with conventional audiometry.

Infants with cerebral palsy

These infants can have varying levels of intellect and the activity chosen must take account of the fact that the child might be quite bright despite having difficulties with communication and with physical co-ordination. A conditioning activity for a performance test using a skittle has already been mentioned above and it is very important to match the response task to the child's cognitive and neuromuscular co-ordination abilities and to seek advice from the parents as to their expectations of the appropriateness of the chosen game. Sometimes, however, parents might underestimate their child's capabilities in the hands of an experienced and skilled tester. Clear demonstration will be needed and the child should be given sufficient time to respond. Often the child's eyes will focus on the response item as soon as the sound stimulus is presented and there will be general postural clues indicating the initiation of effort and determination to perform the task. If given sufficient time to co-ordinate a response success can often be achieved. It can be very rewarding for all parties when the task is eventually performed and on a number of occasions in the author's clinic parents have commented that they did not realize that their child had a sufficient degree of understanding. The golden rules with these children are to allow the luxury of time, to gently persist with conditioning for a task well within the child's capabilities, and to reward correct responses with a method of praise suggested by the parent.

Autistic infants

Of all the children attending audiology clinics autistic infants are by far the most difficult to test. With patience and perseverance it is normally possible to obtain the information required through behavioural testing but it might be necessary to vary the techniques and to clear the room of all unnecessary equipment and distractions because the child can be expected to wander about quite frequently during the test. Some of these children are obsessed with mirrors and it will be desirable to draw curtains across observation windows. The child might show other ritualistic and bizarre behaviour and avoid eye contact or even show total disregard for the tester or for any speech or spoken sound stimuli. Head turn responses are more likely to be obtained to electronically or mechanically generated sounds if the child's attention state is optimal. Spinning activities are usually very good for capturing the child's attention or failing this a bouncing ball will often fascinate the child. Sometimes there may be a fascination for lights and it might be necessary to switch off sets of lights in the clinic and to use a torch or the otoscope light to attract the child's attention to the test area.

Hypersensitivity to sound has been observed in some autistic children and useful pointers may be obtained from the history. Careful note should be taken of any test stimuli that produce adverse reactions so that further use of these can be avoided.

It must be remembered that autistic children can demonstrate amplitude and latency differences in auditory response waveforms compared to normal controls (Mochizuki et al., 1986; Taylor, Rosenblatt and Linschoten, 1982) and the results of ABR investigations must be interpreted with great caution. The author has seen a few unnecessary hearing aid fittings in these children. Behavioural observation tests are particularly important both before and after hearing aid fittings with autistic children.

Concluding comments

The options available for undertaking behavioural audiological assessments have been discussed in this chapter and it has been stressed throughout that the skill and experience of the tester will have a significant bearing on the success of the tests. The expansion of objective test techniques will help to speed up the process of obtaining definitive test results for very young or difficult-to-test children but at the end of an assessment process there will always be the need to determine how well the child uses hearing for communication purposes and nothing can replace good behavioural methods to achieve this objective.

References

Arlinger SD, Jerlvall LB (1987) Reliability in warble-tone sound field audiometry. Scandinavian Audiology 16: 21–7.

Bennett MJ (1975) The auditory response cradle: a device for the objective assessment of auditory state in the neonate. Symposia of the Zoological Society of London 37: 291–305.

Bennett MJ (1979) Trials with the auditory response cradle I. Neonatal responses to auditory stimuli. British Journal of Audiology 13: 125–34.

Bennett MJ, Lawrence R (1980) Trials with the auditory response cradle II. British Journal of Audiology 14: 1–6.

Beynon G, Munro K (1993) A discussion of current sound field calibration procedures. British Journal of Audiology 27: 427–35.

Berg KM, Smith MC (1983) Behavioral thresholds for tones during infancy. Journal of Experimental Child Psychology 35: 409–25.

Bhattacharya J, Bennett MJ, Tucker S (1984) Long term follow-up of newborns tested with the auditory response cradle. Archives of Disease in Childhood 59: 504–11.

Boothroyd A (1984) Auditory perception of speech contrasts by subjects with sensorineural hearing loss. Journal of Speech and Hearing Research 27: 134–44.

Boothroyd A (1991) Assessment of speech perception capacity in profoundly deaf children. The American Journal of Otology 12 (suppl.): 67–72.

Boothroyd A, Cawkwell S (1970) Vibrotactile thresholds in pure tone audiometry. Acta Oto-Laryngologica 69: 381–7.

Boothroyd A, Hanin L, Eran O (1996) Speech perception and production in hearing-impaired children. In Bess FH, Gravel JS, Thorpe AM (eds) Amplification for Children with Auditory Deficits. Nashville, TN: Bill Wilkerson Centre Press, pp. 55–74.

Byrne D, Dillon H (1981) Comparative reliability of warble tone thresholds under earphone and in sound field. Australian Journal of Audiology 3: 12–14.

Carhart R, Jerger JF (1959) Preferred method for clinical determination of pure tone thresholds. Journal of Speech and Hearing Disorders 24: 330–45.

Coninx F, Lancioni GE (eds) (1995) Hearing assessment and aural rehabilitation of multiply handicapped deaf children. Scandinavian Audiology 24: Supplement 41.

Davis AR (1984) The statistical decision criterion for the auditory response cradle. British Journal of Audiology 18: 163–8.

Davis A, Wood S (1992) The epidemiology of childhood hearing-impairment: factors relevant to planning of services. British Journal of Audiology 26: 77–90.

Dawson PW, Nott PE, Clark GM, Cowan RSC (1998) A modification of play audiometry to assess speech discrimination ability in severe-profoundly deaf 2–4 year old children. Ear and Hearing 19(5): 371–84.

De Filippo CL, Scott BL (1978) A method for training and evaluating the reception of ongoing speech. Journal of the Acoustical Society of America 63: 1186–92.

Eisele WA, Berry RC, Shriner TA (1975) Infant sucking response patterns as a conjugate function of change in the sound pressure level of auditory stimuli. Journal of Speech and Hearing Research 18: 296-307.

Ewing IR, Ewing AWG (1947) The ascertainment of deafness in infancy and early childhood. Journal of Laryngology and Otology 59: 309-38.

Fraiberg S (1977) Insights from the Blind. London: Souvenir Press.

Gerber SE (ed.) (1977) Audiometry in Infancy. New York: Grune & Stratton, pp. 71-81.

Gliddon ML, Martin AM, Green R (1999) A comparison of some clinical features of visual reinforcement audiometry and the distraction test. British Journal of Audiology 33: 355-65.

Haggard MP, McCormick B, Gannon MM, Spencer H (1992) The paediatric otologic caseload resulting from improved screening in the first year of life. Clinical Otolaryngol 17: 34-43.

Hammond PD, Gold MS, Wigg NR, Volkmer RE (1997) Pre-school hearing screening evaluation of a parental questionnaire. Journal of Paediatrics and Child Health 33: 528-30.

Harries J, Williamson T (2000) Community-based validation of the McCormick Toy Test. British Journal of Audiology 34: 279-83.

Hoversten GH, Moncur JP (1969) Stimuli and intensity factors in testing infants. Journal of Speech and Hearing Research 12: 689-702.

Hutt SJ, Hutt C, Lenard HG, von Bernuth H, Muntjewerff WJ (1968) Auditory responsiveness in the human neonate. Nature 218: 888-90.

Keefe DH, Bulen JC, Arehart KH, Burns EM (1993) Ear-canal impedance and reflection coefficients in human infants and adults. Journal of the Acoustical Society of America 94: 2617-38.

Kent R, Osberger M, Netsell R, Hustedde C (1987) Phonetic development in identical twins differing in auditory function. Journal of Speech and Hearing Disorders 52: 64-75.

Lancioni GE, Coninx F (1995) A classical conditioning procedure for auditory testing: air puff audiometry. Scandinavian Audiology 24(Suppl 41): 43-8.

Lancioni GE, Coninx F, Brozzi G, Oliva D, Hoogeveen FR (1990) Air-puff conditioning audiometry: extending its applicability with multiply handicapped individuals. International Journal of Rehabilitation Research 13: 67-70.

Lancioni GE, Hoogland GA, Smeets PM, Brozzi G, Scoponi MV, Piattella L, Zamponi N (1985) Hearing assessment in developmentally impaired infants: classical conditioning as a supplement to brainstem evoked response audiometry (BERA). International Journal of Paediatric Otorhinolaryngology 10: 221-8.

Latham AD, Haggard MP (1980) A pilot study to detect hearing-impairment in the young. Midwife, Health Visitor and Community Nurse 16: 370-4.

Lutman ME, McCormick B (1987) Converting free-field A-weighted sound levels to hearing levels. Journal of the British Association of Teachers of the Deaf 11: 127.

Mason S, McCormick B, Wood S (1988) The Auditory Brain Stem Response (ABR). Archives of Disease in Childhood 63: 465-7.

Maw AR, Tiwari RS (1998) Children with glue ear: how do they present? Clinical Otolaryngology 13: 171-7.

McCormick B (1975) Parent guidance: the needs of families and of the professional worker. The Teacher of the Deaf 73 (no.434): 315-30.

McCormick B (1977) The Toy Discrimination Test: an aid for screening the hearing of children above the age of two years. Public Health 91: 67-73.

McCormick B (1983) Hearing screening by health visitors: a critical appraisal of the Distraction Test. Health Visitor 56: 449-51.

McCormick B (1986) Evaluation of a warbler in hearing screening tests. Health Visitor 59:143-4.

McCormick B (1988) Screening for Hearing-Impairment in Young Children. London: Chapman & Hall (republished by Whurr Publishers, London, 1994).

McCormick B (1990) Commentary on Scanlon PE and Bamford JM: Early identification of hearing loss: screening and surveillance methods. Archives of Disease in Childhood 65: 479-85.

McCormick B (1995) History and state-of-the-art in behavioural methods for hearing assessment in low-functioning children. Scandinavian Audiology 24: (suppl. 41) 31-5.

McCormick B (2000) Managing the transition to universal neonatal hearing screening – the missing link (letter to the editor). British Journal of Audiology 34: 67-9.

McCormick B (2002) Assessing audiological suitability of cochlear implants for children below the age of five years. In McCormick B, Archbold S (eds) (2002) Cochlear Implants for Young Children. London: Whurr.

McCormick B, Curnock DA, Spavins F (1984) Auditory screening of special care neonates using the auditory response cradle. Archives of Disease in Childhood 59: 1168-72.

McCormick B, Wood S, Cope Y, Spavins FM (1984) Analysis of records from an open access audiology service. British Journal of Audiology 18: 127-32.

Mendel MI (1968) Infant responses to recorded sounds. Journal of Speech and Hearing Research 11: 811-16.

Mochizuki Y, Ohkubo H, Yoshida A, Tatara T (1986) Auditory Brainstem Response (ABR) in developmentally retarded infants and children. Brain and Development 8: 247-56.

Moore JM, Wilson WR, Thompson G (1977) Visual reinforcement of head-turn responses in infants under 12 months of age. Journal of Speech and Hearing Disorders 42: 328-34.

MRC (2000) Influence of age, type of audiometry and child's concentration on hearing thresholds. British Journal of Audiology 34: 231-40.

Nakisa MJ, Summerfield AQ, Nakisa RC, McCormick B, Archbold S, Gibbin KP, O'Donoghue GM (2001) Functionally equivalent ages and hearing levels of children with cochlear implants measured with pre-recorded stimuli. British Journal of Audiology 35: 183-99.

Nolan M (1978) Guidance on the interpretation of information from a sound level meter. Journal of the British Association of Teachers of the Deaf 2: 169-73.

Nolan M (1987) Letter to the editor. Journal of the British Association of Teachers of the Deaf 11: 128-9.

Nozza RJ, Henson AM (1999) Unmasked thresholds and minimum masking in infants and adults: separating sensory from nonsensory contributions to infant-adult differences in behavioral thresholds. Ear and Hearing 20: 483-96.

Nozza RJ, Wilson WR (1984) Masked and unmasked pure tone thresholds of infants and adults: development of auditory frequency selectivity and sensitivity. Journal of Speech and Hearing Research 27: 613-22.

Olsho LW, Koch EG, Halpin CF, Carter EA (1987) An observer-based psychoacoustic procedure for use with young infants. Developmental Psychology 23: 627-40.

Olsho LW, Koch EG, Carter EA, Halpin CF, Spetner NB (1988) Pure-tone sensitivity of human infants. Journal of the Acoustical Society of America 84: 1316-24.

Orchik DJ, Rintelmann WF (1978) Comparison of pure-tone, warble-tone and narrow-band noise thresholds of young normally hearing children. Journal of the American Academy of Audiology 3: 214-20.

Ousey J, Sheppard S, Twomey T, Palmer AR (1989) The IHR/McCormick Automated Toy Discrimination Test – description and initial evaluation. British Journal of Audiology 23: 245-9.

Palmer AR, Sheppard S, Marshall DM (1991) Prediction of hearing thresholds in young children using an automated toy discrimination test. British Journal of Audiology 25: 351-6.

Reiter LA (1981) Reflex modulation: a new method for measuring hearing in children. International Journal of Paediatric Otorhinolaryngology 3: 79-84.

Rosenfield RM, Goldsmith AJ, Madell JR (1998) How accurate is parental rating of children with otitis media? Archives of Otolaryngology and Head and Neck Surgery 124: 989-92.

Roush J, Bryant K, Mundy M, Zeisel S, Roberts J (1995) Developmental changes in static acoustic admittance and tympanometric width in infants and toddlers. Journal of the American Academy of Audiology 6: 334-8.

Samples JM, Franklin B (1978) Behavioural responses in seven to nine month old infants to speech and non-speech stimuli. Journal of Auditory Research 18: 115-23.

Sinnott JM, Pisoni DB, Aslin RM (1983) A comparison of pure tone auditory thresholds in human infants and adults. Infant Behaviour and Development 6: 3-17.

Sonksen P M (1979) Sound and the visually handicapped baby. Child Health and Development 5: 413-20.

Stoel-Gammon C, Otomo K (1986) Babbling development of hearing impaired and normally hearing subjects. Journal of Speech and Hearing Disorders 51: 33-41.

Summerfield Q, Palmer AR, Foster JR, Marshall DH, Twomey T (1994) Clinical evaluation of test-retest reliability of the IHR-McCormick Automated Toy Discrimination Test. British Journal of Audiology 28: 165-79.

Suzuki T, Ogiba Y (1961) Conditioned Orientation Reflex Audiometry. Archives of Otolaryngology 74: 84-90.

Taylor MJ, Rosenblatt R, Linschoten L (1982) Auditory brainstem response abnormalities in autistic children. Le Journal Canadien Des Sciences Neurologiques 9: 429-33.

Thompson G, Folsom RC (1985) Reinforced and non-reinforced head-turn responses of infants as a function of stimulus bandwidth. Ear and Hearing 6: 125-9.

Trehub SE, Schneider BA, Endman M (1980) Developmental changes in infants' sensitivity to octave-band noises. Journal of Experimental Child Psychology 29: 282-93.

Tyler R, Holstad B (1987) A Closed-set Speech Perception Test for Hearing-impaired Children. Iowa City: University of Iowa.

Watkin PM, Baldwin M, Laoide S (1990) Parental suspicion and identification of hearing-impairment. Archives of Disease in Childhood 65: 846-50.

Weir C (1976) Auditory frequency sensitivity in the neonate : a signal detection analysis. Journal of Experimental Child Psychology 21: 219-25.

Werner LA, Gillenwater JM (1990) Pure-tone sensitivity of 2 to 5-week-old infants. Infant Behaviour and Development 13: 355-75.

Werner LA, Marean GC (1996) Human Auditory Development. Colorado and Oxford: Westview Press.

Werner LA, Mancl LR (1993) Pure-tone thresholds of 1-month old human infants. Journal of the Acoustical Society of America 93: 2367.

Wightman F, Allen P (1992) Individual differences in auditory capacity among pre-school children. In Werner LA, Ruber EN (eds) Developmental Psycholinguistics. Washington DC: American Psychological Association.

Wilson WR, Thompson G (1984) Behavioral Audiometry. In Jerger J (ed.) Pediatric Audiology. London: Taylor & Francis, pp. 1–44.

Wood S, Davis AC, McCormick B (1997) Changing performance of the Health Visitor Distraction Test when targeted neonatal screening is introduced into a health district. British Journal of Audiology 31: 55–61.

Yarnall GD (1983) Comparison of operant and conventional audiometry procedures with multihandicapped (deaf-blind) children. The Volta Review (February–March): 69–82.

Chapter 4
Visual reinforcement audiometry

PAUL SHAW

Introduction

Visual reinforcement audiometry (VRA) is a powerful behavioural assessment technique that can be used to determine frequency- and ear-specific audiological information in the majority of the paediatric population aged between five months and approximately 36 months (developmental age) requiring audiological assessment. It is used extensively around the world and its use in the UK has increased substantially since the mid-1990s. In the majority of hospital-based audiology clinics in the UK it has become an essential technique for assessing young infants. The test is based on the fact that normally developing infants will start to localize to sound at around four to six months of age. With VRA, as the name suggests, a visual reward is used to maintain a child's interest in turning to auditory stimuli. This interest factor enables accurate audiological assessment. Although there has been an important and welcome move towards universal neonatal hearing screening using objective assessment techniques, there still remains the need for simple, accurate and effective behavioural hearing tests which can be performed quickly and reliably on the paediatric population. The reliability of VRA is well established. The American Speech-Language-Hearing Association (ASHA, 1991a) and the National Deaf Children's Society (NDCS, 2000) in the UK recognize the importance of the test procedure and recommend its use as one of a battery of tests available to the paediatric audiologist.

Children who are not developmentally ready for VRA require a combination of objective and behavioural tests to estimate auditory sensitivity. Objective techniques including otoacoustic emission (OAE) tests, auditory brainstem response (ABR) tests, acoustic immittance tests and acoustic reflex threshold tests are used together with behavioural observation audiometry (BOA). Auditory brainstem response has become the test of choice for neonates, babies below five months of age and infants with developmental disorders. For babies above five months of age, ABR can be time-consuming, often requires sedation and sometimes provides only limited information regarding the audiometric configuration and the type of hearing loss.

Behavioural observation audiometry, as the name implies, requires careful observation of infants' responses to sounds (Wilson and Thompson, 1984; Northern and Downs, 1991). Although BOA is a useful technique, it does have numerous limitations. Responses are unconditioned, so they are highly variable, habituate rapidly and depend on the type of stimuli used (Wilson and Thompson, 1984). The distraction test has been commonly used in the UK to assess young infants. This test is a modification of BOA. Gliddon, Martin and Green (1999) compare the distraction test to VRA and discuss the advantages and disadvantages of each technique.

For children capable of performing play audiometry, or indeed conventional audiometry, the task of defining auditory thresholds is somewhat easier. For all infants requiring audiological assessment, a test battery approach including objective and behavioural techniques is least likely to result in over/under estimation of a child's hearing status. Visual reinforcement audiometry plays a central role in this test battery when assessing young infants.

This chapter will look at the development of the procedure, the principles involved, the equipment requirements, calibration issues and how and when to use VRA. It will also explore issues surrounding the use of VRA with premature infants and children with additional disabilities and also at issues surrounding training, research, hearing aid fitting and evaluation and the effects of the test procedure on the families of those children being assessed.

As with any paediatric test procedure, the skill and knowledge of the audiologist is as important as the test itself. The audiologist must understand the principles and be aware of the limitations of visual reinforcement audiometry in order to become proficient in assessing this challenging population.

Awareness of child development and behaviour is also crucial in assessing any child within a holistic framework.

Development of test procedure

The development of the test procedure, which is now widely known as visual reinforcement audiometry, spans a number of decades and countries. Infant assessment techniques were initially based on procedures described by Ewing and Ewing (1944) in England. Dix and Hallpike (1947), also from England, detailed a technique named the 'peep show' test, which was used in pure-tone audiometry with children over three years. A correct response to an auditory stimulus was rewarded with the sight of an interesting picture. Suzuki and Ogiba (1961) from Japan, recognized that a simpler procedure was required for infants below three years of age. Knowing that infants will turn to a new and interesting stimulus (orientation reflex) they developed a procedure named conditioned orientation reflex audiometry (COR). They were able to demonstrate that an infant could be trained to look for a visual stimulus on hearing an auditory stimulus. Two sets of speakers and visual toys were used, with the child positioned midway between them. After training (conditioning) a child by presenting a sound and illuminating a toy together, the test tone was presented on its own and the intensity of this test tone was reduced to determine the quietest level at which the child would look for the illuminated toy. Suzuki and Ogiba realized that only if the infant was correctly conditioned (would turn to look for visual stimulus on hearing test tone) would the assessment be possible. The results of their procedure on over 300 children were very encouraging and suggested that infants could be accurately assessed using this method. This was the first time that a combination of classical and operant conditioning procedures (Suzuki and Ogiba used the terms Pavlovian and instrumental conditioning) had been used in infant audiological assessment.

Liden and Kankkunen (1969) from Sweden modified and simplified Suzuki and Ogiba's technique and named their test visual reinforcement audiometry (VRA). After using Suzuki and Ogiba's method with children with hearing losses, they concluded that the task of locating pure tones was too difficult. The test set-up was different in that the speaker and visual reward were not adjacent. The speakers were positioned at either side of the infant, in close proximity, and the rewards were set in front and at an angle from the infant. Instead of using illuminated toys, slides were projected on frosted glass windows at the desired positions. By positioning the speakers in close proximity to the infants' ears, they hoped to use the head shadow effect (intensity attenuation of a signal due to the obstruction of the head) in an attempt to obtain ear-specific information. The infant was not required to localize correctly to the auditory stimulus but rather to show one of four responses: reflexive behaviour, investigative, orientation or spontaneous response (Liden and Kankkunen, 1969). Results obtained in their initial study demonstrated that the procedure was effective and simple to use. They concluded that children with hearing impairment could be assessed accurately from six to eight months of age and that visual reinforcement audiometry was more effective than COR audiometry in older infants.

Although the above methods had intrinsic design problems, pure tones used in sound fields (see later), and apparatus too close to the infant, the foundations from which modern VRA systems have developed were clearly set. Other workers, notably Haug, Baccaro and Guildford (1967), although not using the term 'VRA', were important in the development of visually reinforced audiological assessment of infants. In the last 30 years there have been developments in the technique, based on well-researched scientific studies, looking at issues such as: complexity of reinforcement (Moore, Thompson and Thompson, 1975); response strength as a function of stimulus (Primus and Thompson, 1985); VRA in infants under the age of 12 months (Moore, Wilson and Thompson, 1977); application of VRA to 'low-functioning children' (Thompson, Wilson and Moore, 1979); VRA with young Down syndrome children (Greenberg et al., 1978); effects of reinforcer duration on response in VRA (Culpepper and Thompson, 1994); effects of prematurity on VRA response (Moore, Thompson and Folsom, 1992); the role of localization in VRA (Primus, 1992); strategies for increasing response behaviour in VRA (Thompson, Thompson and McCall, 1992); VRA results compared with pure-tone audiometry results (Talbot, 1987) and VRA compared to the distraction test (Gliddon, Martin and Green, 1999).

Visual reinforcement audiometry is now regarded internationally as a powerful and effective assessment tool which when coupled with a skilled paediatric audiologist can in most cases provide accurate, reliable, frequency and ear-specific audiological information in the paediatric population aged approximately five months to 36 months.

Equipment requirements

Test room

Ideally a sound-treated room with an observation room and one way window is required (Figure 4.1). The observation room is dimly lit to prevent the infant seeing any activity that may be distracting. It is also useful to have lights in the test room that can be dimmed to facilitate increased awareness of the visual rewards. With this set up, the child being assessed will be positioned in the test area in the test room. The audiologist who will be presenting the auditory and visual stimuli is situated in the observation room. Many clinics do not have the luxury of an observation room and are, nevertheless, successful in obtaining results with the child and audiologist in the same room. Whatever setup is used, there must be minimal distraction from the audiologist presenting the stimuli.

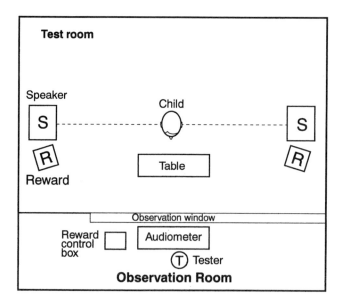

Figure 4.1. Room layout for VRA with observation room. Speakers (S) and rewards (R) at 90° azimuth from forward-facing position of test point.

The test room should be sound-treated and should have very low levels of background noise if sound field assessment and bone conduction assessment are used (most cases of VRA). BS EN ISO 8253-2 (1998) provides further information. Slightly higher levels of noise are permitted if headphones or insert earphones are used (BS EN ISO 8253-1: 1998). The room should be as uncluttered as possible. This may be difficult if the room is frequently used, but every effort should be made to put unused toys away in cupboards and to keep pictures (even if audiologically relevant) off walls. The ideal test room would have a small table, a few chairs, the visual rewards and speakers and a few cupboards for toys. If an observation room is used, it is necessary to fix a microphone in the clinic. This can be placed above the test point and can be fixed into the ceiling. This microphone can then be connected to an amplifier and speaker in the observation room. This enables the audiologist operating the audiometer to hear the proceedings in the clinic.

The document, Health Building Note 12(3): 1994, provides useful information regarding recommended size of audiology clinics and other practical and ergonomic considerations.

Visual rewards

Two visual rewards are required if a two-speaker arrangement is used. As we shall see later, the level of complexity and the variety of the visual rewards used has a direct effect on the success of the VRA test procedure. In simple terms this means the more *attractive* the reward is to infants, the more likely they will keep turning to see it. Furthermore, the greater the variety of the rewards then the greater the likely number of responses. Many different visual rewards are used and these can range from a small teddy with flashing lights attached, to animated flashing toys that appear to dance when activated (Figure 4.2).

Computer monitors are also used that allow the tester endless computer-generated images and pictures. Ideally the rewards should not be visible until activated. This requires housing the rewards in cabinets with darkened glass windows. Care should be taken not to use reflective glass as this often acts as a mirror, which may be appealing to a child. All rewards used should be easily visible when activated and it is useful to have mobile rewards for use with children with motor and/or vision difficulties. Fixing rewards on speaker stands with wheels is one

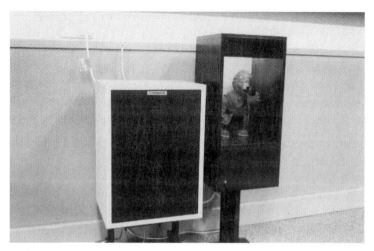

Figure 4.2. Visual reinforcer and speaker.

option. A switch/control box to activate the rewards is positioned in the observation room.

Whichever type of reward is used, the audiologist should be aware of the benefits and limitations of their particular setup.

Audiometer

A two-channel audiometer with options for sound field (SF), headphone (HP), insert earphone (IE) and bone conduction (BC) stimuli will enable full audiological assessment. BS EN 60645-1 (1995) offers guidance. Pure-tone, frequency-modulated (warble) tone and narrow-band noise stimuli should be available.

Audiometers are frequently not capable of providing the very high output levels needed to assess severely and profoundly deaf infants via the sound field. A power amplifier either fitted internally or externally is usually required. The reader is referred to the audiometer operator's manual for further advice.

Transducers

Loudspeakers are required that are capable of delivering high intensity undistorted warble tones over the range of frequencies to be tested. Standards for speakers used in audiometry are difficult to interpret (BS 5942: part 7: 1987). Speakers which have been designed with concentric low, mid and high frequency cones and which operate as a point source will produce the least variable sound field. When calibrating a sound field, the goal is to provide a known intensity, at a defined point, with as little variation in intensity around that point. Speakers that consist of separate speakers within the speaker housing often do not generate a uniform sound field. Careful investigation of the sound field is required before accurate assessment is possible (see calibration section).

Standard headphones used in pure-tone audiometry can be used in VRA.

Insert earphones are often used in VRA. The desired sensation level (DSL) method of amplification selection (Seewald, 1992, Seewald et al., 1997) recommends this transducer for the assessment of infants.

A *standard bone conductor* used in pure-tone audiometry can also be used for VRA and this can provide valuable information in assessing whether the type of hearing loss is sensorineural or conductive.

A collection of preferably soft toys and puzzles is also needed as well as a small low-level table and a collection of differently-sized chairs.

Hearing protection

An important issue discussed by Day (2000) is the area of noise protection at work. The Noise at Work Regulations (1989) outline maximum daily exposure levels above which hearing protection must be used. If assessing a number of children with severe-profound hearing loss then it will be necessary to estimate daily exposure levels. As a guideline, if levels of 85dBA or greater are used in the sound field then hearing protection should be available for both staff and parents/carers.

Calibration

Sound field

Calibrating a sound field requires careful consideration of a number of variables. Size of room, type of room, speaker type, speaker azimuth, stimulus type, background noise levels, test position, available normative threshold data (reference equivalent threshold sound pressure levels (RETSPLs)), measurement scale, dB HL (dB hearing level), dB SPL (dB sound pressure level) or dB A (dB A-weighted), to name a few.

The goal of any hearing test is to define frequency-specific thresholds, which can be related to other test methods across different test centres. For sound field assessment, the issues surrounding calibration are complex. Cox and McCormick (1987), Walker, Dillon and Byrne (1984), Beynon and Munro (1993) and ASHA (1991b), all explore calibration issues, with Beynon and Munro and ASHA providing the most detailed reports. A sound-treated room is required with a position (test point) where frequency-specific stimuli produced by a speaker do not deviate more than 2 dB at positions 15 cm (30 cm if possible) around the point (there should be a sphere around the test point in which accurate assessment can take place). Figure 4.3 provides an illustration of the three axes where signal level is measured.

The test point is usually at the height of the average child's ear when sitting on a parent's/carer's lap or in a small chair. In practice, these two positions may be separated and careful thought has to be given when choosing the test point. The speakers are usually positioned so that the centre of the speaker is at the same height as the test point (Figure 4.3).

Pure tones are only suitable for sound field testing in an anechoic chamber (free field). This is because standing wave patterns are produced in non free field environments and these affect stimulus levels at and around the test point. It is also impossible to keep a child's ear in a specific location and this means that there has to be an area or volume in which the child's ears can move but where sound pressure levels are constant or differ by a very small amount (typically <2dB). The bandwidth of the signal used has to be wide enough to provide a uniform sound field whilst remaining narrow enough to provide frequency-specific information. Frequency-modulated (warble)

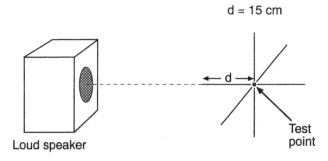

Figure 4.3. Representation of test point and speaker position.

tones and narrow-band noise fulfil these criteria. Frequency modulated (warble) tones are the signal of choice, if the characteristics of the tones comply with recommendations (BS EN ISO 8253-2:1998). Narrow-band noise (NBN) can also be used, if the noise is *narrow* enough. The characteristics of NBN found on most audiometers do not normally permit its use. This is due to the noise being derived from broad-band noise that has been passed through a filter. The noise is often too wide particularly for the higher frequencies. Problems arise due to the rejection rates of the filters, and in most audiometers the bandwidth is too wide for frequency-specific assessment. Digitally filtered noise will overcome this problem.

Physical calibration, biological calibration and RETSPLs

A measurement system including a sound level meter and microphone with calibration traceable to national standards is required. This enables physical calibration and also biological calibration if needed (Beynon and Munro, 1993). It is necessary to place a remote microphone at the test point and to read the sound level meter readings from a position (in the observation room if possible) that will not affect the measurements. The sound field can then be calibrated by adjusting the audiometer dial setting to match the sound level meter reading (dB SPL or dB A calibration). This is usually carried out in the audiometer calibration mode. To calibrate in dB HL requires either a full biological calibration or the use of an appropriate set of RETSPLs. As yet, there are no international standards containing derived normative data (RETSPLs) for frequency-modulated (warble) tone threshold values for use in a typical clinic (quasi-free sound field). BS EN ISO 389-7 (1998) provides normative data for pure-tone stimuli in a free field, and for narrow-band noise in a diffuse field. These two different RETSPL values are very similar across the frequency range 500 Hz to 4 kHz and can be used for warble tones but theoretically only in a free field or diffuse field. Although these RETSPLs were not determined in a quasi-free (semi-diffuse) field found in a typical clinic, they are used routinely and any errors arising from differences in sound field type should be small. If the test signals are to be calibrated in dB HL then, until normative data become available, using stimuli, speaker type, room size, sound field characteristics, infant placement and furniture placement, which are all explicitly defined, the audiologist has the choice of using these suggested (R)ETSPLs or deriving a clinic-specific set of average thresholds (biological calibration). The latter is not easy and requires testing a group of otologically normal young adults both in the sound field and using conventional headphones. From these measurements average sound field threshold values can be derived to enable calibration in dB HL. Noise floor problems (Lutman and McCormick, 1987) and non-linearity of the stimulus at threshold levels may prevent accurate definition of the desired minimum audible field.

Some centres calibrate the sound field in dB SPL others in dB A. Both methods are not ideal (Beynon and Munro, 1993) but can be used with careful consideration of the procedure. It would make sense to report all audiometric findings using a common scale and the measurement scale dB HL would appear most appropriate. This will require the use of appropriate suggested RETSPLs or carrying out a full biological calibration.

It is beyond the scope of this chapter to provide a detailed discussion of sound field calibration, however the reader should be aware of the extremely important issues surrounding this important area and of the need for regular calibration to ensure accurate and meaningful assessment results.

The conclusion to be drawn from the above is that any threshold measured in a sound field is likely to contain some degree of error. The degree of error may be very small but without thorough calibration and evaluation of the sound field and without constant awareness of infant placement in the sound field, errors in threshold determination may occur as a direct consequence.

Headphones, insert earphones and bone conductor

BS EN ISO 389 (1997) provides RETSPLs for the calibration of pure-tone air conduction standard earphones.

For an audiometer calibrated for standard earphones, insert earphones can be plugged directly into an audiometer's standard earphone sockets and by using the manufacturer's correction factors, the insert earphones can be used with only a small possible risk of error. Ideally the audiometer should be calibrated specifically for the insert earphones, if they are to be the most commonly used ear specific transducer. BS EN ISO 389-2 (1997), specifies RETSPLs for two different couplers.

Bone conduction calibration is straightforward with calibration reference levels given in BS EN ISO 389-3 (1999).

It should be noted that all the RETSPLs discussed so far have been derived from determining thresholds in a group of otologically normal young adults with average size adult ears, average-size heads and bodies, and by methodology requiring the listener to attend to auditory stimuli. How this relates to the assessment of small ears on a population not instructed to listen will be discussed in due course.

The reader is referred to the chapter on pure-tone audiometry for further discussion of headphone and bone conduction calibration issues.

Assessment

Introduction

The purpose of the majority of paediatric audiological assessments is to correctly identify the severity, type and configuration of a hearing loss, if present, or to establish normal hearing in the absence of a hearing deficit. The NDCS (2000) document, which outlines best practice for audiological management of a child with permanent hearing loss, details targets for the determination of ear-specific and frequency-specific thresholds by 12 months developmental age. The accuracy of the assessment will determine not only if amplification is necessary but also how much. If amplification is needed then further assessment will be required to evaluate its effectiveness.

At a developmental age of around five months an infant will turn and locate to a sound. Behavioural observation audiometry relies on these reflexive head turns to estimate thresholds. The responsiveness of the child will depend on the stimulus bandwidth (Thompson and Folsom, 1985). A wide-band stimulus containing low to mid frequencies is most likely to generate an infant response. Without reinforcement, a child's responses will soon habituate and may not occur at low intensity levels (Widen, 1990). Furthermore, unconditioned (non-operant) responses are highly variable, imprecise and are not ear specific. Visual response audiometry capitalizes on the natural head turn response of an infant to sound by initially pairing an interesting visual event (bright, animated toy) with the sound stimuli and then by rewarding further auditory-evoked head turn responses with the visual event.

Equipment layout

In the author's clinic, the infant is seated on a parent's lap or in a small chair if mature enough at the test point. The test point is situated midway between two speakers both at 90° azimuth to the child. The visual rewards are adjacent to the speakers (Figures 4.1 and Figure 4.2). Insert earphones and bone conduction transducers are situated inside the clinic (extension cables are required). In front of the child is a small low table with a soft covering. The tester is situated in an observation room directly facing the infant. It is from here that the audiometer and visual rewards are operated. A second tester is usually situated inside the clinic to control the infant's attention if necessary.

Initial conditioning

At this point the author will refer to the tester as the audiologist operating the audiometer and the visual rewards and the second tester as the audiologist in the clinic directing the procedure. It is often useful to use a radio link between the two testers if an observation room is used. The second tester wears a receiver connected to an earpiece with the tester wearing a microphone and radio transmitter. This allows the tester controlling the audiometer in the observation room to relay instructions to the second tester in the clinic. The tester in the observation room hears the proceedings in the clinic by means of a microphone in the test room coupled to an amplifier and speaker in the observation room.

The tester should ensure that the infant can sit with minimal support and that head control is good. The younger infant should be seated on the parent's knees with support around the waist. The child should be facing forwards, sitting upright and not resting on the parent's chest. The older child can sit on a small chair. In the author's clinic a small wooden chair with armrests is used, which serves to secure the child in place. With the infant positioned on a parent's/carer's lap or sitting in a small chair, a supra-threshold auditory signal (narrow-band noise if using sound field) is presented *concurrently* with the visual stimulus. The tester or parent/carer, may need to initially direct the child's attention to the reward (in practice, this is not required if narrow-band noise is used in the sound field). A head turn towards the visual stimulus (and sound source if sound field is used and the speaker is adjacent to the visual reward) represents an orientation reflex. If the conditioning stimulus is not spatially next to the visual reward, the child's attention will have to be directed towards the reward. At this stage, *classical conditioning* is taking place if the child associates the visual stimulus with the auditory stimulus. The assumption here is that the sound is audible. This may not always be the case and the sound may have to be raised in level or transmitted by vibrotactile stimulation to ensure true classical conditioning.

After a couple of these paired presentations, the child is tested to determine if successful conditioning has taken place. The sound stimulus is presented alone, and if the child turns in the direction of the visual reward, then conditioning has been successful (Figure 4.4).

The sound should be presented for approximately two to three seconds. Very young infants often take a little longer to turn than older infants. If the sound is presented for too long then the audiologist may misinterpret a check (false response) for a real response.

If the child correctly turns, the reward is activated for one or two seconds. The parent should also be instructed to praise the child and the second tester can join in by saying 'good boy/girl'. Parental praise will often make the difference, particularly with the older child, between the reward being seen as 'friendly' or 'frightening'. Both parent and audiologist should, however, give sufficient time for the child to see the reward before adding their praise. Only when the child has seen the reward for at least a

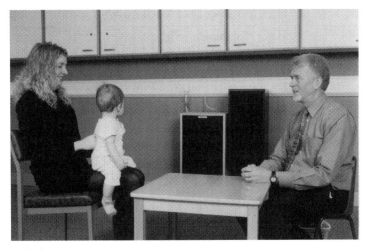

Figure 4.4. Infant turning to sound. Reward to follow.

couple of seconds should the verbal praise be added. If the verbal praise is added too soon, the infant may be prematurely drawn away from the visual reward and this may compromise successful conditioning. If the child has not made the connection between sound and reward then further conditioning trials (sound and reward together) will be necessary. If this proves unsuccessful then the use of higher presentation levels or vibrotactile stimulation should also be used. It is important to remember that the child may have a hearing loss that prevents audition of the initial stimulus.

Occasionally conditioning cannot be achieved and sometimes the child might dislike, or even be frightened by the visual reward. If this happens the test may have to be abandoned and distraction testing may have to be used. If conditioning has been successful, *operant conditioning* is now taking place by only rewarding the child visually following a correct auditory-evoked head turn.

It is vital that the child initially associates the auditory and visual stimuli together. Unless the infant can make an association between the two, the test will not be successful and will function as a non-operant audiometric procedure (BOA). It is also vital that the visual reward is then only operated following a correct head turn. Reconditioning may be necessary (sound and visual reward together) if the child's attention is lost.

Importance of the visual rewards

The more interesting the visual stimulus the greater the success of the test and it is this together with correct conditioning that ultimately achieves accurate results. Furthermore, the use of alternative rewards and/or the use of animated rewards may restore interest in the test and permit further assessment.

Visual rewards should be as interesting as possible with the option of:

- animation (some children are upset by this technique);
- changeable rewards (some children are easily bored);
- flexible positioning (for children with motor or vision difficulties).

Other useful points

A useful method, when assessing a child who wears hearing aids, is initially to condition the child whilst wearing the hearing aids before performing unaided assessment. Conditioning is usually achieved more quickly under the aided condition.

One further point regarding the reward of an auditory-evoked head turn is whether to continue with the auditory stimulus after the child has turned. Does it make any difference to the procedure if the sound and reward are concurrently presented after a head turn? There appears to be no evidence either way but, in the author's clinic, it would appear that for the more difficult-to-test child, continued presentation of the sound stimulus with the reward, following a head turn, serves as further reinforcement of the procedure.

Audiological assessment

Once conditioning has been achieved, the audiologist is in a position to assess the infant's hearing using sound field stimuli, headphone or insert earphone stimuli and bone conduction stimuli if available. Frequencies usually assessed are 500 Hz, 1 kHz, 2 kHz and 4 kHz. Other frequencies are occasionally assessed, particularly 250 Hz, and this stimulus, when presented in the sound field can be used in an attempt to condition a child to vibrotactile stimulation if a child does not condition to sound-field stimuli. The use of an intense 250 Hz sound field stimulus (80 to 110 dB HL) or a low-frequency bone conduction stimulus (250 Hz; 20–40 dB HL: 500 Hz; 55–70dB HL) will produce vibrotactile stimulation (Boothroyd and Cawkell, 1970). The ability or inability to condition to this mode of stimulation may provide important information about the child.

The tester should observe a number of clear true responses before assessing minimal response levels. An ascending/descending (up/down) technique is used in a structured but flexible manner using 20 dB down /10 dB up or 10 dB down/ 5 dB up steps depending on the required accuracy of the assessment. The goal of the assessment is to determine the quietest levels or minimal response levels (MRLs) at which an infant will respond, for frequencies important for hearing speech. Futhermore to determine the type of any hearing loss found and whether it is unilateral or bilateral. The tester should formulate a general but flexible method so as not to start each test session in an ad hoc fashion. It is always important to observe two repeatable responses at the minimal response level and to obtain non-responses at the level below this. For some children, investigation at the high frequencies may be a priority.

For others, low-mid frequency information may be desirable. In most assessments it is necessary to obtain information across the speech frequency range.

Timing of stimulus presentation

The *timing* of presentation of the auditory stimuli is of the utmost importance. The tester must observe the child, be aware of his or her level of activity, and be prepared to wait for a suitable time to present the sounds. If the tester presents sounds when the child is too active or too visually engrossed, then the likelihood of observing a response will be reduced. Experience with the procedure will help the tester to develop his or her skill in determining the periods when a response is most likely to be elicited. Often the tester will have to leave lengthy gaps between presentations, particularly if the child is producing many false responses. Bad timing of stimulus presentation may compound this, and the tester may make the task of identifying true responses very difficult.

In most cases it is unwise to present a sound when:

- a child is reaching for a toy;
- a child is holding a toy (not always true);
- a child is visually engrossed in a toy or a face.

If small toys are used to control the infant's attention it is often useful to keep them out of arm's reach of the infant. A young infant will tend to reach out for anything that is within easy reach.

Presenting auditory stimuli too often is also bad practice. The tester needs to assess quiet periods to enable thorough and accurate evaluation of the child's hearing.

Low-level play activity

It is often necessary to keep a low level of play activity in front of the child. This is usually achieved by the use of a second tester in the room with the child but it can also be the task of a parent/carer on occasions. The play activity can be in the form of moving a soft toy on a table, quietly placing simple toys in front of the child or, for the more mature child, using a soft felt puzzle to keep the child's attention from wandering. There are no hard-and-fast rules for what type of activity is used. For some children who are extremely active and whose attention is poor, it may be necessary to use a wide number of different toys in an attempt to control their attention. What is important is to use as *little activity as is possible.* The ideal would be for a child to sit on a parent's lap and look forwards without any play activity. There is no point performing 'juggling tricks' and exciting the child if it is not necessary. A quiet or shy child might suddenly become excitable and too visually engrossed by an over-enthusiastic tester. The role of the second tester (if used) is as important as the tester controlling the audiometer. Again, experience will allow the correct judgement of the level of play necessary.

Checking behaviour

The child may turn to the visual reward when there is no sound (checking behaviour). The second tester is responsible for guiding the child back to the test position by the use of toys or voice. Once the child's attention is under control again, the tester should revert to using as little play activity as is possible. It may be necessary to leave long gaps between stimulus presentations.

Observation of the child during these quiet periods is important to enable the tester to observe the child's behaviour. Often a child can produce real responses and checking responses, which are almost identical. More frequently, however, a child will turn and wait (true response) as opposed to a quick glance if just checking (false response) for the reward. Delaying the reward for a brief moment may help to differentiate a true response from a checking response. The second tester in the clinic with the child can give valuable information on the general responsiveness of the child to all modes of stimulation. This tester can also observe whether the parent/carer is knowingly or unknowingly giving clues to the child when the sound is presented. In some centres parents/carers are instructed to wear headphones to eliminate any possible clues. This does prevent them from playing a key part in the test session and witnessing the levels at which the child responds. This experience can often be very important, particularly when the loss is mild or restricted to one or two frequencies. Some parents who are in denial of their child's hearing loss might prompt the child and influence the test results. If this behaviour is observed it will alert the audiologist to the possibility that acceptance of a hearing loss may be problematic.

Reconditioning

It might be necessary to *recondition* the child by presenting a supra-threshold auditory signal together with the visual reward. If the child is active and responses are infrequent then it might be because the child has 'forgotten' that a sound is followed by an interesting visual reward. When changing stimulus transducer it is also often useful to present a supra-threshold stimulus and the visual reward together.

Application of the described procedure will, in most cases, successfully enable minimal response levels to be determined for an infant aged five months to 36 months. Each child will present a different challenge and factors such as development, vision, attention and alertness all make up a child's individuality. All of these considerations should be taken into account.

A suggested VRA protocol

It is recognized that alternative protocols will be available and that some audiologists will have developed protocols to suit their particular needs. As long as the fundamental principles of VRA are followed, the use of alternative protocols should result in accurate and consistent results. What follows is one suggested VRA protocol. It represents the method used in the author's clinic.

It is important before and during history taking, and before the test, to interact with the child and the family. A relaxed environment is necessary for both the infant and the parents/carers. It is important to explain the test procedure to the parents/carers and to inform them of their role during the test. For the slightly older child, soft toys or puzzles should be placed on the table in the clinic before entering.

Sound field assessment

1. Explain the procedure to the parents/carers.
2. Condition the child by presenting the sound and reward together (1 kHz narrow-band noise should be used if in a sound field at a level of 60–70 dB HL or higher if hearing loss is suspected or known).Two or more conditioning trials may be necessary. The choice of conditioning stimulus will depend on the audiological information known. Previous assessment results, history of the child's responses to sounds and initial observations are essential in providing an initial signal which can be detected by the child.

3. Present a 1 kHz warble tone at a level judged to be at supra-threshold level (60–70 dB HL). If a head turn is observed then reward with visual reinforcer. If no response then return to NBN to attempt further conditioning trails possibly at a higher level or use bone conductor to attempt vibrotactile conditioning.

4. Following conditioning (head turn to sound alone) determine minimal response levels (MRLs). Use an ascending/descending method (20 dB down, 10 dB up) and attempt to observe two clear responses at each MRL and at least one negative response below this if MRL is not at quietest level tested. (Note that testing below 20–25 dB HL is usually not necessary and may be problematic due to background noise levels.)

5. Attempt to record MRLs at 500 Hz, 1 kHz, 2 kHz and 4 kHz (it may be necessary to omit one mid frequency). Reinforce after each correct head turn.

6. Assess localization if normal hearing is demonstrated. Use NBN or live voice at a level of 10 dB to 20 dB above MRL. Use alternate speakers and rewards.

7. Determine headphone, insert earphone and/or bone conduction MRLs if required.

Insert earphones/headphones

1. Fit inserts or headphones. Child may need to be occupied by the second tester.

2. Recondition with a supra-threshold pure-tone stimulus. If testing opposite ear to the reward used initially, then the use of two rewards may be necessary and may help to obtain further responses. If using only one reward then the child might have to be directed to the reward when reconditioning.

3. Attempt MRLs for pure tones in each ear at as many of the above frequencies as is possible.

Bone conduction

1. If suspicious of a sensorineural hearing loss then attempt bone conduction VRA.

2. Place headband in correct position.

3. Present stimuli and reward together to reinforce the conditioning (use 500 Hz pure tone at 50 dB).

4. Attempt MRLs at as many frequencies as is necessary. Reconditioning of the child may be necessary regardless of transducer used.

This protocol serves only as a guideline and, whatever protocol is used, the audiologist must be prepared to approach each session with a degree of flexibility. The protocol described above is used successfully in the author's clinic with over 2,500 infants per year. A more detailed protocol described by Widen et al. (2000) was used successfully with over 3,000 infants in a controlled trial.

The population being assessed constantly challenges the skills required to perform successful VRA. Experience, together with a willingness to learn, ensure that the paediatric audiologist is constantly evolving and becoming better equipped to assess even the most challenging infant.

Transducer considerations

Sound field

It is usual practice in the author's clinic initially to assess a child in the sound field. This does not require any equipment to be placed on the child and is the least intrusive method of assessment. The initial conditioning of the child requires the use of a narrow-band noise stimulus. If the tester or parent directs the child to the sound and reward then warble tones can be used. A narrow-band, low-mid frequency stimulus will generate a head turn response in the required direction much more easily than a warble tone. It is known that a young infant will respond (when not conditioned) to this type of stimulus more often than to a warble tone or pure tone (Bench and Mentz, 1975; Thompson and Folsom, 1985). Furthermore if a child has even a mild hearing loss, then localization skills are often impaired (Auslander et al., 1991) and narrow-band noise will more likely generate correct localization. Primus (1992) recommends positioning the visual reward adjacent to the speaker. It would therefore seem sensible to use a narrow-band noise signal to condition the child initially, if the speaker and reward are adjacent. The sound is easier to locate initially and it is more 'attention grabbing'. Unless there is any good reason to use a different stimulus, narrow-band noise should be used. The tester, after initially presenting this stimulus, can go on to present a supra-threshold warble tone, at which point the localization of the sound is not important, as the child should be correctly conditioned.

It is important to realize that sound field VRA will test the *better ear* if there is one. Speakers are usually positioned at least one meter from the child's ears and thus only a very small difference in sound intensity will result due to head shadow effects. It is important to report results as binaural response levels if sound field VRA is used.

It is common practice to test down to a set level. Background noise and non-linearity of the test signal at low levels often determines this lower limit. In the author's clinic it is usual to test down to 25 dB HL across frequencies. One must report results in the correct manner, if lower limits are used (that is, ≤25dB HL).

If hearing sensitivity is found to be within normal limits, and if ear-specific transducers are not to be used, it is important to assess localization in an attempt to pick up any problems which may be suggestive of a unilateral hearing loss. Narrow-band noise will most likely elicit a correct localization response. In the author's clinic, the opposite speaker, again at 90°, is used. Some workers argue that a child will not localize a signal if correctly conditioned and that wherever a signal is presented the child will always turn to the visual reward initially used. In a very few cases this is true. In the majority of normally hearing children (both ears within normal limits), correct localization to narrow-band noise is easily observed. The emphasis here is on the child hearing normally. If a child has even a mild hearing loss on binaural testing, then assessing localization in the sound field is of little use. The presence of even a mild hearing loss is known to impair localization skills, which means that unless normal binaural hearing is initially found, accurate localization skills would not normally be expected. Using live voice is also possible to assess localization and the tester may call the child's name from each speaker. If a child demonstrates hearing within normal limits (binaurally), yet shows poor localization skills in the absence of any conductive hearing loss (normal tympanograms), then a thorough evaluation of both ears is necessary. As part of the audiologist's test battery, otoacoustic emission testing can be used at this stage of the assessment if ear-specific transducer VRA is not possible.

Ear-specific transducers are necessary to assess any left/right differences in hearing if asymmetrical hearing is suspected.

Ideally, ear-specific transducers should be used in all assessments and the audiologist should be aware that correct sound field localization of narrow-band noise does not rule out a unilateral hearing loss. Unilateral hearing loss does place a child at risk not only educationally but also environmentally – for example, with regard to awareness of traffic or locating parents' calls.

Headphones

Headphones can be used successfully in VRA. Due to the size of the headband, it is useful to place some covered foam around it to enable comfortable positioning on the child's head. It is also useful, particularly with young children, to hold their arms gently to restrict any attempt to remove the headband. Problems encountered when using headphones include the possible need for masking, the risk of collapsed ear canals and the restriction of movement due to the size of the headphones.

Insert earphones

Insert earphones are more suited to visual reinforcement audiometry. They offer the audiologist several advantages over headphones. These include a reduced need for masking due to greater inter-aural attenuation, elimination of headband, increased attenuation of background noise, prevention of collapsed ear canals and increased effectiveness in hearing aid prescription due to calibration in a 2 cm^3 coupler (Borton et al., 1989; Wright and Frank, 1992; Killion, 1984; Seewald et al., 1999). The Desired Sensation Level (DSL) method of selecting amplification characteristics recommends using insert earphones as the transducer of choice, regardless of which specific paediatric test is being employed (Seewald et al., 1997). By using inserts and obtaining a child's real-ear-to-coupler difference (RECD) (Moodie, Seewald and Sinclair, 1994; Seewald et al., 1999) accurate prediction of ear canal sound pressure level at threshold can be determined. The insert tubes are fitted to foam tips, which are rolled up and inserted into the ear canal. Care has to be taken to ensure correct insertion depth. A more practical method for children with earmoulds is to attach the insert tubes to a child's custom earmoulds (Figure 4.5).

One point to be aware of is that minimal response levels obtained with a child's custom earmoulds might differ slightly from results obtained using foam tips. This is due to the different acoustical properties of the two couplings.

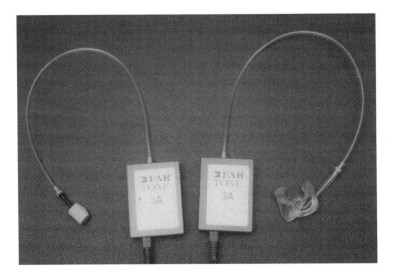

Figure 4.5. Insert earphones connected to a personal earmould and a foam tip.

One advantage of using custom earmoulds is that children who wear hearing aids will often be unaware of the removal of their hearing aids and of the subsequent attachment of the insert earphones. Experience favours using a child's earmoulds if available, rather than foam tips. During assessment the insert transducers can be placed either by use of Velcro or clips on the child's back (Figure 4.6). The insert earphones can be placed in the ears one at a time if necessary, and this is another advantage of using them rather than headphones. Further advantages of both headphone and insert transducers is the possibility of presenting signals up to 110–120 dB HL and also the relaxed positioning of the child due to removal of sound field constraints.

In the author's clinic, it is unusual to attempt insert earphone testing at the infant's initial visit. The first session is usually performed in the sound field with a more detailed assessment at subsequent visits. If however, a child is known to have a hearing loss, then there is no reason not to start with insert earphone testing. A recent report by Widen et al. (2000) demonstrates that ear-specific assessment can be extremely successful but may take more than one visit to the clinic.

Bone conductor

Bone conduction VRA is also possible (Figure 4.7.) and can provide important information regarding type of hearing loss

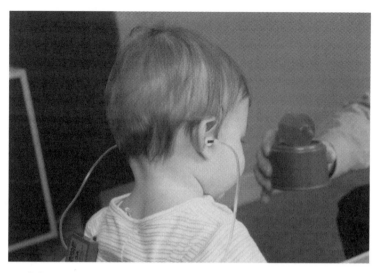

Figure 4.6. Insert earphones worn by infant.

(conductive or sensorineural). Again, as with headphone VRA, it is useful to have some covered foam wrapped around the headband and to possibly modify the headband permanently to enable a better fit on the infant's head. A child may initially appear confused when presenting the sound through the bone conductor, following sound field stimulation, and it is useful and often necessary to recondition the child with a supra-threshold presentation and to direct the child to the visual reward.

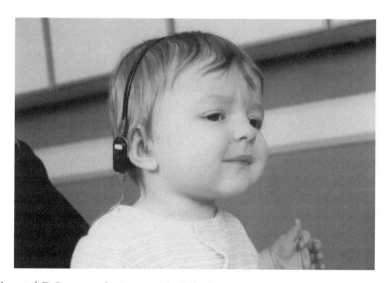

Figure 4.7. Bone conductor worn by infant.

For headphones, insert earphone and bone conduction assessment, masking of the non-test ear may be possible if necessary. As yet there are no standard guidelines for levels of masking to use and it may prove difficult to obtain accurate masked thresholds.

With headphone and insert earphone assessment it is usually possible to test down to 10-15 dB HL, however in practice, testing down to 20-25 dB HL is more commonplace. With bone conduction assessment, as with sound field assessment, background noise levels will determine the minimal levels, which can be used by the audiologist. Testing down to 20-25 dB HL will usually provide enough information to successfully manage the infant being assessed.

Efficacy of VRA

Visual reinforcement audiometry is widely used in most well equipped paediatric audiology clinics for the assessment of infants developmentally aged between five months and 36 months. The procedure is also successful with older children, children with developmental delay, children with some degree of visual impairment and adults with learning disabilities.

There have been numerous studies that have demonstrated the effectiveness and accuracy of the procedure and some of these will be discussed here.

Effect of reinforcer

Moore, Thompson and Thompson (1975) in what is a classic piece of research in VRA, investigated the effects of type of reinforcer (complexity of reward) on the number of responses observed. Four different reinforcers were looked at:

- no reinforcement;
- social reinforcement (smile, verbal praise);
- simple visual reinforcement (flashing light);
- complex visual reinforcement (animated toy bear).

Complex noise was used as the test stimuli, and 48 infants aged between 12 months and 18 months were tested and placed into four groups. Thirty presentations of the auditory stimuli were used (complex noise at 70 dB SPL). No-sound trials were also examined. The mean number of responses in each group are given in Table 4.1.

Table 4.1. Mean number of responses per group.

Groups (n = 12 per group)	Mean no. of responses (30 trials)
1. No reinforcement.	9.7
2. Social reinforcement (smile, verbal praise).	15.2
3. Simple visual reinforcement (flashing light).	20.5
4. Complex visual reinforcement (animated toy bear).	27.3

It is clear from this particular study that the more interesting the reward the greater number of responses observed. The cumulative mean responses from this study are shown in Figure 4.8. The authors, report that the complexity and the familiarity of the reinforcers has a direct effect on the number of head turn responses. What is apparent is that the 'interest' factor of the reward plays a significant role in the success of the technique.

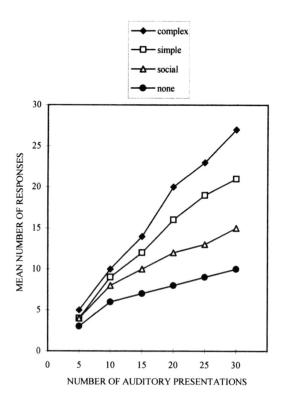

Figure 4.8. Cumulative mean head turn responses in blocks of stimulus trials as a function of reinforcement condition in four groups (N = 12) of infants aged 12–18 months. (From Moore, Thompson and Thompson, 1975.)

Effect of age

Moore, Wilson and Thompson (1977) used the complex reinforcer from the study above to investigate the effect of age on VRA success. Sixty infants between four months and 11 months of age, with no suspected hearing impairment, no developmental delay and no recent ear problems were used in the study. Again, a complex noise stimulus was used as the test signal and presented 30 times to each infant. The children were grouped according to age (seven months to 11 months, five months to six months, and four months of age). Results are shown in Figure 4.9. They also examined the responses of similar control groups who received no reinforcement. It is clear from the study that it is possible to achieve success with infants as young as five months of age, if an interesting reward is used. For children aged four months, VRA did not elicit more responses than unconditioned testing (BOA).

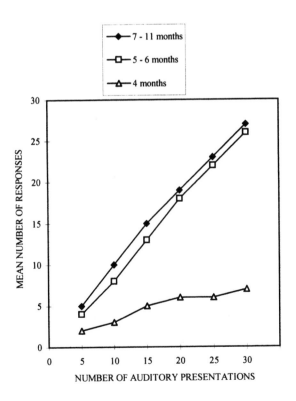

Figure 4.9. Cumulative mean head turn responses in blocks of stimulus trials as a function of age in three groups (N = 10) of infants using complex reinforcement. (From Moore, Wilson and Thompson, 1977.)

Primus and Thompson (1985) investigated the response strength of one- and two-year-olds. They found that both groups of children conditioned at the same rate, however the one-year-old group provided more responses than two-year-olds. They also found that habituation could be delayed in the two-year-old group by introducing novel reinforcers. Thompson, Thompson and McCall (1992) investigated strategies to increase response behaviour in one- and two-year-olds. They again found that two-year-olds habituated more quickly than one-year-olds. They also found that using two rewards led to more responses before habituation. Finally, they found that for the one-year-old group, giving them a break of 10 minutes led to at least five more responses on reassessment.

Thompson and Folsom (1984) compared two conditioning procedures with one- and two-year-old high-risk infants. They used two different conditioning trials but found no difference in the success of the procedure. The only factor of significance was the finding that two-year-olds required less responses to obtain minimal response levels than one-year-olds.

Effect of stimulus bandwidth

It is well known that the complexity of a sound will influence the response rate in non-operant procedures. Thompson and Folsom (1985) investigated the effect of stimulus bandwidth on reinforced and non-reinforced head turn responses on 30 otologically normal one-year-olds. They concluded that although a complex noise (containing low-mid frequencies) would most likely elicit an unconditioned head turn, once an infant was correctly conditioned, using a VRA procedure, the bandwidth of the test signal had no effect on response rate. This finding suggests that the use of frequency-specific (pure-tone or warble-tone) stimuli with conditioned infants does not compromise response behaviour.

Effect of reward and speaker placement

Primus (1992) examined the effect of reinforcer position, relative to sound field speaker position, on the success of VRA. Thirty, one-year-old infants were used with no hearing, visual or developmental problems. Three speaker positions were used. The success of the conditioning is shown in brackets:

- adjacent to the reinforcer (100%);

- directly over the subject's head (70%);
- directly opposite to the reinforcer (40%).

Conditioning was achieved more quickly with the reinforcer adjacent to the speaker. Primus concludes that although localization is not essential to the conditioning process, inappropriate localization cues may reduce performance of the procedure. This finding might have implications for success rates of headphone and insert earphone VRA. Furthermore, if a child suffers from a hearing loss, which disrupts normal localization cues, then it may follow that success rates of sound field VRA may be less in the hearing impaired population.

Accuracy of VRA

Several studies have investigated the ability of VRA to provide minimal response levels, which are accurate, repeatable and can be related to pure-tone audiometry thresholds. So far in this chapter, the terms minimal response levels, hearing levels and thresholds have been used interchangeably. As VRA is a non-directed task - the child is not asked to attend to sounds - the strict use of the term 'threshold' may be unwise. Minimal response level (MRL) would appear to provide the most accurate definition of responses, however care must be taken when reporting these MRLs to other professionals. The term 'minimal response level' can often suggest 'normal hearing' to a professional not working directly with VRA procedures. Comparisons with adult thresholds and longitudinal studies do, however, suggest that VRA results agree well with other directed tests, and the different terms will continue to be used interchangeably. Factors such as attention, motivation, level of activity and background noise levels, will all affect response levels obtained.

Wilson and Moore (1978) examined responses of infants aged six months to 13 months compared with thresholds obtained with young adults. Visual response audiometry was successful in obtaining responses to within 10 dB of the adult thresholds and with slightly closer results at the lower frequencies.

Talbot (1987) performed a longitudinal study to examine the hearing thresholds of a group of 17 hearing impaired infants from initial VRA to subsequent PTA testing. For the VRA assessment, eight infants were initially tested using earphones and nine in the sound field. Play audiometry was performed at an appropriate age. Results demonstrated no significant differences in thresholds between the two procedures, VRA and PTA. Responses were generally within +10 dB of each other at frequencies 0.25, 0.5, 1, 2 and 4 kHz.

Nozza and Wilson (1984) investigated both masked and unmasked pure-tone (1 and 4 kHz) thresholds of a group of 80 infants compared to adults (six-month- and 12-month-old infants, masked and unmasked). A VRA procedure was used for the infants, with a listening procedure for the adults. Masked threshold differences between the infant and adult groups were of the order of 6 dB to 8 dB. Unmasked differences were slightly higher at 5 dB to 14 dB.

Reliability of VRA

Primus (1991) examined the test-retest reliability of both non-operant and operant (VRA) procedures on a group of 20, eight to eleven-month infants. Visual response audiometry demonstrated good threshold repeatability in most infants during one test session (10 dB range for 50% of infants). Threshold deviation was most likely to occur towards the end of the session. Primus concluded that response reliability may be compromised either early on in the session if conditioning is incomplete or towards the end of the session if the child loses interest in the reinforcer.

It is important to investigate the success of threshold determination in the infant population, not only for the normally hearing but also for the hearing impaired. Rudmin (1984), demonstrated the use of VRA with two 11-month-old infants. Both had severe-profound hearing loss and were retested either one day or five months after their initial tests. Although retest variability was higher than reported in normally hearing infants, Rudmin concluded that the procedure was viable even with significantly hearing impaired young infants.

Gravel and Traquina (1992) report their findings with 211 babies, aged six months to twenty-four months, seen in their clinic. One-hundred-and-nine of the infants were considered 'research' infants, due to high risk factors for neurodevelopmental deficits. Most had graduated from the neonatal intensive care unit. A further 102 infants were assessed and these had been referred from a variety of professionals. Thus, the group as a whole contained a typical paediatric audiologist's caseload, including a 'difficult-to-test' population. The 109 at-risk infants were assessed using an automated VRA procedure, with the remaining 102 infants assessed manually (see Gravel and Traquina for further discussion). The results showed that 90% of the total number of infants provided frequency-specific hearing thresholds (headphones or sound field). They also found that 84% of the infants provided ear-specific data (headphones). Out of the at-risk population, 85% provided useful results.

Gravel and Traquina (1992) concluded that ear-specific thresholds are obtainable in the majority of infants in the age group tested. Furthermore, the younger the infant, the more likely the success of headphone placement (<12 months).

A study by Gliddon, Martin and Green (1999) although using a small sample size of 20, compared the clinical features of VRA with the distraction test. The mean age of the 20 infants assessed was 18 months. Both tests were performed a week apart to enable comparison of results. Visual response audiometry provided more information than the distraction test in most infants. The two tests were equally good at demonstrating normal hearing, however, if a hearing loss was present then the distraction test as performed in their clinic often over-estimated the hearing loss. Differences of up to 20 dB HL were recorded, which are significant both statistically and clinically. Furthermore, when parents were questioned as to which test they felt was the better test, 70% preferred VRA.

A recent study reported by Widen et al. (2000) demonstrated that from a population of over 3,000 babies aged between eight and 12 months corrected age, 95% of the infants were reliably tested with their VRA protocol. This protocol determined ear-specific information using insert earphones. Furthermore, 90% provided complete test results (four minimal response levels for both ears).

Experience in the author's clinic where approximately 2,500 infants are assessed by VRA each year confirms these findings. Visual response audiometry is successful with all but the most profoundly hearing impaired infants, so long as other factors such as developmental delay or visual impairment do not prevent correct conditioning of the child.

All these findings are very impressive and set standards for every well-equipped audiology clinic. If a clinic is not achieving these levels of results it would be advisable to evaluate the protocols and VRA setup that are used in that clinic. It is a useful exercise to evaluate any audiological test procedure on a routine basis to determine if there have been changes in success rates and, if so, why. Any attempt to do so would require further long-term evaluation to determine infant thresholds using play audiometry. The success of VRA requires not only the completion of the assessment but also repeatability of results.

Sound field and unilateral loss

Auslander et al. (1991) investigated the use of a four-speaker arrangement to identify unilateral hearing loss. Using a VRA procedure they simulated a mild hearing loss by plugging one ear using a foam E-A-R plug. Twenty-nine infants were assessed using warble tones and speech. They found that significantly more localization errors were observed in the infants with a simulated hearing loss and suggested that a horizontal localization task could be used as a simple screening procedure for detecting unilateral hearing loss. They did however, suggest further research with this speaker arrangement.

Modified VRA

Primus (1988) investigated a modified VRA procedure with 16 11-month-old to 15-month-old infants with normal hearing and development. They used a pre-trial warning, 'listen (child's name)' before presenting the test signal. They recorded an improvement in thresholds of 5.5 dB using the modified procedure compared to conventional VRA. They did, however, find that test sessions were longer and that the infants produced more checking behaviour prior to the test stimulus due to the pre-trial warning.

Premature infants

It is now known that babies born prematurely are at more risk of having permanent sensorineural hearing loss than full term infants. With increasing survival rates, this means that more pre-term babies will present at audiology clinics for assessment. Hearing screening programmes that do not employ universal screening often have *targeted* populations with premature babies making up the majority of this group. Although ABR testing has traditionally been used for initial threshold estimation in the neonatal population, it is obviously important that an infant's audiological profile is evaluated at all stages of development. Two important questions, which need to be addressed, are 'what effect does prematurity have on the success rate of VRA?' and 'what age is the pre-term infant most likely to successfully complete VRA?'

As cited previously (Widen, 1990; Gravel and Traquina, 1992), VRA can be used successfully with the 'at-risk' population including pre-term infants. Culpepper and Thompson (1994), although investigating the effects of reinforcer duration on response behaviour, did so using a group of pre-term infants (gestation age of 34 weeks or less). Conditioning was successful in all infants and their study also provided additional information. They found that by increasing the length of duration of the reinforcer (visual reward), the habituation rate of the infants increased. In other words, providing a short duration (0.5 s) reward, enabled more sound trials to be presented before the child habituated to the task compared to using a longer reward duration (1.5 s and 4 s).

Moore, Thompson and Folsom (1992), looked at the relationship between corrected age, mental age and VRA success. Sixty premature infants were assessed with gestational age 36 weeks or less. All babies were considered to have normal weight for their gestational age. Corrected age was determined by subtracting the estimated number of weeks of prematurity from the infants' chronological age. Infants included in this study had no 'major handicapping conditions'. Results demonstrated that infants with a corrected age of eight months to nine months were successfully assessed (82% success). Infants with a corrected age of six months to seven months performed more poorly (56% success). Infants with a corrected age of four months to five months did not perform well (20% success).

Looking at 'mental' (developmental) age they found that six months was the lower age limit above which VRA was successful. The Bayley scale of infant development (Bayley, 1969) was used to assess developmental age. Thus, a corrected age of eight months to nine months and a developmental age of six months would appear to provide reasonable indicators of the likelihood of success when using VRA with infants born pre-term. The above paper has some further interesting findings regarding 'non-habituation' and 'hyper-responsiveness' of pre-term infants.

A study by Widen et al. (2000) showed that when at-risk infants were assessed using VRA at a corrected age of eight months to 12 months, success was achieved in 95% of infants tested.

Children with developmental delay and other disabilities

Given the high prevalence of hearing loss, both conductive and sensorineural, in the Down syndrome population and given the additional developmental and speech and language problems also found, it is extremely important to accurately determine hearing levels from an early age. In the author's clinic, VRA is successfully used with children with Down syndrome, although the age from which successful conditioning takes place is usually a little higher than in the non-Down syndrome population. Often, children are not interested in the visual reward unless it is highly attractive.

Greenberg et al. (1978), using a group of 41 children with Down syndrome (aged six months to six years) demonstrated that the success of VRA was dependent on a developmental age of around 10 months to 12 months. They also found that not all children with Down syndrome at or above this age could successfully be conditioned.

In a similar study, Thompson, Wilson and Moore (1979) examined the success of VRA with developmentally delayed infants. Again, a developmental age of around 10 months was found to be the lower cut-off age for successful VRA. This would suggest that children with developmental delay will not condition to VRA until at a developmental age of approximately 10 months.

Lancioni, Coninx and Smeets (1989) discuss a novel approach, which can be used in the assessment of 'multi-handicapped persons'. Although not strictly an operant procedure, they used an 'air puff' stimulus to condition the child or adolescent to a sound stimulus. They then compared this procedure with an operant VRA procedure. Condon (1991) also provides further discussion of VRA procedures with challenging populations.

Visual reinforcement audiometry, if approached with a flexible, child-centred philosophy, can in the majority of cases provide useful and meaningful audiological information in the population where hearing loss is most prevalent. Babies born prematurely and children with additional disabilities often have a hearing loss and it is the task of the audiologist, together with parents/carers and other professionals involved, to facilitate the special care and management that each child requires.

In the author's clinic many children with additional difficulties are successfully assessed. Children with visual impairment, cerebral palsy, 'autistic spectrum disorders', motor difficulties and a number of developmental disorders have all been assessed using a flexible VRA procedure.

Automated VRA

In the UK the use of automated VRA procedures is uncommon. There have been successful implementations of computer-based automated procedures (Bernstein and Gravel, 1990; Eilers et al., 1991a, 1991b; Gravel and Traquina, 1992). With the increasing use of technology in audiology it is likely that automated procedures will continue to be developed and used.

Visually reinforced infant speech discrimination (VRISD)

Eilers, Wilson and Moore (1977) investigated using a visually reinforced procedure to assess the ability of infants to detect differences in speech sounds. They presented a speech sound at a rate of one syllable per second and then changed the speech sound. If the infant detected the change the visual reward was activated. They showed that a high proportion of infants in their study, aged six months to 14 months, were capable of discriminating certain speech sounds.

Training

One aspect of VRA, which ultimately affects the success of the test procedure, is training. For large audiology departments with a number of skilled professionals it is usual for trainees to 'sit in' on clinics and initially observe the procedure. When the trainee is familiar with the test procedure it is then usual for the skilled professional to observe the trainee perform the test until a time when competence has been demonstrated. Experience cannot be taught and once competent in the procedure, audiologists must continue to develop their skills. A thorough understanding of the principles behind VRA is a prerequisite before hands-on training. It is useful to have some departmental guidelines and protocols for VRA, not only to ensure some degree of standardization but also to help in training. For a clinic with only one trained professional it is imperative that the procedure is being implemented correctly before attempting to train other professionals. Durham et al. (1994) evaluated a behavioural audiometry simulator for use in teaching VRA. Eight audiology students with little or no experience in VRA testing were split into two groups. One group received no training and the other group were given five hours of time on the simulator. The simulator consisted of a computer, a videodisc player, a video monitor and a custom made audiometer console. All eight individuals then tested an infant. Three skilled professionals rated performance. The group who used the simulator showed a significant improvement in testing compared to the control group who received no training. The study also demonstrated that VRA is complex to learn because the learning must take place in different areas at the same time. Any teaching device that enhances performance for the training audiologist would seem to be a good idea. With the increase in use of VRA there is obvious room for teaching aids.

Holistic family-centred approach

There has been much discussion above regarding the VRA procedure. How it works, when to use it, validity of results, calibration issues to name a few. The most important components of the whole procedure are the child and his or her family or carers. We know that VRA is successful in accurately identifying hearing loss. Whether this is a temporary conductive loss or a permanent sensorineural hearing loss, the audiologist is responsible for making the whole experience as child-centred as possible.

To a parent who might or might not have suspected any hearing loss, the VRA test session may provide the first occasion in which their child is found to have a 'problem'. Inclusion of the parents throughout the session is important. Having explained the procedure clearly to the parents/carers the audiologist can then request their co-operation by playing a part in the test and this often helps in forming a trusting relationship between parent and audiologist. If a child does have a hearing loss then the initial VRA assessment should serve as a foundation for a lengthy, open, trusting and habilitative relationship. Some parents are relieved to find someone confirming their fears that their child does have a hearing problem. Others are totally shocked and are often in denial of their child's hearing loss and it may take several sessions before this denial fades away. Some parents can become quite angry and defensive following an assessment. It is important that the audiologist treats all parents/carers with the utmost awareness of their particular needs. If audiological results are questioned then the audiologist must respect the parents' opinions.

If the audiologist presents the results quickly, immediately followed by a plan of action, before giving the parents time to come to terms with the news, then successful habilitation of the child may be compromised. The parents/carers of the hearing impaired child have to be involved in every step of the habilitation process to ensure a successful partnership with the audiologist.

With infants who have previously undergone ABR testing, with results suggesting a severe-profound hearing impairment, it is absolutely essential to have discussed the initial results in some detail before attempting VRA. High-intensity sound levels will be required to test the infant and earplugs will be necessary for parents. It can be a distressing experience for parents to observe their child not responding to even the most intense auditory stimuli. It may be important to demonstrate vibrotactile conditioning to the parents if possible, and this can help in the acceptance of the lack of response to auditory stimulation.

It is often useful to include one parent (if both are present) with the tester in the observation room. From here the parent should have a clear view of the VRA procedure and can give his or her impressions as to the responsiveness of their child. Similarly the parent in the clinic with the child can also play an important role in the assessment of the child. Although some centres prefer to eliminate parental cues by placing headphones on parents, it is commonplace for parents actively to participate in the VRA test. Joining in the reward when the child turns and commenting on the child's general level of awareness are often important.

For a child who is shy and withdrawn it is often helpful to begin the test with as little fuss as possible. The child may respond better with no audiologist in the test room. The same rule may apply to a child who easily fixates on faces. Some children will require all manner of activities in the room to control their attention. Some children will not position at the test point and will walk around the room. As long as the audiologist is aware of the effects of any unusual behaviour, none of the above should prevent estimation of a child's hearing levels.

VRA can be used with older children who will not co-operate for play audiometry. In fact, the success or not of VRA will often provide valuable information regarding a child's development which may not already be apparent.

Responses to auditory stimuli may not always be typical. Some infants will point to the reward before making a head turn. Some children with severely restricted movement may smile or shift their gaze upon hearing a sound. The important factors with any non-typical response are the repeatability and reliability of the response. Skilled judgements are often required both from the audiologist and the parents.

With children who have been enrolled in a habilitation programme using amplification, VRA serves as an important evaluation and verification technique. Whilst allowing the determination of aided response levels, the procedure can also demonstrate quite effectively the benefits of amplification to parents and carers.

What is important in all audiological assessments is to understand both parents and child as much as possible. Entering every clinic session with a willingness to listen will not only help the audiologist understand the child's history but also the parents' expectations. These two equally important factors could make the difference between a successful habilitation process and simply a valid hearing assessment.

Conclusion

Visual reinforcement audiometry is used extensively in the UK and internationally. Research has demonstrated the effectiveness and accuracy of the assessment procedure in the paediatric population. It is possible to measure ear- and frequency-specific air and bone conduction thresholds in the majority of the infants aged 5 months and 36 months. Developments in areas such as training, sound field calibration and protocol design as well as continued audit of current services will maintain VRA as a powerful procedure for assessing infants and young children.

References

American Speech-Language-Hearing Association (1991a) Guidelines for the audiologic assessment of children from birth through 36 months of age. ASHA 33: 37–43.

American Speech-Language-Hearing Association (1991b) Sound field measurement tutorial. ASHA 33: 25–38.

Auslander MC, Lewis DE, Schulte L, Stelmachowicz PG (1991) Localization ability in infants with simulated unilateral hearing loss. Ear and Hearing 12: 371–6.

Bayley N (1969) Bayley Scales of Infant Development: Birth to Two Years. San Antonio TX: Psychological Corp.

Bench J, Mentz L (1975) Stimulus complexity, state and infants' auditory behavioural responses. British Journal of Communication Disorders 10: 52–60.

Bernstein RS, Gravel JS (1990) A method for determining hearing sensitivity in infants: the interweaving staircase procedure (ISP). Journal of the American Academy of Audiology 1: 138–45.

Beynon G, Munro K (1993) A discussion of current sound field calibration procedures. British Journal of Audiology 27: 427–35.

Boothroyd A, Cawkell S (1970) Vibrotactile thresholds in pure tone audiometry. Acta Otolaryngologica 69: 381–7.

Borton TE, Nolen BL, Luks SB, Meline NC (1989) Clinical applicability of insert earphones for audiometry. Audiology 28: 61–70.

BS 5942-7 (1987) High fidelity audio equipment and systems; minimum performance requirements. Specification for loudspeakers. London: British Standards Institution.

BS EN 60645-1 (1995) Audiometers – Part 1: Pure Tone Audiometers. London: British Standards Institution.

BS EN ISO 389 (1997) Acoustics. Standard reference zero for the calibration of pure tone air conduction audiometers. London: British Standards Institution.

BS EN ISO 389-2 (1997) Acoustics. Reference zero for the calibration of audiometric equipment-Part 2: Reference equivalent threshold sound pressure levels for pure tones and insert earphones. London: British Standards Institutions.

BS EN ISO 389-3 (1999) Acoustics. Reference zero for the calibration of audiometric equipment-Part 3: Reference equivalent threshold force levels for pure tones and bone vibrators. London: British Standards Institutions.

BS EN ISO 389-7 (1998) Acoustics. Reference zero for the calibration of audiometric equipment-Part 7: Reference threshold of hearing under free-field and diffused-field listening conditions. London: British Standards Institutions.

BS EN ISO 8253-1 (1998) Acoustics. Audiometric test methods – Part 1: basic pure tone air and bone conduction threshold audiometry. London: British Standards Institution.

BS EN ISO 8253-2 (1998) Acoustics. Audiometric test methods – Part 2: sound field audiometry with pure tone and narrow-band test signals. London: British Standards Institution.

Condon MC (1991) Unique challenges: children with multiple handicaps. In Geigin J, Stelmachowicz PG (eds) Paediatric Amplification, Proceedings of the 1991 National Conference. Omaha NB: Boys Town National Research Hospital, pp. 183–94.

Cox RM, McCormick VA (1987) Electroacoustic calibration for sound field warble tone thresholds. Journal of Speech and Hearing Disorders 52: 388–92.

Culpepper B, Thompson G (1994) Effects of reinforcer duration on the response behaviour of preterm 2-year olds in visual reinforcement audiometry. Ear and Hearing 15: 161-7.

Day J (ed.) (2000) Visual reinforcement audiometry testing of infants: A recommended test protocol. National Hearing Screening and Assessment Workshop. www.ihr.co.uk.

Dix M, Hallpike C (1947) Peep-show: new technique for pure tone audiometry in young children. British Medical Journal 2: 719-23.

Durham JA, Thelin JW, Muenchen RA, Halpin CF (1994) Evaluation of a behavioral audiometry simulator for teaching visual reinforcement audiometry. Journal of the American Academy of Audiology 5: 417-25.

Eilers RE, Wilson WR, Moore JM (1977) Developmental changes in speech discrimination in infants. Journal of Speech and Hearing Research 20: 766-80.

Eilers RE, Miskiel E, Ozdamar O, Urbano R, Widen JE (1991a) Optimization of automated hearing test algorithms: simulations using an infant response model. Ear and Hearing 12: 191-8.

Eilers RE, Widen JE, Urbano R, Hudson T, Gonzales L (1991b) Optimization of automated hearing test algorithms: a comparison of data from simulations and young children. Ear and Hearing 12: 199-204.

Ewing IR, Ewing AWG (1947) The ascertainment of deafness in infancy and early childhood. Journal of Laryngology and Otology 59: 309-38.

Gliddon ML, Martin AM, Green R (1999) A comparison of some clinical features of visual reinforcement audiometry and the distraction test. British Journal of Audiology 33: 355-65.

Gravel JS, Traquina DN (1992) Experience with audiologic assessment of infants and toddlers. International Journal of Pediatric Otorhinolaryngology 23: 59-71.

Greenberg DB, Wilson WR, Moore JM, Thompson G (1978) Visual reinforcement audiometry (VRA) with young Down's syndrome children. Journal of Speech and Hearing Disorders 43: 448-58.

Haug O, Baccaro MA, Guildford R (1967) A pure-tone audiogram on the infant: the PIWI technique. Archives of Otolaryngology 86: 101-6.

Health Building Note 12. Supplement 3. (1994) ENT and Audiology Clinics: Hearing Aid Centre. NHS Estates. London: HMSO.

Killion MC (1984) New insert earphone for audiometry. Hearing Instruments 35: 45-6.

Lancioni GE, Coninx F, Smeets PM (1989) A classical conditioning procedure for the hearing assessment of multiply handicapped persons. Journal of Speech and Hearing Disorders 54: 88-93.

Liden G, Kankkunen A (1969) Visual reinforcement audiometry. Acta Otolaryngologica 67: 281-92.

Lutman ME, McCormick B (1987) Converting free-field a-weighted sound levels to hearing level. Journal of the British Association of Teachers of the Deaf 11: 127.

Moodie KS, Seewald RC, Sinclair ST (1994) Procedure for predicting real-ear hearing aid performance in young children. American Journal of Audiology 3: 23-31.

Moore JM, Thompson G, Thompson M (1975) Auditory localization of infants as a function of reinforcement conditions. Journal of Speech and Hearing Disorders 40: 29-34.

Moore JM, Thompson G, Folsom RC (1992) Auditory responsiveness of premature infants utilizing visual reinforcement audiometry (VRA). Ear and Hearing 13: 187-94.

Moore JM, Wilson WR, Thompson G (1977) Visual reinforcement of head-turn responses in infants under 12 months of age. Journal of Speech and Hearing Disorders 42: 328-34.

NDCS (2000) Quality Standards in Paediatric Audiology Volume IV. Guidelines for the Early Identification and the Audiological Management of Children with Hearing Loss. London: National Deaf Children's Society.

Noise at Work: Guide 1 (1989) Legal Duties of Employers to Prevent Damage to Hearing. Health and Safety Executive Books.

Northern JL, Downs MP (1991) Hearing in Children. 4 edn. Baltimore, MD: Williams & Wilkins.

Nozza RJ, Wilson WR (1984) Masked and unmasked pure tone thresholds of infants and adults: development of auditory frequency selectivity and sensitivity. Journal of Speech and Hearing Research 27: 613-22.

Primus MA (1988) Infant thresholds with enhanced attention to the signal in visual reinforcement audiometry. Journal of Speech and Hearing Research 31: 480-4.

Primus MA (1991) Repeated infant thresholds in operant and nonoperant audiometric procedures. Ear and Hearing 12: 119-22.

Primus MA (1992) The role of localization in visual reinforcement audiometry. Journal of Speech and Hearing Research 35: 1137-41.

Primus M, Thompson G (1985) Response strength of young children in operant audiometry. Journal of Speech and Hearing Research 28: 539-47.

Rudmin FW (1984) Brief clinical report on visual reinforcement audiometry with deaf infants . Journal of Otolaryngology 13: 367-9.

Seewald RC (1992) The desired sensation level method for fitting children: Version 3.0. The Hearing Journal 45: 36-41.

Seewald RC, Cornelisse LE, Ramji KV, Sinclair ST, Moodie KS, Jamieson DG (1997) DSL v4.1 for Windows: A Software Implementation of the Desired Sensation Level (DSL[i/o]) Method for Fitting Linear Gain and Wide Dynamic Range Compression Hearing Instruments. London, Ontario, Canada: Hearing Health Care Research Unit: The University of Western Ontario.

Seewald RC, Moodie KS, Sinclair ST, Scollie SD (1999) Predictive validity of a procedure for pediatric hearing instrument fitting. American Journal of Audiology 8: 143-52.

Suzuki T, Ogiba Y (1961) Conditioned orientation reflex audiometry. Archives of Otolaryngology 74: 84-90.

Talbot CB (1987) A longitudinal study comparing respones of hearing-impaired infants to pure tones using visual reinforcement and play audiometry. Ear and Hearing 8: 175-9.

Thompson G, Folsom RC (1984) A comparison of two conditioning procedures in the use of visual reinforcement audiometry (VRA). Journal of Speech and Hearing Disorders 49: 241-5.

Thompson G, Folsom RC (1985) Reinforced and nonreinforced head-turn responses of infants as a function of stimulus bandwidth. Ear and Hearing 6: 125-9.

Thompson G, Thompson M, McCall A (1992) Strategies for increasing response behaviour of one-and two-year-old children during visual reinforcement audiometry (VRA). Ear and Hearing 13: 236-40.

Thompson G, Wilson WR, Moore JM (1979) Application of visual reinforcement audiometry (VRA) to low functioning children. Journal of Speech and Hearing Disorders 44: 80–90.

Walker G, Dillon H, Byrne D (1984) Sound field audiometry: recommended stimuli and procedures. Ear and Hearing 5: 13–21.

Widen JE (1990) Behavioural screening of high-risk infants using visual reinforcement audiometry. Seminars in Hearing 11: 342–56.

Widen JE, Folsom RC, Cone-Wesson B, Carty L, Dunnell JJ, Koebsell K, Levi A, Mancl L, Ohlrich B, Trouba S, Gorga MP, Sininger YS, Vohr BR, Norton SJ (2000) Identification of neonatal hearing impairment: hearing status at eight to 12 months corrected age using a visual reinforcement audiometry protocol. Ear and Hearing 21: 471–87.

Wilson WR, Moore JM (1978) Pure-tone earphone thresholds of infants utilizing VRA. Proceedings of the American Speech and Hearing Association. San Francisco CA: USA.

Wilson WR, Thompson G (1984) Behavioural audiometry. In Jerger J (ed.) Pediatric Audiology. London: Taylor & Francis, pp. 1–44.

Wright DC, Frank T (1992) Attenuation values for a supra-aural earphone for children and insert earphone for children and adults. Ear and Hearing 13: 454–9.

Chapter 5
Pure-tone audiometry

SALLY WOOD

Introduction

Pure-tone audiometry is the procedure most commonly used for the measurement of hearing impairment. Pure tones – tones with a single frequency of vibration – are presented via headphones or insert earphones (air conduction) or via a bone vibrator (bone conduction) and the patient's sensitivity at discrete frequencies is measured. For air-conducted stimuli, sound travels through the outer and middle ear – the conducting mechanism – before reaching the cochlea and auditory nerve. Abnormal pathology at any stage in this pathway may affect air conduction sensitivity. For bone-conducted stimuli it is assumed that the stimulus reaches the cochlea through bone and soft-tissue vibration. Abnormal pathology occurring at or beyond the cochlea may affect bone conduction sensitivity. The lowest level at which a pure-tone stimulus is heard through the headphone or insert earphone is known as the air conduction threshold at that frequency and the quietest stimulus that is heard when the bone vibrator is placed on the mastoid bone is known as the bone conduction threshold for that frequency. Threshold is defined precisely later in this chapter. Comparison of air and bone conduction thresholds (the air-bone gap) provides a means of quantifying the amount of conductive hearing impairment. There are some important provisos to the assumptions relating to bone conduction, which will be discussed later.

The purpose of pure-tone audiometry is to measure the threshold of hearing via both air and bone conduction and thus to arrive at a description of the degree and type of hearing impairment.

The audiometer

Audiometers range from simple screening audiometers, with a facility for air conduction measurement at a restricted range of frequencies and intensities, to complex clinical audiometers with facilities for a range of clinical tests in addition to pure-tone threshold measurement. For clinical purposes the frequency range usually extends from 125 Hz to 8 kHz in octave intervals, the octave increase corresponding to a doubling of the previous frequency. The steps are therefore: 125 Hz, 250 Hz, 500 Hz, 1 kHz, 2 kHz, 4 kHz, 8 kHz.

The following intermediate frequencies are also included in most clinical audiometers: 750 Hz, 1.5 kHz, 3 kHz, 6 kHz. The intensity is calibrated in 5 dB steps and extends from –10 dB up to a maximum value that varies with frequency but is most commonly 120 dB in the middle frequencies for air conduction. This decibel scale is known as dB HL (hearing level) and has been especially constructed for pure-tone audiometric measurements. The sensitivity of the human ear varies with frequency, being most sensitive at the middle frequencies. It would be clumsy and inconvenient to have a normal value for threshold that varies with the frequency under test and, therefore, the dB HL scale was constructed such that 0 dB HL corresponds to the normal threshold (for young adults with no history of ear disease or noise exposure) at each frequency. The actual output sound pressure level from the headphone (or bone vibrator) at a dial setting of 0 dB HL will be different at different frequencies. Any pure-tone threshold measurement is, therefore, a statement of how many decibels better or worse the hearing is than normal.

Standards for audiometers

There are a number of different standards that govern the specification of audiometers, audiometric reference levels and calibration equipment.

Specification of audiometers

This is governed by BS EN 60645-1 :1995 which specifies five types of audiometer according to the functions included. For each type the standard defines the test frequencies that should be available, the maximum and minimum hearing levels for air and bone conduction at each frequency, the centre and cut-off frequencies for narrow-band masking noise at each frequency and acceptable deviations from nominal performance in terms of frequency, output, attenuator linearity, harmonic distortion levels and rise and fall time for pure-tone stimuli.

Audiometric reference levels

Parts one to five of BS EN ISO 389 give audiometric reference levels for the range of signal/transducer combinations available in pure-tone audiometers. For air conduction these reference levels are known as reference equivalent threshold sound pressure levels (RETSPL) and vary with frequency. They are specific to the type of signal, the transducer and coupler used for calibration. The bone vibrator is calibrated in terms of the vibratory force levels transmitted to the mechanical coupler when the vibrator is excited electrically at the level corresponding to normal hearing threshold. These values are known as reference equivalent threshold force levels (RETFL). The values refer to a vibrator applied to the mastoid process with a static force of 5.4 N, the non-test ear masked with a narrow-band noise at a level of 35 dB above the pure-tone threshold of that ear and a vibrator with a plain circular driving face with an area between 150 mm² and 200 mm². The Radioear B-71 and B-72 are widely used bone vibrators that comply with the standard. Details of the relevant standards are shown in Table 5.1.

Calibration equipment

The characteristics of the couplers (ear simulator, acoustic coupler, occluded ear simulator) used for calibration of air conduction stimuli and the mechanical coupler (or artificial mastoid) used for calibration of bone conduction stimuli are specified in BS EN 60318, BS 6310 and BS 4009 respectively. Details of these and their IEC equivalents are shown in Table 5.2.

Insert earphones

In recent years there has been increased use of insert earphones (sometimes referred to as tubephones) for air conduction audiometry. Insert earphones do not require the use of a headband, prevent the problem of collapsing ear canals, allow audiometry to be carried out in higher ambient noise levels (Berger and Killion, 1989) and provide increased intra-aural attenuation thus reducing the need for masking (Sklare and

Table 5.1. British and international standards for reference levels for pure-tone audiometry

British standard	International standard
BS EN ISO 389-1: 2000 Acoustics. Reference zero for the calibration of audiometric equipment – Part 1. Reference equivalent threshold sound pressure level 1 for pure tones and supra-aural earphones	ISO 389-1:1998 Acoustics. Reference zero for the calibration of audiometric equipment – Part 1. Reference equivalent threshold sound pressure levels for pure tones and supra-aural earphones
BS EN ISO 389-2:1997 Acoustics. Reference zero for the calibration of audiometric equipment – Part 2. Reference equivalent threshold sound pressure levels for pure tones and insert earphones	ISO 389-2:1994 Acoustics. Reference zero for the calibration of audiometric equipment – Part 2. Reference equivalent threshold sound pressure levels for pure tones and insert earphones
BS EN ISO 389-3:1999 Acoustics. Reference zero for the calibration of audiometric equipment – Part 3. Reference equivalent threshold force levels for pure tones and bone vibrators	ISO 389-3:1994 Acoustics. Reference zero for the calibration of audiometric equipment – Part 3. Reference equivalent threshold force levels for pure tones and bone vibrators
BS EN ISO 389-4:1999 Acoustics. Reference zero for the calibration of audiometric equipment – Part 4. Reference levels for narrow-band masking noise	ISO 389-4:1994 Acoustics. Reference zero for the calibration of audiometric equipment – Part 4. Reference levels for narrow-band masking noise
BS EN ISO 389-5:2001 Acoustics. Reference zero for the calibration of audiometric equipment – Part 5. Reference equivalent threshold sound pressure levels for pure tones in the frequency range 8 kHz to 16 kHz	ISO/TR 389-5:1998 Acoustics. Reference zero for the calibration of audiometric equipment – Part 5. Reference equivalent threshold sound pressure levels for pure tones in the frequency range 8 kHz to 16 kHz

Table 5.2. British and international standards for calibration equipment for pure-tone audiometry

British standard	International standard
BS EN 60318-1:1998 Electroacoustics. Simulators of human head and ear simulator for the calibration of supra-aural earphones	IEC 60318-1:1998 Electroacoustics – Simulators of human head and ear – Part 1. Ear simulator for the calibration of supra-aural earphones
BS EN 60318-2:1998 Electroacoustics. Simulators of human head and ear. An interim acoustic coupler for the calibration of audiometric earphones in the extended high-frequency range.	IEC 60318-2:1998 Electroacoustics – Simulators of human head and ear – Part 2. An interim acoustic coupler for the calibration of audiometric earphones in the extended high-frequency range.
BS EN 60318-3:1998 Electroacoustics. Simulators of human head and ear. Acoustic coupler for the calibration of supra-aural earphones used in audiometry.	IEC 60318-3:1998 Electroacoustics – Simulators of human head and ear – Part 3. Acoustic coupler for the calibration of supra-aural earphones used in audiometry.
BS 6310:1982 Specification for occluded-ear simulator for the measurement of earphones coupled to the ear by ear inserts.	IEC 60711:1981 Occluded-ear simulator for the measurement of earphones coupled to the ear by ear inserts.
BS 4009:1991 Specification for artificial mastoids for the calibration of bone vibrators used in hearing aids and audiometers.	IEC 60373:1990 Mechanical coupler for measurements on bone vibrators

Denenberg, 1987; Frank and Richards, 1991; Munro and Agnew, 1999).

Calibration of audiometers

Regular checks of audiometer performance are essential and should be carried out in accordance with the scheme outlined in BS EN ISO 8253-1. Stage A consists of routine checks and subjective tests that should be carried out daily and weekly. Stage B consists of objective checks to be carried out at regular intervals but not exceeding 12 months. Stage C is a full calibration check, which is required when there is a possibility that the equipment has been damaged or its performance has changed or at five-yearly intervals. Regular subjective checks, as detailed below, should enable problems to be detected early.

Regular (Stage A) checks

The following checks should be carried out on each day of use:

- Switch the equipment on and allow it to warm up in accordance with the manufacturer's recommendation. Check the headphone, insert earphone and vibrator serial numbers. These transducers should be uniquely identifiable to a particular audiometer and must not be exchanged between audiometers without recalibration.
- Listen to the output from all transducers (air and bone) at all frequencies at around threshold to ensure that output is just audible and that no spurious signals or noise are present. (This assumes that the tester has normal hearing and is thus able to check low-level outputs.)
- Repeat the listening check for a high-level output (40 dB bone, 60 dB air) for all signals and transducers; listen for proper function, absence of distortion and intermittency and freedom from spurious signals or clicks. Check that all lamps, indicators and switches are functioning correctly.
- Check that the patient response button operates correctly.

Any other functions provided, such as Stenger tests or wide-band masking should be checked.

Weekly checks should also include a more thorough examination of leads and headbands for wear and tear. Signal attenuators should be checked over the whole intensity range for linearity and silent operation of interrupters and for signal quality.

The audiogram

This is a graphical representation of the results obtained in pure-tone audiometry. Figure 5.1 shows the standard format recommended by the British Society of Audiology (BSA) (1989). The ordinate extends from –10 dB to +140 dB and is marked 'hearing level (dB)'. The marking of the hearing level scale is not specific to a particular calibration standard but a space is included at the bottom of the form to include this information. The abscissa extends from 125 Hz to 8,000 Hz and is marked at octave intervals. Dotted vertical lines represent the frequencies 750 Hz, 1,500 Hz, 3,000 Hz and 6,000 Hz. The scale is marked 'frequency (Hz)'. The symbols recommended by the BSA for use in pure-tone audiometry are shown in Figure 5.2.

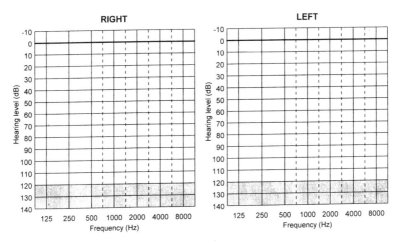

Figure 5.1. The audiogram format recommended by BSA.

	Right	Left
Air conduction, masked if necessary	○	×
Air conduction, not masked (possible shadow point)	●	☓
Bone conduction, not masked	△	
Bone conduction, masked	[	]
In addition, the following symbols may be used on working audiograms		
Air conduction, masked but no change on masking	◒	✕

Figure 5.2. Recommended symbols for use in pure-tone audiometry.

Threshold measurement

The definition of auditory threshold is to some extent arbitrary. As with any psychophysical measurement there will be an intensity above which an individual responds on all presentations and a lower intensity below which the individual will fail to respond on all presentations. Between these two intensities is a region wherein lies the threshold. The precise value of threshold obtained may be affected by a number of variables as discussed below.

Patient variables

The attention, motivation and ability of the patient to concentrate may affect the measurement procedure. It is important that the patient is comfortable. The temperature and ventilation of the test room may affect performance. Wilber (1979) quotes an example of children tested in a room temperature of 90°F whose thresholds were as much as 15 dB poorer than when tested at a more comfortable temperature. The patient should be free from visual and auditory distractions and background noise must be controlled to avoid masking effects.

Equipment variables

Regular calibration and checking of equipment is necessary. The possibility of error when using audiometers with gross calibration errors is obvious (for example, an audiometer whose attenuator is not functioning below a dial setting of 30 dB will result in losses of up to 30 dB being recorded as normal). Cross-talk between earphones may result in false thresholds being recorded in patients with unilateral losses. However, problems may arise even in audiometers that are calibrated to the relevant standard because of the variability that is permitted. For example, at 3 kHz the tolerance on frequency is +3% (for a type 3 audiometer); thus two audiometers, one with an output of 2,910 Hz and one with an output of 3,090 Hz, will both be considered to be within calibration standards. If a patient with a very steeply sloping high-frequency loss is tested the thresholds as measured by the two audiometers at a nominal setting of 3 kHz could be significantly different. In some cases the variability could be as much as 20 dB (Woodford, 1984).

Background noise

Background noise may exert a masking effect resulting in raised (that is, worse) thresholds being recorded. This is dependent upon several factors:

- the frequency characteristics and intensity of the background noise;
- the frequency of the test tones used;
- the lowest threshold it is desired to measure;
- the mode of presentation (air or bone) and the attenuation characteristics of the transducer.

Bone conduction measurements require more stringent criteria for background noise than do air conduction measurements because the supra-aural cushions used in air conduction audiometry have some sound attenuation properties particularly at high frequencies (Berry, 1973). An advantage claimed for the use of insert earphones is the greater attenuation of background noise compared with supra-aural earphones (Berger and Killion, 1989). The effects of background noise are discussed in detail by Shipton and Robinson (1975) who conclude that a frequency analysis of the noise is necessary – a single dB(A) measurement is insufficient as threshold elevation varies greatly with the frequency distribution of the noise. BS EN ISO 8253-1:1998 gives maximum acceptable levels of background noise in audiometric test rooms.

Procedural variables

These include:

- the instructions given to the patient;
- the threshold measurement procedure that is adopted;
- the attenuator step size;
- the criterion adopted for threshold.

Instructions given to the patient can be an important variable. A patient who is instructed to respond only when he or she is sure that the tone is present is likely to respond differently from one instructed to respond if he or she thinks the tone is present.

The numerous ways in which the threshold could be traced vary from a simple descending procedure (starting from a level at which the signal is clearly audible and reducing it until the patient no longer responds) to more sophisticated forced-choice procedures where the patient is instructed that a tone is present in one of two or three intervals and the task is to indicate which interval contains the tone. This forced-choice procedure has been shown to give thresholds that are on average 6.5 dB better than those obtained with a clinical audiological procedure (Marshall and Jesteadt, 1986). However comparison of manual methods of pure-tone audiometry has shown no significant differences in threshold although some methods took significantly longer to establish threshold (Arlinger, 1979; Tyler and Wood, 1980). Time, of course, is an important factor in clinical procedures.

Jervall and Arlinger (1986) compared step sizes of 2 dB and 5 dB in manual audiometry. They found slightly higher (worse) thresholds with the step size of 5 dB but use of the smaller step size resulted in a 30%–40% increase in time required to established threshold. Leijon (1992) points out that the measurement error involved in pure-tone audiometric threshold determination includes a quantization component due to attenuator step size. An increase in step size may decrease the standard deviation of repeated thresholds while at the same time increasing the true measurement error.

It is clear, therefore, that a standard procedure for threshold measurement should be adopted in order to minimize variability. The most commonly used procedure is known at the 'method of limits'. The procedure is based on the Hughson and Westlake ascending technique, which was described by Carhart and Jerger (1959) and modified by the American Speech and Hearing Association (ASHA). This has been adopted as one of two standard procedures by the BSA. The attenuator step size is 5 dB and the criterion for threshold is that the patient respond on 50% of ascending presentations with a minimum of two responses at that level. This procedure is briefly described below. Readers are advised to read the original procedures as described by BSA (1981, 1985).

Determination of threshold in adults

The procedure is explained to the patient, who is instructed to make the desired response whenever he or she hears the test tone, no matter how faintly. Ideally, the patient's response should be silent and indicate the duration of the test tone by, for example, pressing a button (or raising a finger) when the tone appears and releasing the button (lowering the finger) when the tone is no longer heard. Older children and adults are usually tested in a soundproof booth so that auditory and other distractions are kept to a minimum. The tester should be able to observe the patient. The test tones should have a duration of 1 s to 3 s and it is important to avoid a rhythmical presentation, which may allow the patient to anticipate the tone. Equally, it is important to avoid very long silent intervals, which will give rise to false responses.

The better hearing ear is usually tested first at 1 kHz, proceeding to higher and then to lower frequencies with a retest at 1 kHz. If the retest value at 1 kHz is more than 5 dB better than the original threshold the next frequency is retested and so on. The opposite ear is then tested in the same order but without the retest at 1 kHz.

Initially, the tone is presented at about 40 dB above the estimated threshold and the patient's response checked. If there is no response, successive increments of 20 dB are used until there is a response. Once this familiarization has been achieved, measurement of threshold begins. The intensity is reduced in steps of 10 dB steps until the patient no longer responds, at which point the intensity is increased in 5 dB steps until the patient responds. After a positive response the intensity is reduced in 10 dB increments until no response occurs and then again raised 5 dB at a time. Threshold is defined as the lowest level at which a response occurs in at least half of a series of ascending trials with a minimum of two responses at that level: the criterion is met if a patient responds at a particular level on two out of three ascending presentations. This method is often referred to as the '10 down, 5 up' procedure for obvious reasons.

Pure-tone audiometry in young children

Preliminaries

Most normally developing children of 3;6 years and above (and many between 2;6 and 3;6) are able to co-operate successfully with pure-tone audiometric testing using toy material if the tester is sufficiently skilled. The initial approach to the child is very important and he or she should be accompanied into the clinic by the parent or carer. It is not advisable, and rarely necessary, to separate children of this age from the parent for the purpose of audiological assessment. The child should be tested in a clinic room that has been treated to reduce background noise to acceptable levels, or in a soundproof booth that is large enough to accommodate tester, child, parent and equipment. The room should be as free as possible from visual distractions; toys and games should be kept out of sight in cupboards until required as should medical and other equipment not in frequent use. The child is seated in a small chair at a low table with the parent seated next to the child. The tester then sits beside the child with the audiometer placed behind the child and out of his/her vision as shown in Figure 5.3.

Young children can be very adept at picking up extraneous cues and, even with this arrangement, great care must be taken that the child does not see the tester's arm move in activating the signal as this can alert the child to the presentation of a signal. For a skilled tester manipulation of the audiometer controls becomes second nature and their attention can be directed to working with the child.

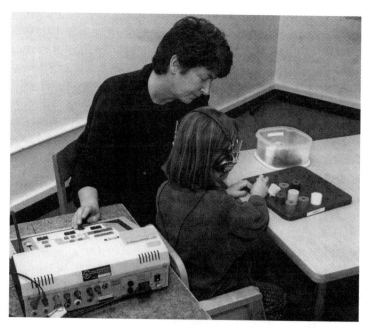

Figure 5.3. Suitable arrangement for pure-tone audiometry with a young child.

This arrangement has the advantage that the tester has direct control over the timing of signal presentation and the reward of valid responses or correction of invalid responses. This optimum synchrony of the stimulus/reward (or correction) is more difficult to achieve if two testers are involved (typically one working with the child and one with the audiometer).

For children between the ages of 3;6 and five years it is a matter for the tester's judgement whether or not to start with a sound-field performance test (see Chapter 4) or with pure-tone audiometry. If the child appears in any way clingy or anxious it is often advisable to start with a sound-field test. This gives the child a chance to relax and co-operate without the added complication of imposing headphones.

Conditioning procedure

The initial stage involves conditioning the child to make a simple response on the presentation of an auditory signal. This initial signal can be a pure-tone or warble-tone produced by a sound-field audiometer or a pure-tone through the headphones, which can be held near the child or worn by the child. Whichever is chosen, it is imperative that this initial signal be well above the child's threshold – a child cannot be conditioned to respond to a signal that he or she cannot hear. Informal observation when the child enters the clinic and during history taking should give some indication of the child's hearing – as will the history and parental opinion. In cases of children with severe hearing loss it is often useful to use a vibratory signal from the bone conductor as the initial signal. The principles of conditioning and response reinforcement using play materials (discussed in Chapter 4) should be applied to pure-tone audiometry at this stage.

Having achieved reliable responses to sound-field stimuli most children will accept the headphones. The tester should wear them for a brief listening check, in case an unexpected fault has developed, and then place each headphone (normally colour coded red for the right ear and blue for the left ear) centrally over the external auditory meatus (after moving the hair out of the way), adjusting the headband to fit. The child is immediately given something (for example, a peg) to hold to occupy the hands and prevent him or her fiddling with head set, and one or two supra-threshold signals are given to remind the child of the task. Some children become upset or worried at this stage and reject the headphones, in which case it may be helpful to have the parent or a co-operative sibling wear the headphones and participate briefly in the task. Alternatively it is possible to detach one headphone and hold it close to the child's ear, encouraging him or her to listen and to make the appropriate response. If thresholds are measured in this way a note should be made on the audiogram as this can introduce some measurement error.

Suitable activities for pure-tone audiometry

When testing children under five years, the most suitable activities involve a simple motor response such as placing a peg in a board or stacking beakers. If the response required is too complicated, or the game is too interesting, the child may become absorbed in the activity rather than listening for the auditory stimulus. The activities should be as simple as possible whilst still providing some interest for the child. A very fiddly response may slow the procedure down and could be difficult for children with poor fine motor skills. For such children a more appropriate response might be to drop an object into a box or to knock it off the table or the arm of a chair. A selection of activities is needed, so that the child's interest and motivation can be maintained by switching to a new activity if necessary. The advantages in using this type of activity (rather than have the child say 'yes' or press a button) are:

- the response in itself is rewarding for the child and this is further reinforced by praise from the tester;
- a false positive response can be corrected by the tester (for example, the peg can be removed from the board);
- the procedure can be carried out without, or with a minimum of, verbal instruction as appropriate for the child's language level.

Threshold measurement in children

Generally speaking, the threshold measurement procedure used with children should be the same as that used with adults (10 down, five up). With young children, however, it is particularly necessary to work rapidly whilst trying to avoid unnecessary sacrifice in accuracy. It is essential to vary the inter-stimulus interval with occasional fairly long intervals (> five seconds) particularly if there is a suspicion that the child is anticipating the signal, but long silent intervals can result in the child losing concentration and it may be necessary to give occasional suprathreshold signals during the process of threshold exploration in order to retain the child's attention. If a child is making a rather hesitant response to a particular signal and the tester is not sure whether this is a genuine response, increasing the dial setting by 5 dB and presenting this signal should result in a very positive response from the child if the previous response was genuine.

If the child's concentration will not permit the measurement of a minimum of three air conduction thresholds for each ear using the standard procedure it may be necessary to modify the procedure by using a '20 down, 10 up' procedure; an alternative is to test down to a level of 15 dB or 20 dB and accept two positive responses at this level, rather than measuring thresholds of 0-5 dB more accurately. If either of these modifications is used the fact should be noted on the audiogram. However, this should not be used as an excuse for sloppy techniques or for using such modifications with children who are capable of carrying out standard threshold measurement procedures: information may be lost in this way, particularly with regard to the need for masking, if true thresholds of –5 dB, for example, are not measured.

Order of test

Older children and adults may reasonably be expected to co-operate for the number of threshold measurements that are deemed to be necessary, but with young children the tester is working with a shorter concentration span and only a limited number of thresholds can be obtained. It is therefore necessary to choose the next threshold measurement on the basis that it may be the last one obtained in that session. It is generally advisable to obtain air conduction thresholds at 500 Hz, 1 kHz, and 4 kHz in both ears first and to fill in other frequencies later depending upon the results obtained. Generally, the convention is to test air conduction first and then bone conduction as required; however, there is room for discretion with young children. For example, if sound-field results have been obtained and show some hearing loss, it may be sensible to test bone conduction first as this will indicate whether there is any sensorineural component in the better hearing ear at each frequency. Experience shows that some young children respond more reliably to bone conduction stimuli than they do to air conduction stimuli. The reason for this is not clear although it seems that the child feels less 'cut off' when wearing the bone conductor than when wearing a set of headphones. If bone conduction measurements are obtained first it also means that vibrotactile conditioning can be used to greater effect. However, if sound-field results have been normal it is more sensible to aim for air conduction thresholds in both ears first, to explore the possibility of a unilateral loss, as this may be missed by sound-field tests.

Other methods

If a child is not developmentally ready for the conditioning and co-operation described above, other methods may be used to obtain pure-tone thresholds. Visual reinforcement audiometry may be carried out with the child wearing supra-aural or insert earphones and/or bone vibrator. Other techniques such as tangible reinforcement conditioning audiometry (TROCA) (Hodgson, 1994) may also be used.

Influence of age on pure-tone thresholds

The deterioration in hearing sensitivity with age (presbyacusis) is well known and standard values for the thresholds of hearing by air conduction as a function of age and sex are available in ISO 7029:1984. This standard gives the median values for otologically normal persons in the age range 18–70 years.

No standard exists for those under 18 years but there has been interest in the question of appropriate normal threshold values for infants and children and in the age at which normal adult values are attained.

It is generally accepted that hearing sensitivity in infants is reduced compared with that of adults (Wilson and Thompson, 1984) and that it improves during childhood. However, there is no consensus on the age at which adult values are attained. Some authors (Fior, 1972; Maxon and Hochberg, 1982; Haapaniemi, 1996) have suggested that adult values are attained at around 10–13 years of age but others (Roche et al., 1978) have demonstrated that improvement continues between 12 and 17 years of age. The mechanism for this improvement is not clear although studies by Elliot and Katz (1980) and Yoneshige and Elliott (1981) appear to have ruled out factors such as mild middle-ear disorders and acoustic leakage due to poor ear/

earphone coupling. It is not clear whether the change results from some form of physiological maturation or maturation of the child in terms of attention and listening skills. The amount of improvement in threshold reported varies across studies that have used different measurement procedures, stimuli and step sizes. Orchik and Rintelmann (1978) used an ascending procedure with a 5 dB step size and reported an improvement of the order of 5 dB between 3;6 and 6;6 year-old children for pure tones at 0.5, 1 and 2 kHz. Buren, Solen and Laukli (1992) found no change in sensitivity in three groups of children aged 10, 14 and 18 years but they did find that mean thresholds differed from the RETSPL values of ISO 389 by up to 4.1 dB in the frequency range 0.5–4 kHz. This raises questions about the choice of population upon which to base standard threshold data.

Reliability of threshold measurement

A number of studies (Hickling, 1966; Robinson and Shipton, 1982; Jervall and Arlinger, 1986; Robinson, 1991) have examined the repeatability of threshold measurement in adults. The general consensus is that for air conduction measurements repeatability is best at 1 kHz and 2 kHz and progressively less good at frequencies outside this range. Threshold measurements in adults typically show test-retest standard deviations of around 5 dB for air conduction and 8 dB for bone conduction (Robinson and Shipton, 1982). Variability at high frequencies is due to the effect of altered earphone placement on standing wave formation whereas variability at low frequencies is thought to be due to leakage of sound through the imperfect seal between the headphone cushion and the ear (Atherley and Lord, 1965). This low-frequency leakage is reduced by the use of circumaural earphones (Shaw, 1966; Dillon, 1977; Lippman, 1981).

Reliability in children

Surprisingly little has been written about the reliability of repeated pure-tone threshold measurement in young children. Lowell et al. (1956) followed a group of 21 hearing impaired children from 3;6 to 6;11 years and compared results of initial and final tests: 66% of threshold pairs were within 5 dB and 89% within 10 dB. During the course of their study with normal hearing children from 3;6–6;6 years of age, Orchik and Rintelmann (1978) looked at test-retest threshold comparisons and found that 93% of threshold comparisons were within 5 dB.

Masking in pure-tone audiometry

One of the main problems in pure-tone audiometry arises from the ability of sound to cross the head: if a sound presented to one ear, the test ear, is sufficiently intense, it may cross the skull and be perceived by the contralateral or non-test ear. If the patient responds positively to this auditory signal a false threshold will be recorded for the test ear. The crucial factor in determining whether this 'cross hearing' is occurring is the amount of sound lost in crossing the skull. This is known as the transcranial transmission loss (transcranial attenuation, inter-aural attenuation) and is different for air and bone conduction stimuli and for different air conduction transducers. If the not-masked thresholds indicate that cross hearing may have occurred then masking procedures should be used. Masking is the process by which the threshold of audibility for one sound is raised by the presence of another sound, the masking sound. In clinical practice the masking sound is introduced to the non-test ear and the test ear threshold redetermined. It is necessary to ensure that the correct level of masking is used; too little and the non-test ear may still perceive the test tone; too much and the masking sound may cross over and raise the threshold in the test ear.

Transcranial transmission loss

Transcranial transmission loss has been investigated for supra-aural earphones and for bone vibrators (Zwislocki, 1953; Coles and Priede, 1970; Snyder, 1973; Smith and Markides, 1981) and more recently for insert earphones (Sklare and Denenberg, 1987; Frank and Richards, 1991; Munro and Agnew, 1999).

There is some inter-subject variability and also variation across frequency. For insert earphones, values also vary with insertion depth with greater transmission loss for deep insertion (outside edge of the ear plug flush with the entrance of the ear canal) compared with shallow insertion (half the plug inside the ear canal). In setting up criteria for masking it is the minimum value of transcranial transmission loss that should be considered. For air conduction stimuli using MX41-AR cushions the minimum value has been found to be 40 dB. Therefore, if any air conduction threshold exceeds the contralateral bone conduction threshold (because it is the contralateral cochlea in which the tone will be perceived) by 40 dB or more, then there is a possibility of cross hearing. This should be indicated on the audiogram by use of the appropriate symbol (✗●) and consideration given as to whether masking procedures are needed. For insert earphones the minimum value is 50 dB for shallow insertion and 55 dB for deep insertion. For bone conduction stimuli the minimum value of transcranial transmission loss has been found to be 0 dB, which means that any bone conduction threshold obtained without masking cannot clearly be attributed to one ear. The necessity for masking procedures is based on an assessment of the significance of any possible air-bone gap. A number of examples are given below to illustrate these points.

Examples of cross hearing

In the examples that follow, the air conduction thresholds have been obtained using conventional TDH-39 earphones with MX41-AR cushions and therefore the appropriate value of transcranial transmission loss for air conduction is 40 dB.

In the audiogram shown in Figure 5.4 the naive tester may well interpret the configuration to show normal hearing in the left ear with a moderate conductive loss in the right ear. However, upon consideration it is clear that the not-masked bone conduction thresholds could refer to either ear and,

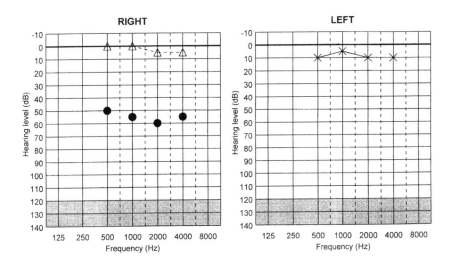

Figure 5.4. Illustration of possible shadow curve.

without masking, it is not possible to assign them to a particular ear. Further, because the left-ear air-conduction thresholds are normal, the left-ear bone conduction thresholds will theoretically be at least as good, and therefore it is possible that the right-ear air conduction thresholds are 'shadow thresholds' from the left cochlea. In this case the true audiogram could be either that shown in Figure 5.5 (a profound loss on the right) or that shown in Figure 5.6 (a moderate mixed loss on the right).

Figure 5.7 shows another audiogram obtained without masking. In this case it is not possible for the air conduction thresholds to be a result of cross hearing because, whichever ear

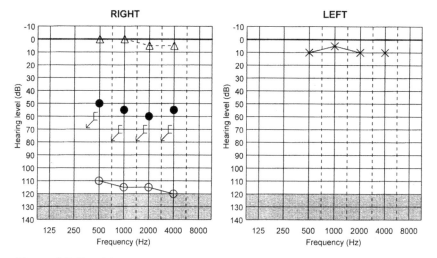

Figure 5.5. Possible true picture – a profound loss on the right.

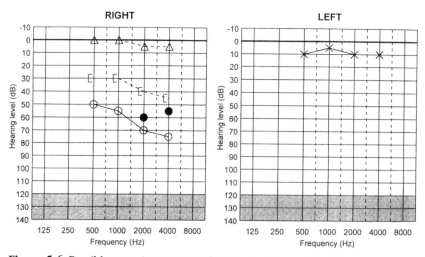

Figure 5.6. Possible true picture – a moderate mixed loss on the right.

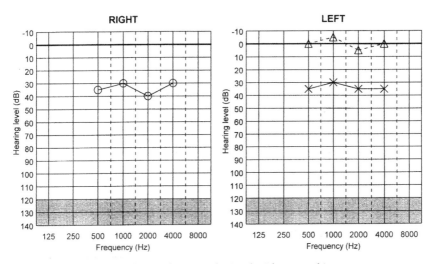

Figure 5.7. Example of an audiogram obtained without masking.

the bone conduction thresholds refer to, there is no difference of 40 dB or more at any frequency. However, without masking it is not possible to assign the bone conduction thresholds to a particular ear. A significant air-bone gap is clearly possible in either ear but without masking it is not possible to quantify the size of the gap. It may be that in one ear the loss is wholly or partly sensorineural.

In measuring masked bone conduction thresholds there is no clear indication about the ear with which to start. Initially, one could decide to obtain masked thresholds for the left ear (masking the right ear). If the masked bone conduction thresholds shift by more than 10 dB it is reasonable to assume that the not-masked thresholds refer to the right ear. However, if they do not shift, it will be necessary to obtain masked thresholds for the right ear (masking the left ear). This situation that necessitates masking both ears for bone conduction arises commonly in bilateral conductive loss.

Another example is shown in Figure 5.8. In this case, having already obtained the not-masked air conduction audiogram, there is no indication to mask at this stage. When the not-masked bone conduction thresholds are obtained at 500 Hz and 1 kHz, a significant air-bone gap could be present in both ears and, therefore, masking is necessary. When the masked bone conduction thresholds are obtained for the right ear it is clear that the not-masked bone conduction thresholds refer to the left ear and, therefore, no further bone conduction masking is

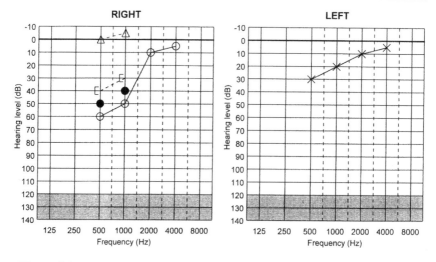

Figure 5.8. Cross hearing in air and bone conduction.

necessary. However, having obtained this information it is now clear that the right ear air conduction thresholds at 500 Hz and 1 kHz could be shadow thresholds from the left cochlea and therefore, masking of the air conduction thresholds at 500 Hz and 1 kHz on the right is necessary.

In the case shown in Figure 5.9, there is the possibility of a significant air-bone gap at all frequencies in the left ear. It is necessary to attempt to obtain masked bone conduction thresholds at 500 Hz and 1 kHz for the left ear. There is no point in masking at higher frequencies because the not-masked

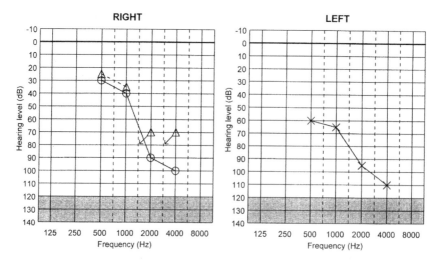

Figure 5.9. A further example of an audiogram obtained without masking.

thresholds for bone conduction are beyond the maximum output of the audiometer (and masked thresholds must be the same as, or greater than, not-masked thresholds).

Summary

The above examples show that consideration of the minimum values of transcranial transmission loss (40 dB for air conduction with supra-aural earphones, 0 dB for bone conduction) together with the not-masked thresholds obtained, indicates when cross hearing may be occurring and therefore when masking is necessary. Masking is necessary in the following circumstances:

- *Air conduction.* Whenever a threshold exceeds the contralateral bone conduction threshold by 40dB or more.
- *Bone conduction.* Whenever a significant air-bone gap may be present. In clinical practice a gap of 15 dB or more is generally considered significant.

Nature of masking stimuli

Masking is the process by which the threshold of audibility for one sound is raised by the presence of another sound – the masking sound. When pure tones are masked by bands of noise only a narrow band of frequencies surrounding the tone – the critical band – contributes to the masking of a tone (Fletcher, 1940). In terms of masking efficiency a bandwidth equal to the critical band is the most efficient. However, this noise would have considerable tonal quality and, therefore, bandwidths of 1/3–1/2 octave are normally used in clinical audiometry. For a further discussion of this see Scharf (1970).

Clinical masking procedures

Studebaker (1979) has classified the approaches to the problem of clinical masking into two groups – psychoacoustic and acoustic methods. The psychoacoustic method is based on the shadow or plateau techniques described by Hood (1960) and is the type most commonly used in the UK. The acoustic or formula method is more often described in American texts (Goldstein and Newman, 1994; Studebaker, 1979). A third method, which involves simply presenting a fixed level of masking to the non-test ear and remeasuring the test ear threshold frequently, gives erroneous results (Coles and Priede,

1970) because it is not possible, with this method, to ensure that insufficient or excessive masking has not been used.

Plateau technique (Hood's Shadow Technique)

A hypothetical masking function is shown in Figure 5.10. The masking stimulus is presented to the non-test ear and its threshold, M, is determined. The masking stimulus is increased in steps of 10 dB and at each increment the pure-tone threshold in the test ear is redetermined. The resulting masking function falls into three phases. In the initial phase, A–B, increases in masking result in equal increments in measured threshold because both stimuli are being perceived in the non-test cochlea. During stage B–C, increases in masking do not produce equal increases in measured threshold. The two are largely independent although a small increase in threshold due to the phenomenon of central masking is often seen. This is the plateau, at which a 20 dB increment in masking results in a change in threshold of 5 dB or less and indicates that the test tone is perceived in the test ear and the masking noise in the non-test ear. At stage C–D further increases in masking produce equal increments in threshold, indicating that both stimuli are now being perceived in the same (test) ear (that is, the masking noise has now crossed over and is being perceived in the test ear). In practice it is not always possible to obtain such a plateau: the maximum masking level may be reached before a plateau is obtained, or the maximum

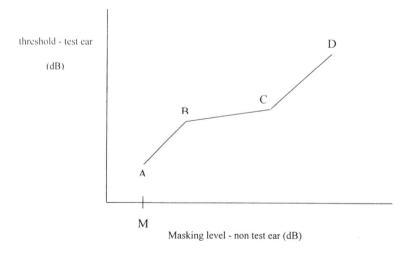

Figure 5.10. Hypothetical masking function.

output of the pure tone may be reached before a plateau is obtained (in this case the masked threshold is designated by the appropriate signal with a downward arrow).

In the case of bilateral conductive losses the so-called 'masking dilemma' can occur. This is because once the masking is of sufficient intensity to mask the non-test cochlea it also reaches the test cochlea and therefore no plateau can be obtained.

Recommended procedure for clinical masking

The method described below is that recommended by the BSA (1986) and readers are advised to refer to the original for full details.

The narrow-band masking noise is presented to the contralateral (non-test) ear via headphone or insert earphone for air conduction audiometry and via insert earphone or insert receiver for bone conduction audiometry. The threshold of masking, M, is determined in the usual way. If no interrupter switch is provided for the masking channel an ascending threshold is established. The patient is next instructed to respond to the test tone as usual and to ignore the masking noise. The masking is increased by 10 dB to ensure effectiveness, and the pure-tone threshold redetermined. The results are plotted on a masking chart as shown in Figure 5.11.

This procedure is continued until the masking function and a plateau are obtained. This is usually defined as the level over which a 20 dB change in masking results in an increase in

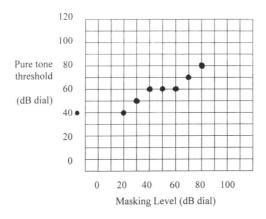

Figure 5.11. Example of a masking function.

threshold of 5 dB or less. In the example shown in Figure 5.11 the true pure-tone threshold is 60 dB. In some cases it may be necessary to check intermediate steps until a plateau can be clearly defined.

In cases of more severe loss the limit of masking may be reached before a clear plateau is defined. This should be indicated on the masking chart and no clear conclusion about the threshold can be drawn. In other cases the pure-tone threshold may exceed the maximum output of the audiometer before a plateau is obtained and the conclusion in such a case is that the threshold exceeds this level: this should be indicated on the audiogram.

Minimum effective masking level

This is the level of masking, above the threshold of masking, which is required to ensure that the masker is effective (that a 10 dB increase in masking will result in a 10 dB increase in threshold). The value has been shown to vary between individuals (Coles and Priede, 1970; Barret and Rowson, 1982) but generally a level of 10–20 dB SL is sufficient to ensure effective masking.

Effective masking

Effective masking refers to the level of the test tone that the masker will *just* mask – for example a narrow-band noise masker set to 40 dB effective masking should just mask a pure-tone signal at 40 dB HL. Some audiometers have masking dials that are claimed to be calibrated in effective masking. Before relying upon this it is wise to check the calibration of this using one of the methods described by Studebaker (1979) or Coles and Priede (1970).

Masking procedures for children

Many children who are able to co-operate sufficiently to obtain reliable pure-tone audiograms will also be able to respond reliably when masking procedures are used. The age at which children will respond reliably in this way is quite variable but between three and five years of age an increasing number of children are able to do this.

First, the threshold for the masking noise in the non-test ear (M) must be determined. The child is instructed to listen for the 'rushing noise' or the 'noise like the sea' and when this is presented at a supra-threshold level the child is guided in making an appropriate response and rewarded for doing so. When he or she is responding reliably at supra-threshold levels the threshold of masking can be measured. If several masked thresholds are required it is advisable to obtain M at all frequencies first to avoid constantly changing the listening task and possibly confusing the child. Once M has been obtained the child is instructed to listen for the 'whistle' and ignore the masking noise. The masking noise is presented at a level of 10 dB above the recorded threshold. At this point the child is likely to respond to the masking noise and needs to be reminded to wait for the 'whistle' which is then presented at a supra-threshold level and the child guided/rewarded for the correct response. Two or three responses at this level will retrain the child to respond upon presentation of the pure tone.

The threshold for the pure tone can now be redetermined in the normal way, again using the technique of demonstrating and guiding the child in the correct response with appropriate reward. This is more likely to be successful than giving complex verbal instructions about ignoring one sound and listening for another, which tend to confuse young children. As the masking levels are increased it is important to observe the child carefully because high levels of masking may cause distress: if this occurs the procedure should be terminated and an appropriate note made on the masking chart and the audiogram.

Frequencies to be masked

A clear understanding of the mechanism of cross hearing and the levels at which it may occur is necessary for the correct interpretation of audiometric results. However, a literal adherence to the masking rules can result in a very large number of frequencies that require masking. This is rarely possible in children and it is preferable to obtain a small number of masked thresholds reliably. The frequencies and mode of presentation will depend upon the possibilities presented by the not-masked audiogram and when testing children it is often useful to carry out impedance measurements before deciding which frequencies to mask.

Impedance measurements are not a substitute for bone conduction measurements; they can show the existence of a conductive problem but not its magnitude. For example, consider the audiogram shown in Figure 5.7. If middle-ear impedance measurements showed a normal tympanogram and stapedial reflexes in the right ear but a flat tympanogram in the left, it would be advisable to obtain masked bone conduction thresholds for the right ear first, because this ear is more likely to have a sensorineural loss. Without the impedance results there is no clear indication to mask one ear rather than the other; if masked bone conduction thresholds were obtained first for the left ear and these were no different from the not-masked thresholds, this would indicate a need to obtain masked bone conduction thresholds for the right ear. However, by this time the child is likely to have lost concentration. Although this example may be unlikely in practice it illustrates the potential usefulness of impedance measurement in making informed decisions about masking.

Interpretation of audiograms

The purpose of pure-tone audiometry is to quantify the degree, and if possible the type, of hearing loss based upon comparison of the air and bone conduction thresholds for each ear at each frequency (assuming that all necessary masking has been carried out). However a number of factors must be considered in order to ensure that results are interpreted correctly.

Collapse of the ear canal during audiometry

Collapse of the ear canal is caused by pressure of the supra-aural cushion on the pinna resulting in some degree of occlusion of the canal, which gives rise to artefactually depressed air conduction thresholds. The higher frequencies (1 kHz and above) are usually affected and threshold shifts of the order of 15 dB are common, although shifts as large as 30 dB have been observed (Ventry et al., 1961). The problem has been demonstrated in children with one study showing that this occurred in 3.5% of 282 six- to nine-year-old children who underwent pure-tone audiometric testing at school (Creston, 1965). The solutions that have been suggested include:

- use of circumaural earphones;
- sound-field audiometry;
- holding the supra-aural cushion and phone against the child's ear;
- use of rubber inserts to maintain canal patency;
- use of insert earphones.

In children, indications of a conductive problem on pure-tone audiometry with absence of such indication on either sound-field testing or impedance measurement should alert the tester to this problem: it may be more common than has been previously thought.

Vibrotactile thresholds in air and bone conduction

The phenomenon of vibrotactile perception of auditory stimuli has been known for many years and has been investigated in a number of studies (Nober, 1964, 1967, 1970; Boothroyd and Cawkwell, 1970). It is generally agreed that the phenomenon does not occur at frequencies above 1,000 Hz and is dependent upon transducer type. The phenomenon may occur with conventional supra-aural earphones at high output levels but is virtually eliminated by the use of insert earphones. For bone conduction measurement the level at which tactile perception occurs depends upon placement (mastoid or forehead) and upon oscillator type (Dean and Martin, 1997). These studies show considerable inter-subject variability in tactile thresholds and therefore it is not possible to simply draw a line on an audiogram that will separate tactile and auditory thresholds. Rather, it is necessary to be aware that there is a range of values over which the possibility of vibrotactile perception must be considered. These are shown in Table 5.3 for supra-aural headphones and for mastoid placement of the bone conduction oscillator.

Table 5.3. Vibrotactile thresholds (dB HL)

Transducer	Frequency (Hz)		
	250	500	1000
Supra-aural earphones	80–110	100–120	120–130
Bone vibrator (mastoid placement)	20–40	50–70	75–85

The audiogram shown in Figure 5.12 illustrates the problem. This audiogram could well be interpreted as showing a mixed loss at low frequencies when in fact the bone conduction thresholds could be vibrotactile rather than auditory and the loss entirely sensorineural.

This is another example where impedance measurements can contribute to the interpretation of pure-tone audiometric results.

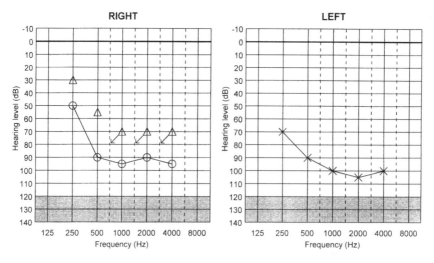

Figure 5.12. Example of vibrotactile thresholds.

Bone conduction measurements

Measurements of hearing by bone conduction are generally more problematic and subject to error than air conduction measurements. These problems arise from the difficulties associated with calibration and other equipment variables. There has been debate about the relative merits of forehead and mastoid placement of the bone vibrator and although forehead placement results in better test-retest reliability and smaller inter-subject variability, the differences are not large enough to be of great practical advantage (Dirks, 1994). It has also been suggested that bone conduction measurements at the forehead are less influenced by the status of the middle ear than are mastoid measurements. The main advantage of mastoid placement is its greater sensitivity; a less intense signal is needed to reach threshold, which means that a greater dynamic range is available and therefore a greater range of hearing levels can be measured.

The force with which the vibrator is applied and its surface area may also affect measured thresholds. BS ISO 389-3 (1999) specifies a bone vibrator of 150–200 mm² applied with a force of 5.4 (+ 0.5) N. Despite these requirements, techniques for making these measurements are not widely available (Smith and Foster, 1997) and there are few data regarding the effect of headband force on pure-tone thresholds. It is likely that headbands designed for adults may not apply the vibrator with the required force when used with small children but this has not been investigated in any detail.

The limited accuracy of bone conduction audiometry is discussed in detail by Coles, Lutman and Robinson (1991). Their prime concern is with the significance and interpretation of air-bone gaps in medicolegal assessment. They point out that bone conduction thresholds have a greater degree of variability compared with air conduction thresholds and calibration is more problematic for bone conduction than for air conduction. The mechanical coupler is required to be stabilized at a temperature of 23°C – a condition that can be difficult to achieve in practice – and a deviation of 2°C can produce a calibration error of about 1 dB. Bone conduction calibration standards are based on thresholds obtained with 35 dB of effective masking in the non-test ear to ensure a strictly unilateral measurement; inevitably an element of central masking is introduced, which tends to elevate the measured threshold. If masking is then not used in the clinical situation there is inevitably a bias towards better (lower) thresholds.

Airborne radiation in bone conduction audiometry

Airborne radiation of sound can be a problem during bone conduction measurements at high frequencies (3 kHz and 4 kHz) (Lightfoot, 1979; Shipton, John and Robinson, 1980; Bell, Goodsell and Thornton, 1980). Airborne sound may enter the normal pathway of external and middle ear and if it is subjectively louder than the vibratory sensation a false bone conduction threshold and hence a false air-bone gap will be recorded. This problem may be overcome by the use of sound attenuating earplugs in the test ear at these frequencies. However, the plugs should not be in place for all bone conduction testing because at lower frequencies the occlusion effect (an improvement in bone conduction thresholds when the test ear is occluded) may occur.

Influence of the middle ear on bone conduction

In some instances the influence of the middle ear status on bone conduction measurements is well known. Carhart (1962) first described the depression in bone conduction thresholds in patients with otosclerosis and the subsequent improvement in these thresholds after stapes mobilization. He quantified the artefactual depression of bone conduction thresholds as 5 dB at

500 Hz, 10 dB at 1 kHz, 15 dB at 2 kHz and 5 dB at 4 kHz; this is now known as the Carhart notch.

Other types of middle-ear impairment including secretory otitis media have been shown to influence bone conduction thresholds with an improvement in low-frequency bone conduction response and a depression of the high frequency response in the presence of middle-ear problems (Hulka, 1941; Huizing, 1964; Carhart, 1962; Dirks and Malmquist, 1969). Improvements of up to 25 dB in bone conduction thresholds before and after treatment for otitis media with effusion have been reported (Kobayashi et al., 1988).

Similarly, experimental work in animals has shown that various alterations to the middle and external ear (such as loading the tympanic membrane, pressure changes in the external canal or fixation of middle-ear structures) result in changes in bone conduction thresholds (Huizing, 1960; Tonndorf, 1966).

The occlusion effect

The occlusion effect is the improvement in bone conduction threshold obtained when the external auditory meatus is occluded. It occurs in ears with normal hearing or sensorineural losses but is absent in conductive losses. The improvement in threshold is about 25 dB at 250 Hz, 20 dB at 500 Hz, 5-10 dB at 1 kHz and is generally absent at frequencies above this. It is often seen clinically when masked bone conduction thresholds are measured. Initially, the bone conduction threshold is not masked and not occluded but insertion of the insert receiver or earphone provides occlusion and therefore the not-masked threshold may improve. It is advisable to re-measure the not-masked occluded bone conduction threshold with the insert receiver in place before proceeding with masking.

The occlusion effect is another example of the ability of changes in the external canal and middle ear to influence bone conduction thresholds. For a fuller discussion of the mechanisms of bone conduction and the way in which these mechanisms are influenced by the external and middle ears readers are referred to Dirks (1994) or Tonndorf (1972).

Limited output on bone conduction

The maximum output available from the bone vibrator is limited, particularly at low frequencies, because of problems in producing high level outputs without distortion. Typically, the maximum output at 500 Hz is 60 dB and at 1 kHz it is 70 dB. Care should be taken not to exceed the maximum output (many audiometers permit the dial setting to be increased beyond this level with no comparable increase in output). This limited output means that in children with more severe losses bone conduction measurements may not contribute much useful information. In such cases impedance measurements are extremely useful in identifying conductive problems although they do not provide any measure of the degree of any conductive loss.

Conclusion

Obtaining and interpreting pure-tone audiograms from young children is a skilled activity. In practice it is often not possible to carry out extensive masked threshold measurement but because of this it is essential to have a thorough understanding of the problems and pitfalls in order to interpret correctly the results from pure-tone audiometric testing.

References

Arlinger SD (1979) Comparison of ascending and bracketing methods in pure tone audiometry. Scandinavian Audiology 8: 247-51.

Atherley C, Lord P (1965) A preliminary study of the effect of earphone position on the reliability of repeated auditory threshold determination. International Audiology 4: 161-6.

Barret H, Rowson V (1982) Normal variation in the masking effectiveness of the narrow band noises of one audiometer. British Journal of Audiology 16: 159-65.

Bell I, Goodsell S, Thornton ARD (1980) A brief communication on bone conduction artefacts. British Journal of Audiology 14: 73-5.

Berger EH, Killion MC (1989) Comparison of the noise attenuation of three audiometric earphones with additional data on masking near threshold. Journal of the Acoustical Society of America 86: 1392-403.

Berry BF (1973) Ambient Noise Limits for Audiometry. National Physical Laboratory Acoustics Report AC60.

Boothroyd A, Cawkwell S (1970) Vibrotactile thresholds in pure tone audiometry. Acta Otolaryngologica 69: 381-7.

British Society of Audiology (1981) Recommended procedures for pure-tone audiometry using a manually operated instrument. British Journal of Audiology 15: 213-16.

British Society of Audiology (1985) Recommended procedures for pure-tone bone-conduction audiometry without masking using a manually operated instrument. British Journal of Audiology 19: 281-82.

British Society of Audiology (1986) Recommendations for masking in pure tone threshold audiometry. British Journal of Audiology 20: 307-14.

British Society of Audiology (1989) Recommended format for audiogram forms. British Journal of Audiology 23: 265–6.

BS EN 60645-1:1995 Audiometers Part 1: Pure Tone Audiometers. London: British Standards Institution.

BS EN ISO 389:1997 Acoustics. Reference Zero for the Calibration of Pure Tone Air Conduction Audiometers. London: British Standards Institution.

BS EN ISO 389-2:1997 Acoustics. Reference Zero for the Calibration of Audiometric Equipment – Part 2. Reference Equivalent Threshold Sound Pressure Levels for Pure Tones and Insert Earphones. London: British Standards Institution.

BS EN ISO 389-3:1999 Acoustics. Reference Zero for the Calibration of Audiometric Equipment – Part 3. Reference Equivalent Threshold Force Levels for Pure Tones and Bone Vibrators. London: British Standards Institution.

BS EN ISO 389-4:1999 Acoustics. Reference Zero for the Calibration of Audiometric Equipment – Part 4. Reference Levels for Narrow-Band Masking Noise. London: British Standards Institution.

BS EN ISO 389-5: 2001 Acoustics. Reference Zero for the Calibration of Audiometric Equipment – Part 5. Reference Equivalent Threshold Sound Pressure Levels for Pure Tones in the Frequency Range 8 kHz to 16 kHz. London: British Standards Institution.

BS EN 60318-1:1998 Electroacoustics. Simulators of Human Head and Ear. Ear Simulator for the Calibration of Supra-aural Earphones. London: British Standards Institution.

BS EN 60318-2:1998 Electroacoustics. Simulators of Human Head and Ear. An Interim Acoustic Coupler for the Calibration of Audiometric Earphones in the Extended High Frequency Range. London: British Standards Institution.

BS EN 60318-3:1998 Electroacoustics. Simulators of Human Head and Ear. Acoustic Coupler for the Calibration of Supra-aural Earphones used in Audiometry. London: British Standards Institution.

BS 6310:1982 Specification for Occluded-ear Simulator for the Measurement of Earphones Coupled to the Ear by Ear Inserts. London: British Standards Institution.

BS 4009:1991 Specification for Artificial Mastoids for the Calibration of Bone Vibrators used in Hearing Aids and Audiometers. London: British Standards Institution.

BS EN ISO 8253-1:1998 Acoustics. Audiometric Test Methods – Part 1: Basic Pure Tone Air and Bone Conduction Threshold Audiometry. London: British Standards Institution.

Buren M, Solem BS, Laukli E (1992) Threshold of hearing (0.125–20 kHz) in children and youngsters. British Journal of Audiology 26: 23–31.

Carhart R, Jerger JF(1959) Preferred method for clinical determination of pure tone thresholds. Journal of Speech and Hearing Disorders 24: 330–45.

Carhart R (1962) Effect of stapes fixation on bone conduction. In Ventry IM, Chaiklin JB, Dixon RF (eds) Hearing Measurement. New York: Appleton-Century-Crofts, pp. 116–29.

Coles RRA, Priede VM (1970) On the misdiagnoses resulting from incorrect use of masking. Journal of Laryngology and Otology 84: 41–63.

Coles RRA, Lutman ME, Robinson DW (1991) The limited accuracy of bone conduction audiometry: its significance in medicolegal assessments. The Journal of Laryngology and Otology 105: 518–21.

Creston JE (1965) Collapse of the ear canal during routine audiometry. Journal of Laryngology and Otology 79: 893–901.

Dean M, Martin FN (1997) Auditory and tactile bone-conduction thresholds using three different oscillators. Journal of the American Academy of Audiology 8: 227–32.

Dillon H (1977) Effect of leakage on the low frequency calibration of supra-aural headphones. Journal of the Acoustical Society of America 61b: 1383–6.

Dirks D (1994) Factors related to bone conduction reliability. Archives of Otolaryngology 79: 551–8.

Dirks E, Malmquist CM (1969) Comparison of frontal and mastoid bone conduction thresholds in various conductive lesions. Journal of Speech and Hearing Research 12: 725–46.

Dirks D (1994) Bone conduction testing. In Katz J(ed.) Handbook of Clinical Audiology. Baltimore: Williams & Wilkins, pp. 132–46.

Elliott L, Katz D (1980) Children's pure tone detection. Journal of the Acoustical Society of America 67: 343–4.

Fior R (1972) Physiological maturation of auditory function between 3 and 13 years of age. Audiology 11: 317–21.

Fletcher H (1940) Auditory patterns. Review Modern Physics 12: 47–65.

Frank T, Richards WD (1991) Hearing aid coupler output level variability and coupler correction levels for insert earphones. Ear and Hearing 12: 221–7.

Goldstein BA, Newman CW (1994) Clinical masking: a decision making process. In J Katz (ed.) Handbook of Clinical Audiology. Baltimore: Williams & Wilkins, pp. 109–31.

Haapaniemi J (1996) The hearing threshold levels of children at school age. Ear and Hearing 17: 469–77.

Hickling S (1966) Studies on the reliability of auditory threshold values. Journal of Auditory Research 6: 39–46.

Hodgson R (1994) Testing infants and young children. In J Katz (ed.) Handbook of Clinical Audiology. Baltimore: Williams & Wilkins, pp. 465–76.

Hood JD (1960) The principles and practice of bone conduction audiometry. Laryngoscope 70: 1211–28.

Huizing EH (1960) Bone conduction, the influence of the middle ear. Acta Otolaryngolgica (Suppl.) 155: 1–99.

Hulka J (1941) Bone conduction changes in acute otitis media. Archives of Otolaryngology 33: 333–46.

IEC 60318-1:1998 Electroacoustics. Simulators of Human Head and Ear – Part 1: Ear Simulator for the Calibration of Supra-aural Earphones. Geneva: IEC.

IEC 60318-2:1998 Electroacoustics. Simulators of Human Head and Ear – Part 2: An Interim Acoustic Coupler for the Calibration of Audiometric Earphones in the Extended High Frequency Range. Geneva: IEC.

IEC 60318-3:1998 Electroacoustics. Simulators of Human Head and Ear – Part 3: Acoustic Coupler for the Calibration of Supra-aural Earphones used in Audiometry. Geneva: IEC.

IEC 60711:1981 Occluded-ear Simulator for the Measurement of Earphones Coupled to the Ear by Ear Inserts. Geneva: IEC.

IEC 60373:1990 Mechanical Coupler for Measurements on Bone Vibrators. Geneva: IEC.

ISO 389-1:1998 Acoustics. Reference Zero for the Calibration of Audiometric Equipment Part 1: Reference Equivalent Threshold Sound Pressure Levels for Pure Tones and Supra-aural Earphones. Geneva: ISO.

ISO 389-2:1994 Acoustics. Reference Zero for the Calibration of Audiometric Equipment – Part 2. Reference Equivalent Threshold Sound Pressure Levels for Pure Tones and Insert Earphones. Geneva: ISO.

ISO 389-3:1999 Acoustics. Reference Zero for the Calibration of Audiometric Equipment – Part 3. Reference Equivalent Threshold Force Levels for Pure Tones and Bone Vibrators. Geneva: ISO.

ISO 389-4:1994 Acoustics. Reference Zero for the Calibration of Audiometric Equipment – Part 4. Reference Levels for Narrow-band Masking Noise. Geneva: ISO.

ISO/TR 389-5:1998 Acoustics. Reference Zero for the Calibration of Audiometric Equipment– Part 5: Reference Equivalent Threshold Sound Pressure Levels for Pure Tones in the Frequency Range 8 kHz to 16 kHz. Geneva: ISO.

Jervall L, Arlinger S (1986) A comparison of 2 dB and 5 dB step size in pure tone audiometry. Scandinavian Audiology 15: 51–6.

Kobayashi K, Kodama H, Takezawa H, Suzuki T, Kataura A (1988) Elevation of bone conduction threshold in children with middle ear effusion. International Journal of Paediatric Otorhinolaryngology 16: 95–100.

Leijon A (1992) Quantization error in clinical pure-tone audiometry. Scandinavian Audiology 21: 103–8.

Lightfoot GR (1979) Air-borne radiation from bone conduction transducers. British Journal of Audiology 13: 53–6.

Lippman PR (1981) MX41/AR ear phone cushions versus a new circumaural mounting. Journal of the Acoustical Society of America 69: 589–92.

Lowell E, Rushford G, Hoversten G, Stoner M (1956) Evaluation of pure tone audiometry with pre-school age children. Journal of Speech and Hearing Disorders 21: 292–302.

Marshall L, Jesteadt W (1986) Comparison of pure tone audibility thresholds obtained with audiological and two interval forced choice procedures. Journal of Speech and Hearing Research 29: 82–91.

Maxon A, Hochberg I (1982) Development of psychoacoustic behaviour: sensitivity and discrimination. Ear and Hearing 3: 301–8.

Munro KJ, Agnew N (1999) A comparison of inter-aural attenuation with the Etymotic ER-3A insert earphone and the Telephonics TDH-39 supra-aural earphone. British Journal of Audiology 33: 259–62.

Nober EH (1964) Pseudoauditory bone conduction thresholds. Journal of Speech and Hearing Disorders 29: 469–76.

Nober EH (1967) Vibrotactile sensitivity of deaf children to high intensity sound. Laryngoscope 77: 2128–46.

Nober EH (1970) Cutile air and bone conduction thresholds of the deaf. Exceptional Children 56: 571–9.

Orchik DJ, Rintelmann WF (1978) Comparison of pure tone, warble tone and narrow band noise thresholds of young normal hearing children. Journal of the America Audiology Society 3: 214–20.

Robinson DW (1991) Long-term repeatability of the pure-tone hearing threshold and its relation to noise exposure. British Journal of Audiology 25: 219–36.

Robinson DW, Shipton MS (1982) A standard determination of paired air- and bone-conduction thresholds under different masking noise conditions. Audiology 21: 61–2.

Roche AF, Siervogel RM, Himes RM, Johnson JH (1978) Longitudinal study of hearing in children: baseline data concerning auditory thresholds, noise exposure, and biological factors. Journal of the Acoustical Society of America 64: 593–1601.

Scharf B (ed.) (1970) Critical bands. In Tobias JV (ed.) Foundations of Modern Auditory Theory. London: Academic Press, pp. 159–202.

Shaw E (1966) Ear canal pressure generated by circumaural and supra-aural earphones. Journal of the Acoustical Society of America 39: 471-9.

Shipton MS, Robinson DW (1975) Ambient noise limits for industrial audiometry. National Physical Laboratory Acoustics Report AC 69.

Shipton MS, John AJ, Robinson DW (1980) Air radiated sound from bone vibration transducers and its implications for bone conduction audiometry. British Journal of Audiology 14: 86-99.

Sklare DA, Denenberg LJ (1987) Interaural attenuation for tubephone insert earphones. Ear and Hearing 8: 298-300.

Smith BL, Markides A (1981) Interaural attenuation for pure tones and speech. British Journal of Audiology 15: 49-54.

Smith PA, Foster JR (1997) Audiometer calibration: two neglected areas. British Journal of Audiology 31: 359-64.

Snyder JM (1973) Interaural attenuation characteristics in audiometry. Laryngoscope 83: 1847-55.

Studebaker GA (1979) Clinical masking. In Rintelmann WF (ed.) Hearing Assessment. Baltimore: University Park Press, pp. 51-100.

Tonndorf T (1966) Bone conduction studies in experimental animals. Acta Otolaryngologica Suppl 213: 1-132.

Tonndorf J (1972) Bone conduction. In Tobias JV (ed.) Foundations of Modern Auditory Theory. Volume 2. New York: Academic Press, pp 197-237.

Tyler RS, Wood EJ (1980) A comparison of manual methods for measuring hearing levels. Audiology 19: 316-29.

Ventry IM, Chaiklin JB, Boyle WF (1961) Collapse of the ear canal during audiometry. Archives of Otolaryngology 73: 727-31.

Wilber L (1979) Pure tone audiometry. In Rintelmann WF (ed.) Hearing Assessment. Baltimore: University Park Press, pp. 1-38.

Wilson WK, Thompson G (1984) Behavioural audiometry. In Jerger J (ed.) Paediatric Audiology. San Diego: College Hill, pp. 1-44.

Woodford CM (1984) The effect of small changes in frequency on clinically determined estimates of auditory threshold. ASHA (April): 25-30.

Yoneshige Y, Elliott LL (1981) Pure tone sensitivity and ear canal pressure at threshold in children and adults. Journal of the Acoustical Society of America 70: 1272-6.

Zwislocki J (1953) Acoustical attenuation between the ears. Journal of the Acoustical Society of America 25: 752-9.

Chapter 6
Electric response audiometry

STEVE MASON

Introduction

Recording of electrical activity from the neural pathways of the auditory system, evoked by auditory stimulation, is an essential tool in the audiological management of infants and young children. Electric (or Evoked) response audiometry (ERA) is the term that encompasses different types of auditory evoked potential (AEP) of which the auditory brainstem response (ABR) is the most valuable in the paediatric population. These investigations enable an 'objective' assessment of hearing when reliable behavioural testing is not appropriate or is unreliable. The recordings can also provide valuable information about the origin of pathology.

Historical perspective

The electroencephalogram (EEG) of the brain was first recorded from the intact scalp in humans by Berger in 1929 and in the following year he described changes in the rhythm of the EEG to loud sounds (Berger, 1930). This was the birth of ERA. The next significant contribution to the field was by P.A. Davis (1939) and H. Davis and co-workers (1939) who described more specific changes in the EEG. All these early investigations, however, encountered the problem of detecting the response to a stimulus when the background noise was high. The only method of detection available to these workers was a simple superimposition of 10 to 20 EEG traces in order to identify the response. It was the introduction of signal averaging by Dawson in 1951, and the subsequent development of the electronic averaging computer (Clark, 1958), which completely revolutionized the field of ERA. The power of this technique is clearly demonstrated by the fact that over 50 years later we still employ the same signal-averaging technique for acquisition of evoked potentials

The auditory pathway

The functioning of the auditory system at different levels of the pathway has been extensively investigated both in man and animals using electrophysiological techniques (Abbas, 1988; Pickles, 1988). A range of auditory evoked potentials (AEPs) can be recorded, which represent electrical activity from almost all the different stages of the auditory pathway; cochlea and auditory nerve (electrocochleography), brainstem (auditory brainstem response), mid-brain/cortex (middle latency response) and cortex (auditory cortical response) (Picton et al., 1974). The following sections briefly summarize the anatomical and functional aspects of the pathways relevant to the AEPs recorded in ERA.

Cochlea

The external auditory canal and middle ear serve to transmit sounds into the cochlea of the inner ear, which is the receptor organ for hearing. The cochlea is a membraneous spiral structure (2.5 turns) within the temporal bone. Along its length on the basilar membrane lie the sensory inner and outer hair cells and their supporting structures, known as the organ of Corti (Figure 6.1). There are approximately 15,000 hair cells in the human cochlea. At the basal end of the cochlea there are three rows of outer hair cells to each row of inner hair cells; towards the apical end the ratio of inner to outer hair cells increases to five. On each hair cell there are stereocilia, which project upwards. The stereocilia on the outer hair cells are imbedded into the underside of a jelly-like structure called the tectorial membrane whereas those on the inner hair cells are free to move. Sound waves are converted into pressure changes in the fluid in the scala vestibuli of the cochlea by the action of the stapes and oval window. This provides the mechanical drive for the basilar membrane, which results in stimulation of the hair cells.

The mode of fluid vibrations in the cochlea is a travelling wave pattern (Bekesy, 1947), beginning at the base of the cochlea and travelling towards the apex. The envelope of the travelling wave pattern is not symmetrical, rising slowly on the basal side and falling abruptly on the apical side. The point of maximum excursion of the wave occurs at progressively more apical locations along the basilar membrane as the frequency of a steady-state stimulus is lowered. A transient stimulus produces a travelling wave that starts at the basal end and moves up the cochlea. The most apical point reached by the wave depends upon the rise time, duration and frequency content of the stimulus. The wave takes about 5 ms to travel from the base to the apex in the human cochlea. This broad mechanical tuning is the result of the physical properties of the basilar membrane. However, in addition to this broad tuning there is a 'second active process' that makes the neuronal response of the auditory nerve fibres more specific to one characteristic frequency (fine tuning) than would be expected from just the simple travelling wave theory, as described later. This is sometimes referred to as the 'cochlear amplifier'.

The auditory (VIII cranial) nerve fibres and spiral ganglion cells, of which there are about 30,000 in man, connect to the hair cells along the length of the basilar membrane. About 90% to 95% are radial fibres innervating the inner hair cells and form

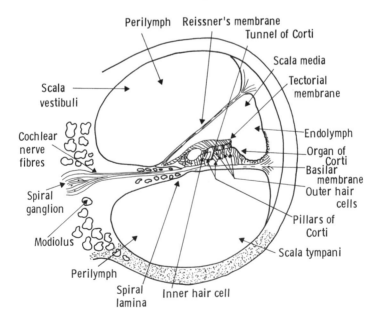

Figure 6.1. Cross-section through the basal turn of the cochlea showing the organ of Corti and the inner and outer hair cells.

the main afferent pathway into the brainstem. The remaining 5% to 10% of fibres provide efferent innervation to the more numerous outer hair cells along the basilar membrane and are known as spiral fibres. It is the electromotility of the outer hair cells and their complex interaction with the inner hair cells (Brownell, 1986), controlled by the efferent system (Sahley et al., 1997), which generates the fine frequency tuning associated with the afferent auditory nerve fibres. Overall the afferent neurones can be described by a tuning curve, which is sharply tuned to a characteristic frequency for low intensity tones and broadly tuned for high intensity tones.

Electrical activity associated with functioning of the hair cells (receptors) and the auditory nerve fibres can be recorded using electrocochleography (ECochG). The AC and DC receptor potentials are known as the cochlear microphonics (CM) and the summating potential (SP) respectively. The first true neurogenic response that can be recorded is the compound auditory nerve action potential (AP)

Auditory brainstem pathways

The three main structures that make up the brainstem are the medulla oblongata, pons and mid-brain. The auditory brainstem response consists of components originating from nuclei and tracts in these structures as electrical activity ascends the auditory pathway up to the cortex (Figure 6.2). The auditory nerve leaves the cochlea through the internal auditory meatus and subsequently reaches the ipsilateral cochlear nuclei, which lie at the dorsolateral border of the ponto-medullary junction. All incoming auditory nerve fibres terminate on cells within the cochlear nucleus complex. This structure acts as the first coding and sorting centre for auditory impulses helping to isolate the most important impulses and dispatch them to various other centres in the brainstem. The dorsal region of the nucleus projects a number of fibres to the lateral lemniscus and inferior colliculus directly, whereas the ventral region communicates with the superior olivary complex. There are both contralateral and ipsilateral projections although the contralateral are more numerous. The medial superior olive has remarkable sensitivity to the relative time of arrival of stimuli from the two ears leading to the suggestion that this nucleus is concerned especially with the processing of directional information. This is the first level at which interaction can occur between the two ears. The short

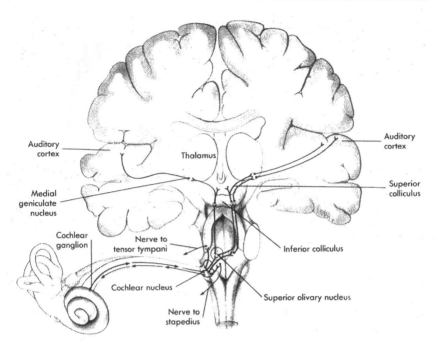

Figure 6.2. The auditory pathway including the cochlea, brainstem and cortex (from Seeley et al., 1992).

tract of the lateral lemniscus delivers the main fibres to the inferior colliculus; these are at least third-order neurones from the cochlea. The inferior colliculi then give rise to nerve fibres, the majority of which pass to the medial geniculate body of the same side. A few, however, cross over to the opposite side, the highest level at which fibres cross in the auditory pathway. The inferior colliculus acts as a relay station, but also has a role in the localization of sounds. The medial geniculate body is functionally part of the thalamus and its main output is an ordered tonotopic distribution of nerve fibres to the primary auditory cortex. The middle latency response (MLR) has its origins in the thalamus and primary auditory cortex.

Cortex

The primary auditory cortex (AI) in man lies in the superior gyri of each temporal lobe and its function is to analyse auditory information in terms of discrimination of pitch and intensity, and the perception of auditory sequence and pattern. Secondary auditory areas (AII) are present in parts of the temporal, parietal and frontal cortex. The main language processing cortex (Wernicke's area) is usually located in the superior part of the left temporal lobe adjacent to the primary auditory cortex, whereas the cortex responsible for the generation of language (Broca's area) is located in the posterior part of the inferior frontal gyrus. Understanding of language and the production of speech depend on highly integrated cortical activity within the primary and secondary auditory cortices. The auditory cortical response (ACR) and event related potentials (ERPs) are responses that can access this electrical activity in the brain in response to a stimulus.

Origin of hearing loss

The two most common causes of hearing loss are pathology in the middle ear (conductive loss) and damage to the receptors (for example, hair cells) in the cochlea (cochlear or sensorineural hearing loss). Although a hearing loss may arise beyond the cochlea in the brainstem (retrocochlear) or in the cortex of the brain itself (central hearing loss), the number of these cases is very small when compared to other types of hearing loss. A conductive loss arises when there is a reduction in the transmission by the middle-ear bones and may be caused for example by infection and fluid in the middle ear cavity, for example glue. The hearing loss in these cases may be slight to moderate but a patient is never totally deaf. However, hair cell damage in the cochlea may be slight or severe, or in worst cases the patient may be profoundly or even totally deaf. The type and severity of hearing loss will influence the characteristics of the auditory evoked potential as described later.

Types of auditory evoked potential

Evoked potentials arising from the auditory pathway are often described in terms of the time at which the response occurs following the auditory stimulus; early (0–10 ms), middle (10–60 ms) or late (60–1,000 ms) latency responses as shown in Figure 6.3. Each time period represents electrical activity from progressively higher levels of the auditory pathway. Electrocochleography (ECochG) and the auditory brainstem response (ABR) are classed as early latency responses, the middle latency response (MLR) as middle latency, and the auditory cortical response (ACR) and event related potentials (ERPs) as late latency.

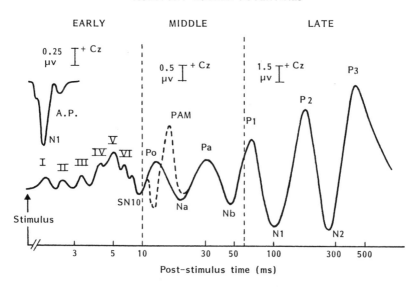

Figure 6.3. Early, middle and late latency components of the auditory evoked potential. The time axis following presentation of the stimulus is displayed on a logarithmic scale.

The above terminology for the different types of AEP will used throughout this chapter and is typical of that described in the literature. However, alternatives are in evidence – particularly for the brainstem and cortical responses. The ABR is sometimes described as the brainstem evoked response (BSER), or brainstem electric (or evoked) response audiometry (BERA). The term 'slow vertex response' (SVR) also describes the ACR, which can also be documented as cortical electric (or evoked) response audiometry (CERA).

Electrocochleography (ECochG)

There are two commonly used locations for the recording electrode in ECochG. The trans-tympanic method, first described by Portmann et al. in 1967, involves the placing of a needle electrode through the tympanic membrane coming to rest on the promontory in the middle ear. This technique gives large well-defined responses, but it is invasive. An alternative method is the extra-tympanic technique, which involves the positioning of an electrode in the external auditory meatus close to the tympanic membrane (Mason et al., 1980). This technique is non-invasive and has wider applicability compared to the trans-tympanic method. However, in practice both techniques require a general anaesthetic in young children.

Three response components are recorded in ECochG; cochlear microphonics (CM), summating potential (SP), and the compound auditory nerve action potential (AP), as shown in Figure 6.4. The CM and SP are predominantly receptor potentials, and reflect activity of the hair cells. The AP is the summation of electrical activity from a large number of individual nerve fibres originating from close to the cochlea. It is the only component from ECochG that has good threshold sensitivity and that can be used for assessment of hearing acuity. The supra-threshold SP can be used as a diagnostic indicator of

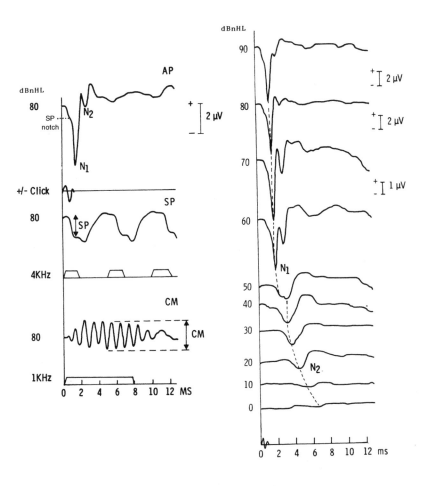

Figure 6.4. Electrocochleography showing recordings of the compound auditory action potential (AP), summating potential (SP) and cochlear microphonics (CM).

endolymphatic hydrops. The CM is a direct measure of hair cell activity and is useful in assessment of auditory neuropathy and retrocochlear pathology.

Auditory brainstem response (ABR)

The electrical activity evoked in the auditory nerve and brainstem pathways is known collectively as the auditory brainstem response (ABR). The first definitive description of the ABR in humans was given by Jewett and Williston (1971), although Sohmer and Feinmesser first recorded these neurogenic responses in 1967. Jewett showed that the response evoked by a high-intensity click stimulus and recorded from a vertex and ipsilateral mastoid electrode configuration, consists of a series of up to seven waves (designated I to VII in the Jewett classification), occurring in the first 10 ms post-stimulus (Figure 6.5). These waves are a far-field recording of the electrical activity from sequentially activated neural tracts and nuclei in the ascending auditory nerve and brainstem pathways.

The precise origins of these waves are difficult to define and are complicated by the interaction between different generator sites. Proposed origins are based largely on either studies in animals (Achor and Starr, 1980), patients with brainstem disorders (Stockard and Rossiter, 1977) or comparative studies of surface and depth recorded ABRs in patients undergoing surgery (Moller and Janetta, 1984). An extensive review of neural mechanisms of the ABR is reported by Moller (1999).

Wave I is known to be the compound action potential of the auditory nerve and is the far-field equivalent of the AP component in ECochG. Wave II is thought to arise predominantly from proximal regions of the auditory nerve and wave III from the cochlear nucleus. The superior olivary complex is considered to be the main source of wave IV and the lateral lemniscus wave V. Waves VI and VII are thought to arise mainly from the inferior colliculus. These proposed generator sites for waves II to VII are slightly more distal compared to early studies of the ABR.

As well as these fast individual waves of the ABR, as described by Jewett and Williston, there is a slow wave associated with wave V and a negative component at a latency of about 10 ms. This slow negative response is often called SN10 after Davis and Hirsh (1979) and is thought to originate in the mid-brain, probably representing post-synaptic activity within the inferior colliculus (Hashimoto, 1982).

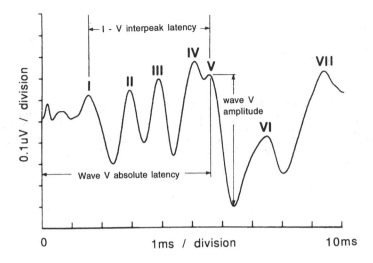

Figure 6.5. The ABR waveform as described by Jewett and Williston (1971) showing the classic wave I to VII.

Short latency component (SLC)

In addition to the well-documented waves I to V on the ABR an SLC can sometimes be observed on waveforms evoked by either acoustical (Mason et al., 1996) or electrical stimulation (Mason et al., 1997). Using a high-intensity click stimulus (typically 100 dB nHL or more) the SLC is predominantly a vertex-negative component at a latency of about 3 ms and can be identified clearly when there is no obvious response from the auditory sensory pathway, as in the case of profound hearing loss (Figure 6.6). This response has also been termed an N3 component by Kato et al. (1998). The SLC can also be evoked by electrical stimulation at the promontory and is similar to the acoustical response except the latency of the negative component is earlier as expected (typically 2 ms). The presence of the SLC appears to be unrelated to the conventional components of the ABR because it is present both with and without a wave V or eV component. It is believed to arise from stimulation of the vestibular system with the response arising primarily from the vestibular nuclei in the brainstem.

Middle latency response (MLR)

Components of the middle latency responses (MLR) were first reported by Geisler in 1958. They are generally accepted as

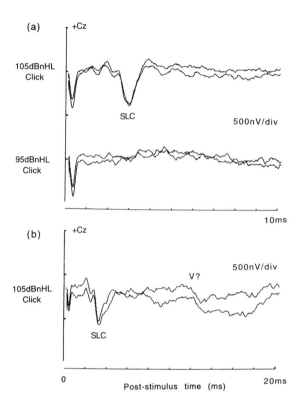

Figure 6.6. An example of the short latency component (SLC) evoked by acoustical stimulation in profound hearing loss (from Mason et al., 1996).

being neurogenic in origin but can easily become contaminated with myogenic components (Bickford et al., 1963). Many studies suggest that the MLR arises mainly from the thalamus and primary auditory cortex (Parving et al., 1980; Kraus et al., 1982). The typical MLR waveform consists of three sequential waves with peaks and troughs labelled Po, Na, Pa, Nb and Pb at latencies of 12, 20, 30, 45 and 60 ms respectively, as shown in Figure 6.7. It is recorded from a standard electrode configuration of vertex (active) and ipsilateral mastoid (reference) using a click or tone-pip stimulus. Early reports of the MLR often demonstrated a waveform having sinosoidal characteristics that were produced by using a restricted-filter bandwidth. However, with a wide-filter bandwidth the peak latencies are shortened and the waveform becomes less rounded. The slow wave V and SN10 components of the ABR, which contribute to the MLR, are then apparent.

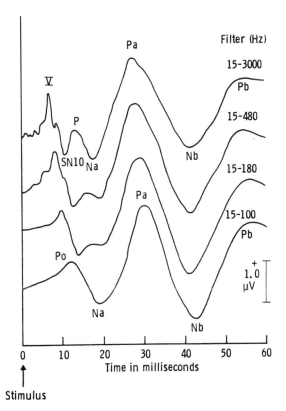

Figure 6.7. Components of the ABR and MLR evoked by a 60 dB nHL click stimulus showing the effects of different high frequency filter settings.

In awake subjects, particularly older children and adults, the MLR can be used reliably for assessment of hearing acuity. However in young children and infants it must be employed with caution because sleep and sedation significantly reduce response amplitude, particularly the Pa, Nb and Pb components (Brown, 1982; Okitsu, 1984). The MLR, in conjunction with other AEPs, can also be used as a diagnostic tool to assist with identification of the site of lesions in the auditory pathway.

Post-auricular myogenic response (PAM)

Myogenic activity can also be recorded from muscles in the body that react to sound in the middle time period (Bickford et al., 1963). The most clinically useful is the post-auricular muscle, which attempts to move the pinna in order to localize a sound. It generates the post-auricular myogenic response (PAM) first described by Kiang in 1963. This is a near-field response recorded from an electrode positioned directly over the muscle. It is a reflex response resulting from the passage of neural impulses through a reflex arc involving afferent pathways in the cochlea and brainstem and an efferent pathway in the facial nerve.

The PAM response comprises a complex waveform with five positive and negative peaks occurring between 10 ms and 24 ms. However, when recorded on the ABR waveform there is typically a positive peak at about 11 ms and a negative component at about 14 ms as shown in Figure 6.8. At high click stimulus intensities a large amplitude response can often be recorded. However, close to hearing threshold the response becomes small, variable, and more difficult to identify (Gibson, 1978). Most reduction and variability in amplitude can be related to loss of muscle tone. Some workers have recorded the

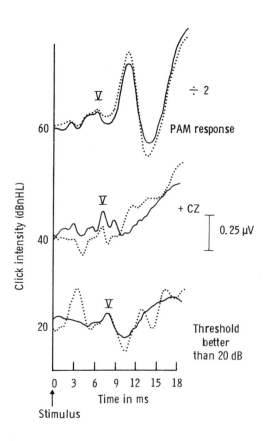

Figure 6.8. The typical configuration of the PAM response when recorded on the ABR waveform.

response from both right and left post-auricular muscles simultaneously (the crossed acoustic response) in an attempt to improve the detection of the response (Douek et al., 1975). Both muscles are often activated even if only a monaural stimulus is presented. In audiological practice the presence of a PAM response confirms a functioning cochlea and lower brainstem at the delivered stimulus intensity. However, an absent response is non-diagnostic.

Auditory cortical response (ACR)

A frequency-specific tone-burst stimulus can be employed to elicit the ACR in contrast to the earlier responses, which require a transient stimulus such as a click or tone-pip. The typical adult response, recorded from a standard electrode configuration of vertex (active) and mastoid (reference), consists of a small positive peak (P1) at approximately 50 ms post-stimulus, a large negative peak (N1) at about 100 ms and a large positive peak (P2) at around 175 ms. There is sometimes a low amplitude negative component (N2) at about 300 ms, which is inconsistent in adults but often dominates the immature response (Beagley and Kellogg, 1968), as shown in Figure 6.9. Picton et al. (1999) showed that the dominant intra-cerebral sources for the late components, including the N1 component, were in the supratemporal plane and lateral temporal lobe, in or close to primary auditory cortex. The analyses also suggested the possibility of additional sources in the frontal lobes.

Recording the ACR in young children and infants is difficult because of a problematic EEG signal baseline and a poorly defined ACR waveform (Figure 6.9), both being the result of lack of maturation of the auditory system (Davis et al., 1967). Reliable audiological application of the technique is therefore restricted to older children and adults. Even in these subjects the level of attentiveness or habituation to the stimulus can cause problems of consistency in the measurements.

Steady state AEP (SSAEP)

One of the earliest reports of the SSAEP was published by Galambos in 1981 and described the averaged waveform as the '40 Hz' response because the stimulus rate employed for the test was 40 stimuli per second. At this repetition rate there is an in-phase overlap of the ABR and MLR components during signal averaging, to produce a 40 Hz compound sinusoidal waveform.

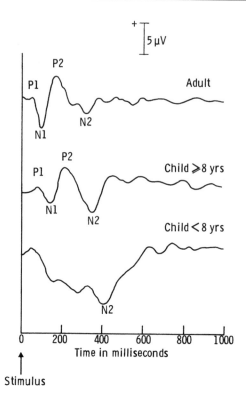

Figure 6.9. Typical effects of maturation on the ACR showing the dominance of the N2 component in children.

However, because the response is dominated by the middle latency components it is reduced in amplitude by the effects of natural sleep and sedation (Brown, 1982). For this reason the 40 Hz response never fulfilled the role as an objective measure of hearing threshold in infants.

More recently there has been a revival of interest in SSAEPs elicited by amplitude and frequency modulated tonal stimuli where modulation frequencies of 80 Hz to 100 Hz are employed (Lins et al., 1995; Aoyagi et al., 1999; Rance et al., 1998). At these modulation frequencies the response is dominated by brainstem components and is more resistant to the effects of sleep and sedation than the 40 Hz response. Data collection and analysis of the signal generated by the modulated tonal stimulus requires the measurement of an online frequency spectrum rather than conventional signal averaging. This approach to the analysis is ideal for applying automated statistical tests for assessing the presence or absence of a response. A combination of different modulation and tone frequencies into one complex stimulus may enable four or even eight thresholds to be determined simultaneously (John and Picton, 2000). This SSAEP is potentially a very attractive technique for objective audiological assessment in the routine clinic, however, some issues relating to sensitivity and reliability still need to be addressed.

ERA in the paediatric population

Children are referred for electric response audiometry (ERA) because conventional behavioural audiometric tests have failed or are unable to provide reliable or adequate information about hearing acuity. There are a number of reasons for this:

- a child may be developmentally delayed or mentally handicapped and unable to co-operate with the test procedure;
- sedation or anaesthesia may be required to achieve a satisfactory level of compliance for testing;
- reflex pathways in very young infants, typically less than five to six months of age, are simply too immature for reliable behavioural testing;
- behavioural testing is inherently difficult in some children due to lack of compliance or co-operation with the test procedure even though there may be no underlying clinical problems.

The decision of which type of AEP to implement in a young child or infant is influenced by a number of factors:

- practical aspects of the test procedure such as electrode application;
- threshold sensitivity and reliability of the response;
- the level of patient co-operation required for the test;
- effect of sleep or sedation on the response;
- maturation of the response waveform;
- information required from the test.

Auditory brainstem response

The response that addresses these factors the best overall is the ABR and this is the preferred response for objective audiological assessment in young children (Davis, 1976; Mokatoff et al.,

1977; Klein, 1983; Jacobson, 1985; Glasscock et al., 1987; Mason et al., 1988; Hall, 1992; Hood 1998). The ABR plays a major role in both newborn screening of hearing and in the early follow up of babies who fail the screening test. This role will be enhanced in the near future as we move towards screening all newborn babies: universal neonatal hearing screening (UNHS). A congenital or acquired hearing loss is a significant threat to normal development of speech and language skills and social integration.

The ABR is recorded using conventional surface scalp electrodes, in contrast to the ear canal and trans-tympanic needle electrodes required for ECochG. The wave V and SN10 components of the ABR are stable and can be recorded reliably with stimulus levels close to the threshold of hearing (Figure 6.10). These components are resilient to the effects of adaptation and habituation and are not affected significantly by

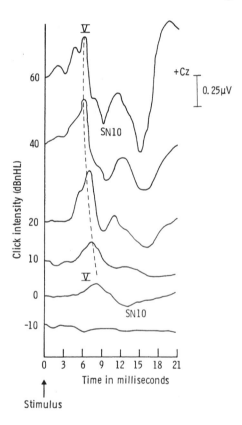

Figure 6.10. Click-evoked ABR waveforms recorded down to hearing threshold in a normally hearing child.

sleep, sedation or anaesthesia. This is in contrast to the ACR and to some extent the MLR. However, in the operating theatre it is important to be aware of possible effects of surgical intervention. Mason et al. (1995) reported temporary threshold shifts with the ABR when recorded immediately after myringotomy and aspiration of glue in young children. Although the amplitude and latency of the ABR is affected by lack of maturation of the peripheral and brainstem pathways, particularly below the age of 18 months, it can still be detected reliably in very young infants and neonates. The main disadvantage of the click-evoked ABR is its limited relationship to specific frequencies on the pure-tone audiogram, however this can be improved through the use of tone-pip stimuli (Stapells and Oates, 1997).

Role of electrocochleography

Historically, ECochG has been used extensively for assessment of hearing acuity in children (Gibson, 1978; Abramovich, 1990). However this role has now been largely superseded by the ABR. Nevertheless, ECochG is still a valuable tool for investigation of difficult and complex cases.

Assessment of older children

The MLR and ACR have the potential to provide reliable objective estimates of hearing threshold in older children (typically above eight years of age) and adults but are generally unreliable in young children (Okitsu, 1984; Stapells et al., 1988). This is the result of poorly defined response waveforms and active EEG signal baselines. Reduction and variability of response amplitude are also observed during sleep and sedation. The MLR and ACR therefore have limited application as threshold tests in young children. However, recordings of the ACR evoked by high supra-threshold levels of stimulation, when combined with the ABR, can provide valuable information to help in the differential diagnosis of cochlear and central hearing loss.

Future role of SSAEP

The SSAEP, using amplitude and frequency-modulated tonal stimuli, has the potential to be a valuable clinical tool to estimate objectively frequency-specific thresholds of hearing. The technique is currently undergoing development and investigation is taking place on research-oriented systems. Its full potential or limitations should soon be realized now that clinically oriented equipment is becoming available from the manufacturers.

ABR methodology

Equipment for ERA can be essentially divided into two strands: (1) an auditory stimulator to provide the necessary sounds to evoke the response, (2) the data collection system consisting of the headbox, signal amplifier, processor and display facilities. A schematic diagram of the set-up of this equipment is shown in Figure 6.11. The headbox (differential pre-amplifier) is the important stage of the system that interfaces the patient to the rest of the evoked potential system. It must provide a high level of electrical isolation of the patient from the mains-driven equipment and should comply with current safety standards as documented in IEC 60601 series. The whole equipment must have periodic safety inspections and electrical safety tests to check that it complies with the standards.

It is important to establish the purpose for recording the ABR in a patient. Audiological application (assessment of hearing threshold and screening for hearing loss) requires different

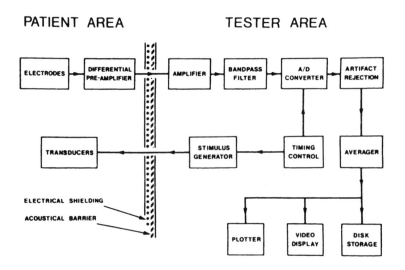

Figure 6.11. A schematic diagram of the stimulating and recording equipment for ERA (from Lightfoot et al., 2001).

stimulus and recording parameters when compared to an otoneurological investigation (detection and localization of lesions). This is illustrated in Figure 6.12. The slow components associated with wave V and the SN10 are reliable indicators of the response close to threshold, whereas the supra-threshold latencies of the faster components (waves I, III and V) provide a measure of brainstem transmission. Optimal differentiation of these two applications is affected primarily by three parameters: signal filter bandwidth, stimulus repetition rate and sweep time (Hood, 1998; Lightfoot et al., 2002) and is summarized later in this section. Recommended test protocols for recording ABR thresholds in neonates have been reported by Stevens et al. (2001b) for the click and by Mason et al. (2001a) for the tone-pip.

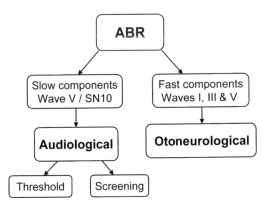

Figure 6.12. A flow diagram of applications of the ABR that necessitate appropriate stimulus parameters and data collection techniques.

The auditory stimulus

The optimum stimulus characteristics for evoking an AEP depend on the recording level of the auditory pathway. The stimulus to evoke a well-defined response from the cochlea and brainstem pathways must have a fairly fast onset (for example a click stimulus or tone-pip) so as to produce a high level of synchronization of firing of nerve fibres. A much slower stimulus (tone burst) can be used to elicit the ACR since the response represents high level cortical activity.

Characteristics

Two types of stimulus are routinely used to elicit the ABR; the click and tone-pip (Figure 6.13). The click stimulus has a fast rise time and evokes a well-defined response waveform because a large number of auditory nerve fibres are fired in close synchrony. It is generated by passing a short-duration electrical pulse (100 µs) through a headphone transducer. It can be presented as either a predominantly condensation pressure wave (+) or rarefaction wave (-), depending on the polarity of the electrical pulse presented to the transducer. In some cases the + and - click stimuli elicit small differences in amplitude and latency of the fast waveform components of the ABR. However, the slower components of the ABR are generally resistant to any polarity effects (Mason, 1985; Sininger and Masuda, 1990) and a train of stimuli with alternating polarity is usually employed for audiological application. An alternating stimulus also has the advantage of cancellation of stimulus artefact at high intensity levels during signal averaging.

The disadvantage of the click stimulus, however, is its poor frequency specificity. There is acoustical energy across a wide

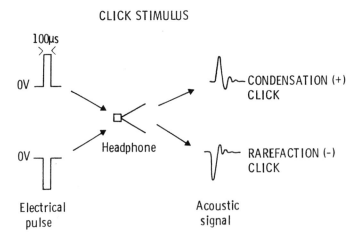

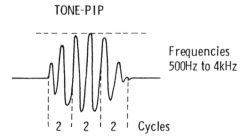

Figure 6.13. The typical click and tone-pip stimuli.

range of frequencies and the spectrum depends to a large extent on the characteristics of the headphone transducer. An improvement in the frequency specificity can be achieved using a short burst of pure tone (tone-pip) that concentrates more energy at one acoustical frequency. The typical configuration of a tone-pip is a rise and fall time of 2 cycles of the tone with a plateau of 1 or 2 cycles (Figure 6.13). However, this improvement in the frequency specificity is at the expense of loss of clarity of the ABR waveform when compared with the click stimulus, particularly for tone frequencies below 2 kHz and with stimulus levels close to threshold. This is caused primarily by the slower rise time of the tone-pip stimulus resulting in a reduction in the synchronization of firing of nerve fibres (Hawes and Greenberg, 1981).

Presentation of the stimulus

The click or tone-pip stimulus is commonly presented by air conduction techniques using either Telephonics type headphones (for example TDH39 or 49) or inserts. When using headphones only light pressure should be applied in very young babies in order to avoid collapsing of the ear canal (Hosford-Dunn et al., 1983). Bone conduction stimulation is also used to evoke the ABR (Kramer, 1992; Yang et al., 1993; Cone-Wesson, 1995) and recently there has been renewed interest in this technique as a means of identifying conductive loss, particularly in very young babies (Stevens et al., 2001a). A Radioear B71 or B70 bone vibrator can be used to present the stimulus via the mastoid. The ABR can also be evoked by a stimulus presented through a hearing aid in a deaf child (Mahoney, 1985) and this technique has been employed in the evaluation of children prior to cochlear implantation (Garnham et al., 2000a). Air and bone conduction techniques will be addressed in this chapter.

Stimulus repetition rate

Selection of the stimulus repetition rate is a compromise between a fast rate to minimize the recording time, and a slow rate to maintain the required characteristics of the response. The slow wave V and SN10 components of the ABR are very resilient to increased rates of stimulation, as shown in Figure 6.14 (Hyde et al., 1976; Mason, 1985); in contrast to the fast waves I, II and III. Typically a rate of 30 pps or more is employed

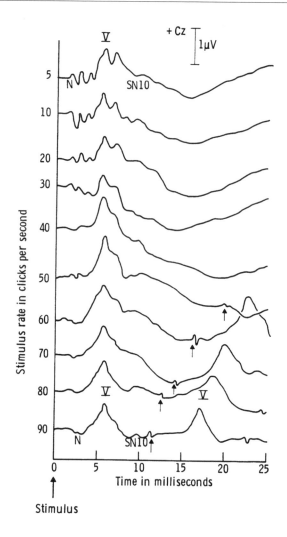

Figure 6.14. Effects of stimulus rate on the ABR waveform at a click intensity of 60 dB nHL.

for audiological application of the ABR and about 10 pps for otoneurological. An exact fraction or multiple of 50 should not be used otherwise a time-locked signal arising from the 50 Hz mains interference may be recorded.

Very high rates of stimulation (greater than 100 pps) can be employed to record the ABR using the maximum length sequence (MLS) technique (Picton et al., 1992). A psuedo-random train of stimulus and no-stimulus conditions is presented and the resultant overlapping responses are unscrambled to produce a final averaged waveform. The technique is more efficient at increasing the signal-to-noise ratio than simple signal averaging since stimuli can be presented far more rapidly. However, the level of this increase will be affected by any adaptation of the ABR due to high rate stimulation and also by adding noise to the final MLS waveform when there has been no response present (a no-stimulus condition). Application of the MLS technique has the potential to reduce test time and investigate adaptation of the neural system. In audiological application there is a need to establish the degree of sensitivity and efficiency that can be achieved with the MLS ABR compared to conventional signal averaging with stimulus levels close to hearing threshold.

Stimulus intensity and calibration: air conduction

The auditory stimulus must be accurately calibrated in terms of its characteristics (for example rise and fall time) and its intensity level. For short duration transient stimuli, such as clicks and tone-pips, the psychoacoustic threshold is raised compared to a continuous pure tone with the same sound pressure level (SPL). Temporal summation and spectral spread are the primary causes of this shift. An in-house biological calibration of the transient stimulus in at least 10 otologically and audiologically normal subjects is performed so as to establish normal hearing threshold (0 dB nHL). Sound pressure level of the biologically calibrated transient stimulus can then be compared to the SPL of a continuous pure tone using the term 'peak-to-peak equivalent sound pressure level' (ppeSPL) as described in the standard BS EN 60645-3 (1995). The equipment and technique are illustrated in Figures 6.15 and 6.16 respectively. The click has a recommended reference value of +33dBppeSPL for hearing threshold (Stevens et al., 2001b); for example a 60 dB nHL click has a ppeSPL value of 93 dB. The ppeSPL measures for tone-pip stimuli are smaller than the click because of their longer duration and are dependent on tone frequency. For example the reference ppeSPL for a 1 kHz tone pip is typically 22 dB (Mason et al., 2001a). Routine calibration of the transient stimuli can be maintained by checking the ppeSPL relationship.

Stimulus intensity and calibration: bone conduction

The temporal characteristics of the click and tone-pip stimuli for bone conduction, such as stimulus duration and rate, are similar

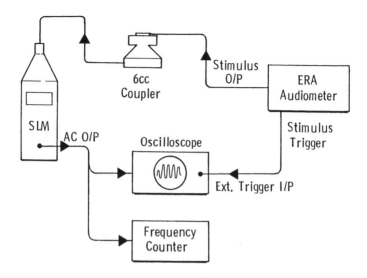

Figure 6.15. Equipment for calibration of auditory stimuli in ERA.

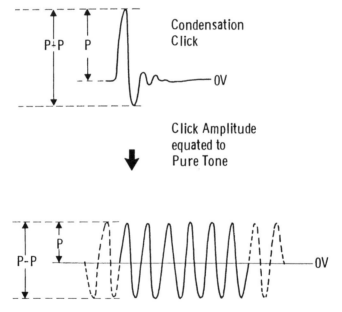

Figure 6.16. The relationship of the click to a pure tone for the purposes of calibration showing the difference between peak-to-peak and peak measurements.

to those employed for air conduction. The intensity of the bone conduction stimulus also needs calibrating in a similar way to air conduction using an in-house study of normally hearing adult subjects. In this way a reference level of force that relates to normal hearing threshold (dB nHL) can be established. However, there is an increase in the effective intensity of this stimulus in young infants when compared to adults and a correction factor needs to be applied as described by Stevens et al. (2001a). For example, a 30 dB nHL stimulus as biologically calibrated in adults would be equivalent to 40 dB nHL in a full term newborn baby, a correction factor of 10 dB.

Contralateral masking

The possibility of crossover of the test stimulus to the non-test ear exists in ERA as it does in behavioural audiometry. In patients with a profound unilateral hearing loss, delayed but repeatable click-evoked ABR waveforms have been observed from stimulation of the deaf ear, which were subsequently absent when masking was presented to the non-test normal ear (Chiappi et al., 1979). Inter-aural attenuation for the air-conducted click is typically 50 dB (Reid and Thornton, 1983) and therefore contralateral masking of the non-test ear should be employed when there is 50 dB or more difference in hearing loss between the test ear and the bone conduction thresholds across 2000 Hz to 4000 Hz in the non-test ear. Using bone conduction stimulation there is evidence of an inter-aural attenuation of 20 dB in young babies (Stevens et al., 2001a), probably the result of lack of skull growth and fusion. However, this reduces significantly in older children and adults. A white noise masking sound is usually employed for the click stimulus and a narrow-band noise for the tone-pip centred at the tone frequency.

Reliable behavioural thresholds are generally not available in children referred for ERA so there is a dilemma about the application of masking. There are two schools of thought: either use it for all investigations or just when the evoked response thresholds on each ear differ by 50 dB or more. There are also the practical aspects of presentation of the masker to consider. There is a risk of disturbing a sleeping baby when positioning the transducer on the non-test ear. Typically, contralateral masking is presented at about 30 dB down on the test stimulus in order to reduce the risk of any over-masking. The level of masking is directly related to the intensity of the test stimulus, so that any adjustment of the stimulus must be accompanied by a similar change in the masking level.

Data collection

The auditory evoked potential (AEP) is measured as the difference in a signal recorded from a pair of surface scalp electrodes using a differential amplifier (the pre-amplifier headbox). One electrode is positioned over an area of high response activity (active) and a second electrode over an area of low response activity (reference). When the active electrode is positioned close to the site of generation of the response, this is termed a near-field recording whereas an active electrode that is sited some distance away is often called far field. The ABR is a far-field recording of brainstem activity. All AEPs are invariably small when compared to the background electrical noise, a repetitive stimulus is required so that the response-to-noise amplitude ratio can be improved using signal averaging. The following data collection techniques for the audiological ABR are very similar for both air and bone conduction stimuli using either the clicks or tone-pips.

Recording electrodes

There are a number of different types of electrode for recording the ABR from the surface of the scalp but the following two are most commonly used: silver/silver chloride discs (available in either disposable or reusable forms) or disposable pre-gelled tab electrodes. There is significant advantage in using disposable electrodes in order to avoid the need for cleaning and sterilization.

The single, most common source of problem associated with ERA is electrode application. Low and balanced contact impedance (<5 kΩ) are essential for optimum performance of the pre-amplifier. The standard procedure to achieve this is:

- thoroughly clean the skin with surgical spirit;
- use a skin-preparation gel to reduce contact impedance;
- securely attach the electrodes with the recommended procedure depending on the type of electrode;
- apply conductive electrode jelly as required.

It is important to remember that skin preparation gels are not conductive and must be removed before application of the electrode. Conductive electrode jelly provides a low impedance bridge between the electrode and the scalp. In very young babies and neonates particular care should be taken concerning application of the electrodes. Some types of skin preparation gel are fairly harsh and must be used cautiously in order to avoid flaring the skin. The use of collodion glue and blunted-ended needles for application of disc electrodes is not recommended in very young babies.

Electrode configuration

An active electrode is positioned at the vertex of the scalp (or high forehead) where there is a high level of response activity (wave V and SN10) and a reference electrode on either the ipsilateral earlobe or mastoid (or nape) where there is low response activity, as shown in Figure 6.17. A third electrode, the earth or guard, is required for proper functioning of the amplifier and is often positioned on the forehead or contralateral mastoid. A high forehead electrode (active site) which is outside the hairline is particularly convenient in young children and infants and also avoids the fontanelle area in very young babies. There is only a small reduction in response amplitude at a high forehead site (18%) when compared to the vertex (Mason, 1985).

In ABR recordings the reference electrode site (ipsilateral mastoid or earlobe) is not completely inactive and records the early waves I and II, and to some extent wave III. This is generally the prefered reference site for many clinics. The

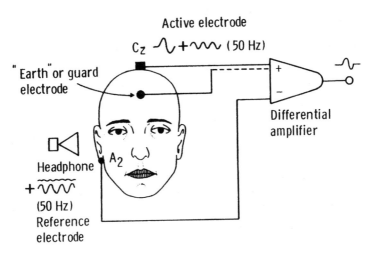

Figure 6.17. The standard electrode configuration for recording the ABR and connection to the pre-amplifier.

general configuration of the ABR waveform is affected using a nape or contralateral mastoid/earlobe reference.

Pre-amplifier headbox

The function of the pre-amplifier in the headbox is to detect small differences in signals across the recording electrodes (active and reference) whilst rejecting interference that is common to all its inputs (for example 50 Hz mains). Other important operating characteristics are a low level of amplifier noise and a high input impedance. The headbox is positioned close to the patient so that the length of the electrode lead does not exceed about one metre in length. It is at this stage, before amplification, that the signal is easily contaminated with interference. Normally the active electrode is connected to the 'positive' or red input of the headbox, reference to 'negative' or black input, and the third electrode to the 'common/ground' or green input. This configuration will normally result in wave V being displayed as a positive going wave, which is the convention used throughout this chapter. However, some clinics prefer to display wave V as negative going which can be achieved by simply reversing the electrode leads in the 'positive' and 'negative' inputs of the pre-amplifier.

Signal amplification and filtering

Amplitude of the ABR is typically in the range 0.1 µV to 1 µV and is often superimposed on a background signal (EEG and noise) of between 20 µV to 50 µV. An amplifier gain of around 100,000 (sometimes described as sensitivity in units of µV per display division) is required in order to bring the overall amplitude up to a few volts which is typical of the input range of the analogue-to-digital converter in the signal processor. When adjusting the gain it is important to remember that in some ERA systems the level of amplitude artefact rejection is determined by the gain of the amplifier.

The signal from the patient will contain a wide spectrum of frequencies relating to the ABR waveform, EEG activity, and noise. Filtering is therefore required in order to exclude signals that have frequency components outside the lower and upper limits of the spectrum of the ABR. This has the effect of improving the response-to-noise amplitude ratio. In most ERA equipment this is an analogue filter where a low and high cut-off frequency can be specified for the filter bandwidth. The cut-off frequency is usually the point at which the signal is attenuated by 3 dB, and the rate of attenuation outside the pass-band is typically in the range of 12 dB to 24 dB per octave. Some systems have digital filtering available which eliminates problems of phase distortion and better attenuation outside the pass-band. However, this type of filtering can often only be applied off-line after the ABR has been recorded.

For audiological application of the ABR using either clicks or tone-pips it is important to record the slow components of the ABR associated with wave V and SN10 (Yamada et al., 1983). To achieve this a low cut-off frequency in the range 20 Hz to 50 Hz must be employed in contrast to 100 Hz for otoneurological investigation as shown in Figure 6.18. The optimum low cut-off frequency is dependent on the attenuation slope (dB/octave) of the filters in the amplifier. A 20 Hz cut-off is optimum with a fairly steep filter slope of 36 dB/octave (Mason, 1984a) whereas 30 Hz or 50 Hz is more suited to a shallower filter slope (12 dB/octave). If the cut-off frequency is too low then large amounts of slow EEG activity can contaminate the signal

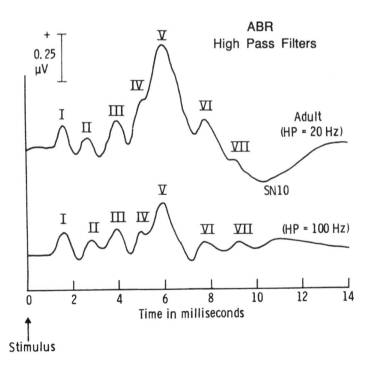

Figure 6.18. A comparison of click-evoked ABR waveforms recorded for audio-logical (HP = 20 Hz) and otoneurological (HP = 100 Hz) application.

baseline. The high cut-off frequency is less critical and 1 kHz or 3 kHz is typical (Davis and Hirsh, 1976; Klein 1983). High-frequency noise on the averaged waveform can also be removed to some extent using a three or five-point smoothing routine, which is available on most ERA systems.

Artefact rejection

Large fluctuations of the online signal baseline, arising from movement, myogenic activity and excessive EEG activity, can be excluded from the signal average using amplitude artefact rejection. If the amplitude of a sweep of incoming signal exceeds a pre-determined level it is excluded thereby avoiding contamination of the averaged waveform. The rejection level is chosen so as to allow through all normal baseline signals but to reject high levels of activity. For the ABR this is typically in the range ±10 μV to ±5 μV when referred to the input signal. In an active child the signal may frequently exceed ±25 μV. If the number of rejected sweeps exceeds about 50% of those collected then it may be necessary to discontinue testing. The artefact rejection must not be increased to overcome rejection of the signals. The quality of the collected sweeps (averaged waveform) in this situation will be poor. In a sedated or sleeping child the signal may be less than ±10 μV resulting in very few rejected sweeps.

Analysis window

The period of time for which the signal is recorded is termed the analysis window, sweep time or epoch. An analysis window of 18 ms to 25 ms is required for audiological application of the ABR. The upper limit of 25 ms will keep the slow SN10 component of the waveform well within the window particularly when using low frequency tone-pips with stimulus levels close to threshold. This contrasts with the otoneurological ABR where a time window of 12 ms is typical.

Signal averaging

The primary technique for detection of the ABR response amongst the background noise is signal averaging. This technique relies on the evoked potential being synchronised to the stimulus whereas the noise is randomly distributed. Individual sweeps of the signal are averaged which results in enhancement of the response relative to the background noise. Theoretically, the response-to-noise amplitude (R/N) ratio is improved by a factor equal to the square root of the number of sweeps taken into the average. However, this increase in R/N ratio will only be strictly adhered to if there is an invariant response and normally distributed random noise. In most situations for the ABR these assumptions are sufficiently satisfied. One notable exception, however, is when the stimulus rate accidentally locks onto some residual interference, such as the 50 Hz mains. For this reason exact multiples or fractions of 50 Hz for the stimulus rate should not be used.

In theory it is possible to infinitely improve the R/N ratio by acquiring more and more sweeps. However, the most efficient increase is in the early stage of the averaging process due to the square root of N relationship and there is a trade-off between the time taken to acquire the averaged waveform and the relative improvement in the response-to-noise ratio. This is often referred to as the law of diminishing returns. With the ABR it is common practice to record 2,000 sweeps because this will enable identification of a close-to-threshold response under most test conditions. However, if the signal baseline is fairly active or amplitude of the response is very small then the number of sweeps can be increased. It is not advisable to exceed 4,000 sweeps in a single averaged waveform as the signal-averaging process becomes inefficient at this stage. In a sedated or sleeping child it may be possible to stop the average at 1,000 or 1,500 sweeps when a well-defined response is present. However, caution is advised if the averaging process is stopped early because of the risk of interpreting residual noise on the averaged waveform as a genuine response.

Audiological versus otoneurological application

Optimization of the ABR for audiological or otoneurological application involves primarily the selection of different values for three test parameters as summarized in Table 6.1.

Recording environment

Careful consideration must be given to the site of the test room in the clinic in order to provide low levels of background electrical interference and acoustical noise. It is necessary to sound treat the room or to install a soundproof enclosure to the

Table 6.1. Optimization of ABR test parameters for audiological and otoneurological application.

	Audiological	Otoneurological
Amplifier filter bandwidth	20 Hz or 30 Hz to 1 kHz or 3 kHz	100 Hz to 3 kHz (or 5 kHz)
Sweep time	18 ms to 25 ms	10 to 15 ms
Stimulus repetition rate	31 pps to 49 pps	11 pps

same standard as for conventional audiological investigations. When a child is sedated or anaesthetized on the ward or in the operating theatre, higher levels of interference and noise may have to be addressed. It essential to keep levels of noise to a minimum through co-operation of local staff. Ideally use a quiet side room for tests performed on the ward.

In a hospital environment there are many sources of electrical interference particularly related to the 50 Hz mains arising from transformers, wiring, fluorescent lights, and adjacent plant machinery such as lifts. Hospital 'bleep' systems can also introduce significant levels of high-frequency interference. In order to reduce the problems of electrical interference care should be taken regarding the siting of the clinic. Tungsten filament lights should be used rather than fluorescent tubes, and a filtered mains supply for the clinic taken as a spur off the ring main is preferable. Good attachment of the recording electrodes, with low and balanced contact impedances, will significantly improve the performance of the pre-amplifier in rejecting this interference.

Interpretation of the ABR

Reliable identification of a true response in the averaged waveform can be a challenging task in ERA and highly dependent on the quality of the recording conditions. When reporting the results of ERA careful attention should therefore be paid to the level of reliability that can be attached to the interpretation.

Data collection procedures

Reliability can be improved by adopting appropriate recording procedures. Two or more averaged waveforms recorded with the same stimulus intensity (Figure 6.19) will check the reproducibility of the response waveform and will help to identify random noise components. This replication process is essential in ERA – even more so when attempting to identify small mid- to low-frequency tone-pip responses. Addition and subtraction of two averaged waveforms may help further in the differential identification of residual noise and true response components. Although two averaged waveforms can be recorded sequentially, an alternative technique is to record them almost simultaneously by averaging the odd and even numbered individual sweeps separately (Mason, 1985).

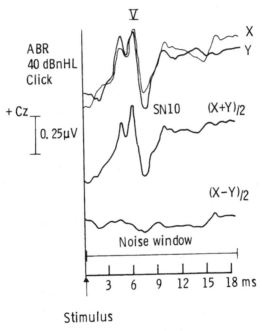

Figure 6.19. Replication of the averaged ABR recording to assist with the differentiation of true response from residual noise.

Waveform scores

Scoring waveforms for the presence or absence of a response is an interactive process that should be carried out during ERA by an experienced tester. In threshold measurements the result of the interpretation at one stimulus intensity will influence the choice of the stimulus for the next run, and so on. From the point of view of efficiency and reliability it is valuable to have in mind specific decision categories. For example in Nottingham we have four waveform scores:

- definite response present (++);
- possible response present (+);
- no response (−);
- unreliable recordings (?).

Threshold protocol

A time-efficient ERA test requires the minimum number of averaged waveforms, at both supra-threshold and sub-threshold stimulus intensity, in order to accurately determine the threshold of the ABR. A protocol that controls the order at which runs at different stimulus intensities are presented to the child will help to achieve this (Mason, 1984b). The following protocol is used in Nottingham.

The stimulus intensity for the first run of a threshold is set at 40, 30 or 20 dB above the suspected hearing threshold, depending on the degree of hearing loss. For example, +40 dB for suspected thresholds of better than 40 dB HL, +30 dB for hearing loss up to 50 dB HL, and +20 dB for a loss of 60 dB HL or more. It is advisable not to exceed 80 dB nHL or possibly 90 dB nHL for the first stimulus run at the risk of disturbing a young child or baby. High intensity stimuli should be used cautiously throughout the investigation in order minimize discomfort, particularly if a recruiting-type cochlear loss is suspected.

The order of stimulus intensities for subsequent runs is then dependent upon previous waveform scores. In general the stimulus intensity is decreased by 20 dB after a ++ score, 10 dB after a + score, and increased by 20 dB following a − score. These changes are then modified close to threshold until a clear no response and positive response are observed across a 10 dB interval, as shown in the stimulus sequences in Figure 6.20. In routine ERA, there is usually insufficient time to record at intensity intervals of 5 dB and therefore an interpolation procedure needs to be adopted to estimate the threshold to the nearest 5 dB. If the waveform score immediately above the response threshold is a + score the threshold is positioned at that stimulus level, whereas a ++ score gives a threshold which is 5 dB better (Figure 6.20). In routine ERA investigations a ++ response at 20 dB nHL is usually acceptable to define normal hearing without proceeding to lower stimulus levels.

Observer scoring of the waveforms and interpretation of response threshold is greatly assisted by displaying the averaged waveforms in order of descending stimulus intensity. This

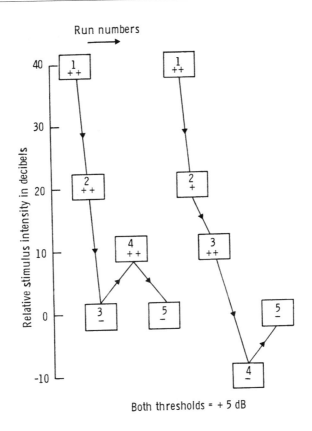

Figure 6.20. Two typical sequences of stimulus runs and subsequent waveform scores in order to define the threshold of the response.

enables identification of the characteristic changes in amplitude and latency of the response as threshold is approached. These changes are known as the input/output functions of the response and are discussed in more detail later.

Accuracy of the threshold

A high percentage (>90%) of click-evoked ABR thresholds should be within 10 dB of the behavioural threshold with good recording conditions. In a study of 25 normally hearing adults (Mason 1985), 92% of the click-evoked ABR thresholds were within 10 dB of the behavioural click threshold. The recording conditions in that study of adults were equivalent to a child sitting quietly for the test. It might be expected that in a sleeping or sedated child the agreement would be higher.

The ABR evoked by tone-pip stimuli is not as well defined and as easy to identify as the click ABR, particularly for mid to low tones. Nevertheless, it is reported that more than 90% of tone-pip ABR thresholds are within 20 dB of the pure-tone behavioural threshold, and a high proportion within 10 dB, as reviewed by Stapells and Oates (1997). They also reported that the accuracy in estimating pure-tone behavioural thresholds appears even better for the hearing impaired population versus subjects with normal hearing. This is probably the result of the effects on the ABR characteristics of a recruiting type cochlear hearing loss.

Effects of maturation

The ABR is affected systematically by a complex process of maturation of the peripheral and brainstem pathways (Eggermont and Stein, 1996). Typical click-evoked ABR waveforms and wave V latency changes in the neonate are shown in Figures 6.21 and 6.22 respectively. There are maturational effects in both the conductive mechanism and the neural pathways,

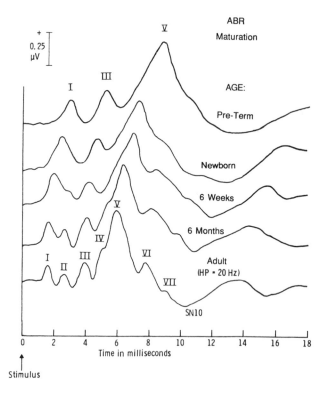

Figure 6.21. Effects of maturation on the amplitude and latency of the ABR waveform.

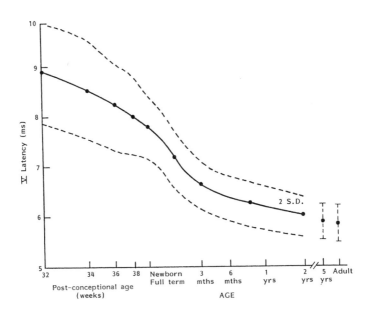

Figure 6.22. The relationship between wave V latency and age for a 60 dB nHL click stimulus.

whereas many aspects of cochlear function are fully developed at birth (Sininger and Abdala, 1996; Moore et al., 1996). Both axons and synapses are likely to be involved in this process of maturation with the level of myelination of nerve fibres playing an important role.

Waves I, III and V are most apparent at birth and these components are delayed and broadened. The waveform begins to resemble the adult response by the age of 18 months with waves II, IV, VI and VII becoming identifiable (Salamy and McKean, 1976). There is a progressive decrease in the latencies and inter-peak latencies of waves I, III and V with maturation. Hawes and Greenberg (1981) reported that the latency of the SN10 component in newborns was about 12.5 ms, compared with 10 ms in adults. The ABR can be recorded at birth in both normal newborns and pre-term babies but the threshold of the response is elevated when compared to normal adult responses. Sininger and Abdala (1996) showed an elevation in threshold of between 5 dB and 25 dB. The largest elevation, and hence lack of maturity, was recorded with high-frequency stimuli, such as the click. Since there is maturational effect on response threshold it is advisable to avoid very early assessment of hearing thresholds with the ABR. The follow-up of neonates referred from screening tests of hearing is usually performed at a corrected age of 4 to 6 weeks so that consistently reliable thresholds of better than 20 dB nHL can be achieved in normally hearing infants.

Measurement of the ABR: input / output functions

The peak-to-trough deflection on the waveform is usually recorded as the amplitude of wave V, as shown in Figure 6.23. Latency of wave V represents the time from onset of the stimulus to the peak of the component. Typical amplitude and latency input/output (I/O) functions for wave V of the click-evoked ABR in normally hearing infants and young children, showing the effects of maturation, are presented in Figures 6.24a and 6.24b. In general there is a reduction in response amplitude and increase in latency with reduced stimulus intensity. The rate of this change is dependent on the relative level of the stimulus intensity; rapid increase in wave V latency is observed close to threshold in normal hearing. Changes in these characteristics can sometimes assist with the differential diagnosis of conductive and recruiting type cochlear loss as discussed later.

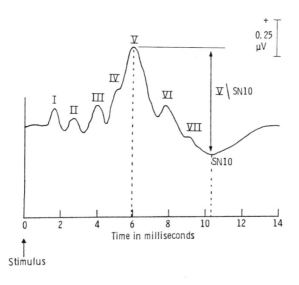

Figure 6.23. Measurement of the amplitude and latency of the wave V and SN10 components of the ABR.

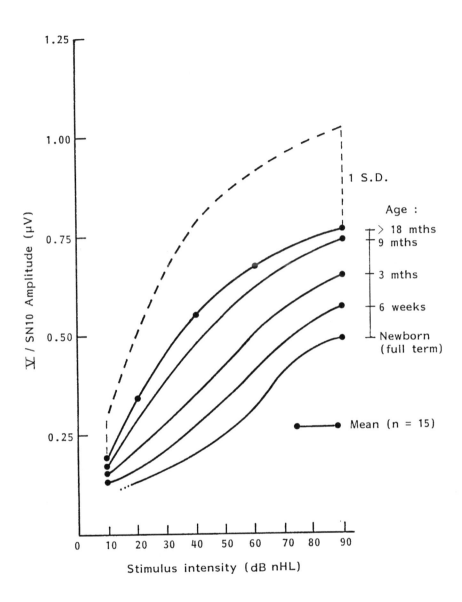

Figure 6.24a. Input/output (I/O) functions of the amplitude for wave V of the click-evoked ABR showing the effects of maturation.

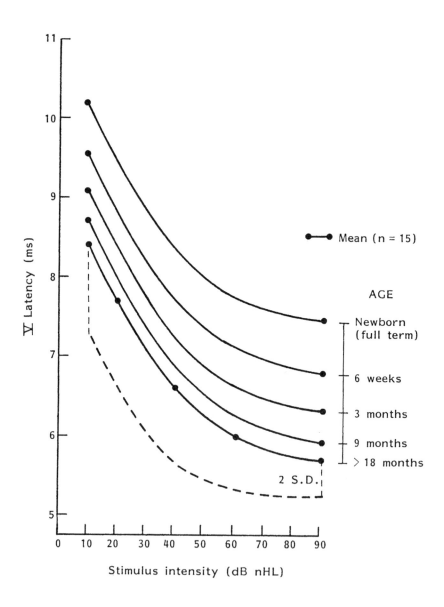

Figure 6.24b. Input/output (I/O) functions of the latency for wave V of the click-evoked ABR showing the effects of maturation.

Frequency specificity

The relationship of the ABR threshold to behavioural audiometric frequencies is very important when the technique is to be used to objectively predict hearing thresholds. Click stimuli, by their very nature, have limited frequency specificity. The use of tone-pips go some way towards improving this relationship but at the expense of clarity of the response waveform. Frequency specificity of the ABR is dependent on the characteristics of the auditory stimulus and the subsequent generation of the response by the cochlea. Since the ABR is evoked predominantly by the onset of the stimulus rather than by the continuation of it, the rise time of the stimulus is an important characteristic. A slower rise time results in better stimulus frequency specificity but results in loss of synchronization of firing of auditory nerve fibres and hence degradation of the response waveform.

Click-evoked ABR

The click generates maximal response activity from the basal, high-frequency turn of the cochlea and the resultant ABR threshold generally correlates with behavioural hearing across 2 kHz to 4 kHz (Coats and Martin, 1977; van der Drift et al., 1987). Figure 6.25 shows an approximate representation of the frequency specificity of the click-evoked ABR on the behavioural pure-tone audiogram. Since there is a spread of energy outside the 2 kHz to 4 kHz region, this may result in activation of

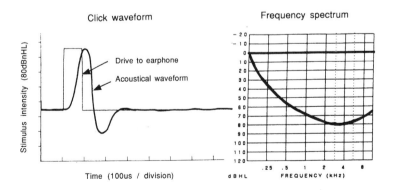

Figure 6.25. The frequency spectrum of the click stimulus represented schematically on the pure-tone audiogram graph (from Lightfoot et al., 2002).

neuronal activity from these higher and lower frequencies of hearing. This is more likely to occur with high levels of stimulation and when there is sloping loss on the PTA, as discussed later.

Tone-pip ABR

An improvement in frequency specificity of the ABR threshold can be achieved using a tone-pip stimulus that concentrates more energy at the tone frequency, as shown in Figure 6.26. The configuration of the frequency spectrum depends on the characteristics of the tone-pip (rise/ fall time, plateau and tone frequency). Typical configurations of the tone-pip ABR waveforms at tone frequencies of 1 kHz and 4 kHz are shown in Figures 6.27a and 6.27b respectively. The slower components dominate the response waveform particularly at mid- to low-tone frequencies (for example at 500 Hz and 1 kHz) and at intensity levels close to threshold. The response is smaller and much broader when compared to the click-evoked ABR. The latency of wave V becomes longer with lower tone-pip frequencies. This change in latency is the result of a slower rise time of the auditory stimulus with lower frequency tones and the time taken by the travelling wave to reach the more apical regions of the cochlea. Reliable interpretation of tone-pip ABR requires knowledge of these waveform characteristics, which in practice are different to those experienced with the click-evoked ABR.

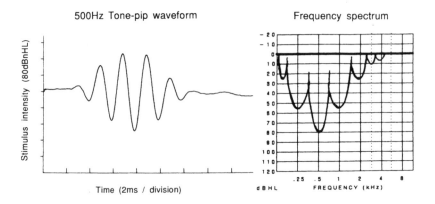

Figure 6.26. The frequency spectrum of a 500 Hz tone-pip stimulus represented schematically on the pure-tone audiogram graph. A pip with higher tone frequency and/or slower time characteristics would have less spread of energy across the PTA (from Lightfoot et al., 2002).

(a)

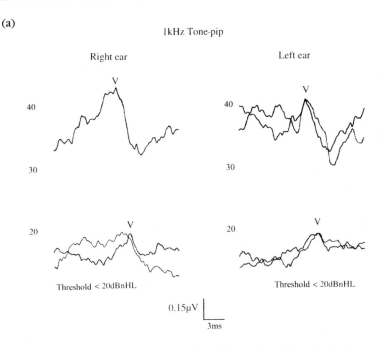

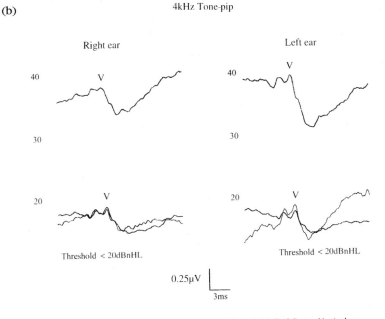

Figure 6.27. Typical configuration of the tone-pip ABR waveform in a young child for tone frequencies of (a) 1 kHz and (b) 4 kHz.

Tone-pip ABR with ipsilateral masking

There is still a spread in frequency content with the tone-pip and the resultant travelling wave in the cochlea. High intensity, low-frequency tone-pips evoke an ABR that is probably mediated to some extent by the high-frequency region of the cochlea. This spread of energy away from the nominal frequency of the tone-pip tends to become sub-threshold as the stimulus intensity is decreased, resulting in better frequency specificity towards threshold, particularly in normal hearing. Studies by Klein (1983) and Folsom (1984) suggest that good frequency specificity of the ABR can be achieved when the intensity of the tone-pip is less than about 60 dB nHL at tone frequencies of 1 kHz and above.

Presentation of ipsilateral masking noise, simultaneously with the stimulus, will help to prevent the spread of excitation in the cochlea (Picton et al., 1979; Fjermedal and Laukli, 1989, Stapells and Oates, 1997). Two types of masking noise can be used: high frequency and notched noise. High frequency (or high pass) noise will selectively mask the response from high-frequency fibres. The cut-off frequency of the high pass filter is adjusted to be just above the frequency of the tone-pip. Notched noise is a masker where a narrow-band of frequencies has been stopped or rejected from a broad-band noise. Theoretically this allows response from the tone-pip, which is matched to the frequency of the notch, but activity at frequencies outside the notch are masked.

The choice of which type of masking to use needs to be debated and to some extent depends on the tone frequency of the stimulus. Responses to low-frequency tone-pips are probably best recorded with high-frequency masking because there is minimal spread of masking into the lower frequency region of the cochlea in contrast to notched noise. For high-frequency tone-pip responses the optimal type of masker is notched noise. Although low-frequency noise might at first appear the best choice, the specificity of this type of masker is poor because of spread of energy into the high frequency, basal end of the cochlea.

Some workers recommend the use of tone-pips with notched noise (Picton et al., 1979; Stapells and Oates, 1997) whereas others consider that tone-pips without masking are acceptable for routine ERA (Davis et al., 1985). There is no doubt that the use of tone-pip represents a significant improvement in frequency specificity over the click stimulus, with or without ipsilateral masking. However, the move from click to tone-pip ABR measurements is at the expense of ease of application of the technique. The tone-pip ABR is generally smaller and broader than the click response. It requires very good recording conditions and often more replications of individual runs in order to achieve reliable identification. This obviously extends the time that is required for a child to be in a quiet state for testing. This may result in the need for wider application of sedation in order for a child to be in a suitable state for testing.

Application in the routine clinic

Test conditions

Reliable measurement of the ABR requires good recording conditions. A quiet, good-quality signal baseline is achieved when a child is asleep. This will minimize noise on the signal baseline arising from myogenic activity and movement artefacts. A co-operative, awake child might sit in a comfortable chair or lie on a couch for the test, and a younger child or infant may sit still on a parent's lap, or be cradled. In this situation it is possible to achieve acceptable recording conditions, particularly when using click or high frequency tone-pip stimuli.

Infants should be disturbed as little as possible when they arrive in the clinic. If they are asleep in a pram or pushchair on arrival then attempts should be made to carry out the test without moving them. However, in some children it will not be possible to achieve reliable recording conditions without the use of sedation or even general anaesthesia. It is valuable to establish with other professionals how co-operative a child might be and liaise with the parents regarding the requirements for the test – for example, to try to keep young children or infants awake prior to the test so that they fall asleep soon after arrival in the clinic.

The frequency of use of sedation in the routine ERA clinic varies considerably between different centres. Some centres use sedation and even a general anaesthetic for all young children whereas others are more selective. The age range of one to three years is the most difficult period. In Nottingham, children are selected as to whether they are likely to require sedation and typically 75% of children in this age range are sedated. Infants up to 12 months of age are not sedated without special guidance from the paediatrician or anaesthetist. We use trimeprazine (Vallergan Forte) with an oral dose of 3 mg/kg body weight together with Droperidol, 0.2 mg/kg body weight. Chloral hydrate is one of a number of alternative sedatives. The sedation is administered on the ENT ward and the ERA test is carried out in a quiet side room on the ward when the child is asleep. Usually the child is admitted to the ward the day before the test and is given the sedative the following morning. In our experience the overnight stay makes the child more receptive for sleeping during the test compared to admission on the same day. Usually children recover sufficiently to be allowed home by around mid-afternoon. A general anaesthetic, normally administered in the operating theatre, is an alternative choice to sedation. In some centres it may be the preferred procedure but is more widely employed for children in whom sedation has been problematic.

When reporting the results of ERA it is important to document the level of reliability that can be attached to interpretation of the waveforms and hence the estimation of response threshold. The ABR evoked by click and high-frequency tone-pips (2 kHz to 4 kHz) is more clearly defined than mid- to low-frequency stimuli (such as 500 Hz and 1 kHz). A signal baseline that is satisfactory for high-frequency stimuli may still be too active to record a reliable low-frequency tone-pip ABR. This information needs to be included in the report.

Interpretation of hearing loss

Conductive hearing loss

The external and middle ear comprise the conductive mechanism. Developmental and pathological conditions of the external and middle ears can interrupt the efficiency of the transfer of sounds into the inner ear and impair the generation of an evoked potential. Audiometrically a conductive loss is characterized by elevated thresholds for air-conducted sounds and relatively normal bone conduction thresholds. A conductive loss can be investigated objectively by recording the ABR to both air and bone conduction stimuli and from examination of the input/output functions of the air-conducted ABR. Tympanometry at the time of ERA will also provide valuable information about the status of the middle ear. In infants younger than about three or four months of age, it is important to employ a high frequency probe tone in order to achieve reliable interpretation (Sutton et al., 2001).

The effect of conductive pathology on the air-conducted ABR is to prolong the latencies of all components of the ABR, including wave V (Hecox and Galambos, 1974). This results in the latency input/output (I/O) function for the wave V being shifted from the normal curve by an amount equivalent to the level of conductive hearing loss but maintains the same profile, as shown in Figure 6.28. Although the amount of this shift is an approximate indication of the level of hearing loss (Fria and Sabo, 1980), the most accurate assessment is derived from measure of response threshold (Eggermont, 1982). The amplitude I/O function for wave V/SN10 shows a similar characteristic shift.

The most prevalent middle-ear disorder in young children is otitis media and results from inflammation of the mucoperiosteal lining in the middle ear. The build-up of fluid and thicker glue initially causes an audiometric configuration

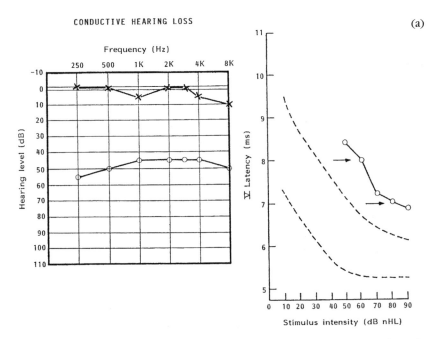

Figure 6.28. An example of the I/O functions of wave V latency (a) and amplitude (b) with the click-evoked ABR in conductive hearing loss. The dashed lines indicate the upper and lower limits in normal hearing (+/- 2SD).

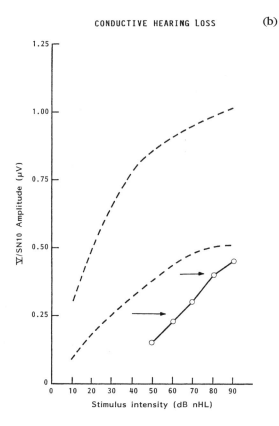

Figure 6.28. (contd).

which has increased hearing loss at lower frequencies but this subsequently develops into a flat loss as the fluid increases and thickens. In many cases of acute and chronic otitis media the threshold of the click-evoked ABR can be raised by 30 dB or more because frequencies of 2 kHz to 4 kHz are affected to some extent. However, a lower frequency tone-pip stimulus, typically 1 kHz, can help define the slope of the loss. A conductive hearing loss at 1 kHz can easily approach levels of 40 db HL to 50 dB HL.

Bone conduction ABR

Bone-conducted stimuli can be used to evoke an ABR (Schwartz and Berry, 1985) and a recommended test protocol has been reported by Stevens et al. (2001a). The technique is a valuable tool in the differential diagnosis of conductive and sensorineural hearing loss, particularly in patients with a severe mixed hearing loss or in complex cases of external and middle ear malformations. A comparison of the air- and bone-conducted ABR in a young child with conductive hearing loss is shown in Figure 6.29. Although variability in the characteristics of the response, particularly latency measurements have been reported (Finitzo-Hieber and Friel-Patti, 1985) the technique is reliable and consistent for clinical application. The air-conducted ABR is employed first for assessment of hearing acuity with the bone conduction stimulus available for cases of suspected conductive loss.

Cochlear hearing loss

Malformation or damage to the delicate hair cell structures in the cochlea will result in a cochlear hearing loss. The intensity and frequency characteristics of the loss will depend on the degree of damage and its position along the basilar membrane. The shape of the PTA varies widely, although most commonly the hearing loss is relatively flat across all frequencies or more pronounced at high frequencies. The characteristics of the ABR will depend on the level and frequency pattern of this hearing loss.

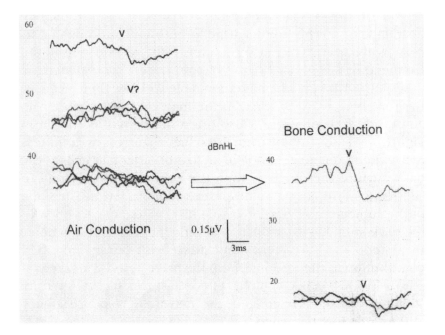

Figure 6.29. An example of recordings of air and bone conduction ABR in a young child with conductive hearing loss.

The effect of cochlear hearing loss on the ABR waveform is more complex than for a conductive loss. In many flat cochlear losses, the threshold latency of the click-evoked ABR waveform is shorter than that observed in normal hearing as shown in Figure 6.30, whereas in a conductive hearing loss the threshold latencies are similar (Hyde, 1985). The latency I/O functions often lie within the normal range but have a different profile to the normal curve. At high stimulus intensity the latency of wave V is similar to that in normals but may become delayed as threshold is approached. There is also often a rapid decrease in response amplitude associated with. These features in the response are consistent with a compression of the range of loudness often observed in cochlear hearing loss (loudness recruitment) which arises predominantly from a selective loss of outer hair cells in the cochlea. The sharp tips of the tuning curves of the auditory nerve fibres at low stimulus levels are lost and this results in a rapid increase in the number of fibres activated as the stimulus level increases above the raised threshold of the fibres.

In high-frequency cochlear hearing loss the patterns of the I/O functions to a click stimulus will depend on the active region of the basilar membrane. A severe high-frequency hearing loss, arising from damage to both inner and outer hair cells, will suppress any contribution to the response from the basal end of the cochlea. This will introduce a general increase in response latency, which is compatible with the time taken for the travelling wave to traverse the inactive basal region. The amplitude I/O function is also often depressed as shown in Figure 6.31. If the hearing loss has features of loudness recruitment, due to a predominant loss of outer hair cells at the basal turn of the cochlea, then the latency will still tend to shorten towards normal values at high stimulus levels. The slope of the audiogram across 2 kHz to 4 kHz, where excitation with the click stimulus is maximal, will influence the I/O functions. In a steep, high-frequency loss there will be an increased contribution to the response from the more apical 2 kHz region with a low-level click stimulus in contrast to a higher intensity stimulus. This tends to enhance the increase in response latency as threshold is approached.

The configuration of the I/O functions can assist in the differential diagnosis of a conductive and cochlear hearing loss in addition to the bone conduction ABR and tympanometry.

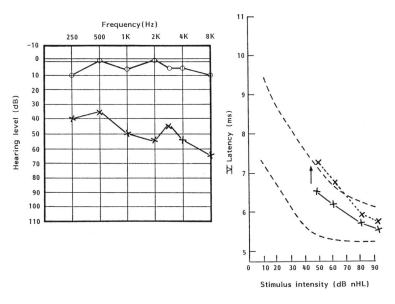

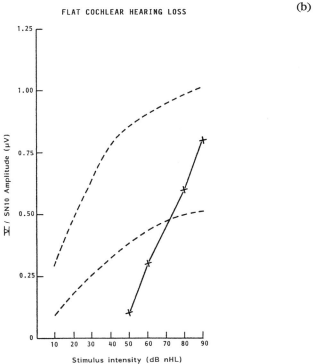

Figure 6.30. An example of the I/O functions of wave V latency (a) and amplitude (b) with the click-evoked ABR in flat cochlear hearing loss. The dashed lines indicate the upper and lower limits in normal hearing (+/- 2SD).

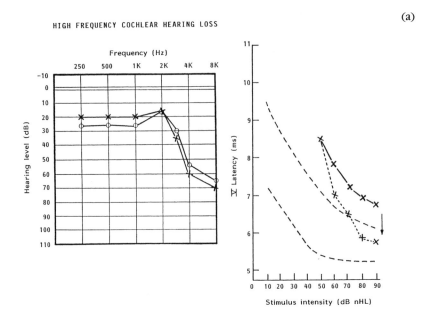

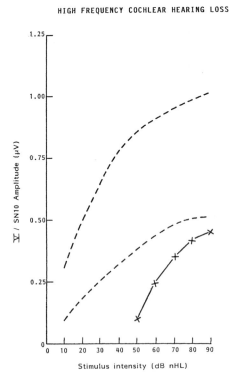

Figure 6.31. An example of the I/O functions of wave V latency (a) and amplitude (b) with the click-evoked ABR in high frequency cochlear hearing loss. The dashed lines indicate the upper and lower limits in normal hearing (+/– 2SD).

However, caution must be exercised in reporting I/O functions due to the variation in their profile, particularly in cases of high-frequency and mixed losses. Responses must be recorded over a wide range of stimulus intensity in order to examine the I/O profile and to accurately define the threshold of the ABR otherwise the results may be misleading.

Retrocochlear and central hearing loss

The most common origin of hearing loss in infants and young children is middle-ear disorder or cochlear damage. However, the possibility of more central pathology at higher levels of the auditory pathway, the brainstem or cortex, should not be overlooked. The ABR only examines the status of hearing up to about the level of the lateral lemniscus and any pathology affecting hearing beyond that point will not be detected. In these cases it may be useful to record a supra-threshold MLR or ACR, in addition to the ABR, in order to assess the integrity of the pathway. Although reliability of the thresholds of these responses is poor in young children and infants, a response can often be detected at raised stimulus levels.

In some cases it may be valuable to measure the amplitudes and latencies (absolute and inter-peak) of waves I, III and V of the ABR in order to assess the possibility of retrocochlear pathology. Also some clinical conditions, such as hydrocephalus, may affect the amplitude and/or the latency of these individual components and this may or may not influence the interpretation of the response threshold (Hall, 1992; Hood, 1998). Fortunately, infants and children referred for ABR investigation are likely to have already been diagnosed or classified as being at risk for these types of pathology from their clinical history. Nevertheless, its presence is likely to complicate the assessment and management of hearing loss.

Auditory neuropathy

Early screening and detection of hearing loss using ABR and evoked otoacoustic emissions (OAE) has highlighted a category of pathology known as auditory neuropathy (Starr et al., 1996; Wood et al., 1998; Rance et al., 1999, Sininger and Starr, 2001). It is characterized by the presence of an OAE (or receptor activity in ECochG) and an absent or poorly defined ABR. The likely causes of auditory neuropathy are either selective loss of inner hair cells, synaptic dysfunction, demyelination of auditory nerve fibres or possibly axonal loss, combined with intact outer hair cell function. It has been subdivided into two types: type I where neuropathy exists in both peripheral and auditory nerves, type II where the neuropathy is specific to the auditory nerve. In neonates and young children the presence of auditory neuropathy has serious implications regarding management and the provision of hearing aids.

Relationship of the ABR threshold to the PTA

The threshold profile of hearing is, of course, unknown when young children and infants are referred for ERA. The expected relationships of the click (plotted at 3 kHz) and tone-pip ABR thresholds to the threshold profile of the pure-tone audiogram (PTA) are shown in Figure 6.32 for different levels and profiles of hearing loss. These relationships are based on reports by Davis et al. (1985), Stapells et al. (1985), Gorga et al. (1985), Keith and Grenville (1987) and experiences in the Evoked Potentials Clinic in Nottingham.

ABR threshold: click

In cases of flat or shallow sloping hearing losses (a, b and c in Figure 6.32), the click-evoked ABR threshold is in good agreement with the PTA. However problems arise when the hearing loss has a steep slope in the region of 2 kHz to 4 kHz (d) and there is a tendency to underestimate the degree of hearing loss present, being biased towards better hearing at 1 kHz and 2 kHz. In some cases of severe to profound loss the click may slightly underestimate the level of hearing loss present (Mason et al., 1990). This is probably the result of a relatively faster growth in loudness for wide-band sounds, such as the click, when compared to narrow-band pure tones (Moore, 1989).

ABR threshold: tone-pip

In flat or shallow sloping hearing losses, particularly with only mild to moderate hearing loss as shown in (b) and (c), the tone-pip ABR provides good estimates of frequency specific thresholds. However, with a severe low-frequency hearing loss, as in (a), the degree of loss may be underestimated for the 500 Hz and 1 kHz tone-pip ABRs because high-intensity low-frequency stim-

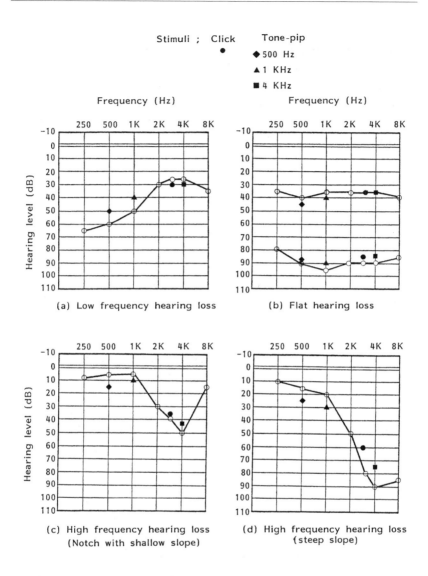

Figure 6.32. The expected relationships of the click and tone-pip ABR thresholds to the shape of the pure-tone audiogram.

uli may initiate activity in the basal region of the cochlea (Stapells et al., 1985). A similar problem also exists with the PTA when using high-intensity low-frequency pure tones. In very steep high-frequency hearing loss (d) the 4 kHz tone-pip ABR may underestimate the threshold, with activity arising from regions of better hearing at 3 kHz.

ABR threshold: tone-pip with ipsilateral masking

An excellent review of the estimation of the PTA by ABR can be found in Stapells and Oates (1997). This paper demonstrates the limitations of the click-evoked ABR and the practical application of the tone-pip ABR, including the use of ipsilateral masking noise. It shows that the tone-pip ABR can provide sufficiently accurate estimates of pure-tone hearing sensitivity from 500 Hz to 4 kHz. The frequency specificity of these thresholds being improved for steeply sloping losses and high-intensity stimulation by using ipsilateral masking such as notched noise. Although there is limited availability of these masking techniques on commercial evoked potential equipment, this should not restrict application of ABR measurements using tone-pips alone. The technique without masking is still a significant improvement in frequency specificity when compared to the click ABR.

Click and tone-pip protocols

The number of either air- or bone-conducted ABR thresholds that can be recorded from an infant or young child in a routine clinic session are limited by time factors and test conditions. It is important to have a formal protocol that controls the order of testing so that it maximizes the efficiency of the test. However, in the clinic, deviations from the protocol are inevitable because of test conditions, accessibility to the test ear, and the clinical history and information requested.

Ideally at least two air-conducted thresholds on each ear will provide valuable information about the general profile of the hearing loss. In the Nottingham protocol, the ABR thresholds to 4 kHz and 1 kHz tone-pips are recorded whenever possible. In difficult recording situations the more robust identification of the click ABR is preferred combined with a 1 kHz tone-pip if test conditions permit. Inclusion of bone conduction ABR testing is dependent on the results of tympanometry, history of middle-ear pathology, and if there are raised air-conducted ABR thresholds. In contrast, Stapells and Oates (1997) describe a protocol that focuses initially on the use of air- and bone-conducted 2 kHz tone-pips with ipsilateral notched noise masking. This is followed by the use of 500 Hz tone-pips and other frequencies, as required and time permitting.

Screening hearing

Early detection and management of hearing loss in infants will assist the development of speech, communication and social skills (Ramkalawan and Davis 1992; Yoshinaga-Itano, 1999). The ABR has a major role to play in the process both at the time of screening, also including evoked otoacoustic emissions (OAE), and in the early follow-up of referred babies. Screening an at-risk population of babies shortly after birth has been widely adopted in the past but we are now moving towards the early screening of all newborn babies (universal neonatal hearing screening; UNHS). The prevalence of bilateral severe to profound permanent childhood hearing impairment (PCHI) in the at-risk population (for example, NICU) is typically 1% to 2% compared with 0.1% to 0.2% in the general newborn population (Davis et al., 1997).

Development of screening techniques

Several different types of response to sound stimuli have been identified and investigated as a means of assessing the status of hearing in young infants: behavioural, electrophysiological and otoacoustic emissions. Early techniques for screening involved multi-behavioural measurements in automated screening devices such as the Auditory Response Cradle (Bennett, 1975) and the Crib-O-Gram (Simmons and Russ, 1974). In more recent years attention has focused on the use of the ABR (Alberti et al., 1983, Mason, 1998) and the evoked otoacoustic emission (EOAE) (Kemp et al., 1990; Stevens et al., 1990; Lutman et al., 1997).

Automated ABR

Over the last few years there have been major developments in the ABR aimed at providing a simple-to-use, quick and objective screening test of hearing. This technique of recording the ABR has now become known as the automated auditory brainstem response (AABR). A definition of the AABR has been reported by Mason et al. (2001b):

> Recordings of the ABR performed with a highly automated and standardized procedure for data collection for the purpose of screening for hearing loss. The presence of a response (pass) or absence (refer) at the screening intensity level of the stimulus is determined primarily by a clinically proven machine scoring algorithm operating online.

The aim of the AABR is to provide an effective tool for neonatal hearing screening programmes that can be used reliably by staff who are relatively inexperienced in ERA measurements. In order to satisfy these aims an AABR system often has the following features:

- easy application and checking of recording electrodes;
- quick and user-friendly test procedure;
- portability for flexible implementation;
- objective (machine) pass and refer test results on each ear;
- high sensitivity and high specificity;
- printout of test results;
- availability of recorded waveforms for skilled review and audit.

Technical aspects of the AABR

Many of the stimulus and data collection parameters implemented on AABR equipment are similar to those employed on conventional ERA equipment. A click stimulus with intensity in the range 35 dB nHL to 50 dB nHL is widely used and is presented through inserts, headphones or ear shells. The resultant signal is recorded from disposable electrodes on the scalp and is subjected to signal filtering and averaging in much the same way as conventional ABR recordings. The major differences are in the automated test procedure and the introduction of machine scoring to achieve a completely objective interpretation. These machine scoring techniques to determine whether or not a response is present are often based on template methods (Thornton et al., 1985; Kileny, 1987), FSP analysis (Don et al., 1994; Sininger et al., 2001) or measurements of correlation and response-to-noise ratio (Mason, 1984b). The automated ABR has been implemented on a number of commercially available systems such as the Algo IIe (Natus), ABaer (Biologic Corporation), SABRe (SLE Ltd), and on in-house equipment (Nottingham ABR Screener) (Mason, 1988). Typical neonatal ABR waveforms recorded on the Nottingham ABR Screener are shown in Figure 6.33.

Screening tests in neonates

It is common practice to perform the neonatal screening test of hearing shortly before a baby is discharged home. The most successful time is soon after a feed, which is often a very settled

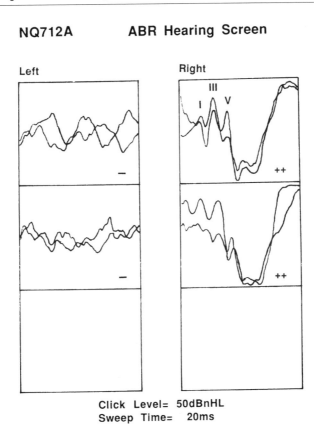

NQ712A   ABR Hearing Screen

Left   Right

Click Level= 50dBnHL
Sweep Time= 20ms

Figure 6.33. Recordings of the ABR in a pre-term neonate from NICU who has unilaterally failed the screen at a click level of 50 dB nHL. The test was performed on the Nottingham ABR screener.

period. It is important to avoid disturbing the baby as little as possible and so approaches such as testing in their cot or recording initially from the ear that is most accessible should be adopted.

In at-risk screening, the ABR, rather than the OAE, is often the preferred choice of test as it provides a high level of sensitivity and specificity. However, any baby that refers the ABR screen should then have an OAE test in order to exclude the possibility of auditory neuropathy. In newborn hearing screening of well babies, a two-technology screen is widely employed. One or two OAE tests are performed first, followed by ABR for babies that refer on the OAE tests (Gravel et al., 2000). These approaches to screening are recommended in the UK national protocol for the newborn hearing screening programme (NHSP).

Follow-up assessment of babies

All babies that refer the newborn hearing screen must be followed up with a comprehensive assessment of hearing thresholds using the ABR. This is typically carried out at a corrected age of four to six weeks, which gives time for sufficient maturation of the ABR in order to achieve stable and reliable estimates of hearing threshold. It is at this stage that objective frequency-specific thresholds are important and where the use of tone-pip stimuli for ABR is so valuable. In the future, the steady state AEP may play an important role in this part of the assessment process.

Performance of the ABR

The number of babies failing a neonatal screening test is affected by factors such as the criteria for referral (unilateral and bilateral, or bilateral only), test conditions, prevalence of middle-ear pathology, stimulus level and the level of any hearing loss. In Nottingham the typical number of referrals for at-risk screening are in the range of 5% to 7% when both unilateral and bilateral failures are followed up. These data are based on a screening level for the click of 50 dB nHL using the Nottingham ABR Screener. If only the bilateral failures are investigated then the referral rate falls to about 2%. In the NHSP with a two-technology screen the referral rate for combined unilateral and bilateral failures is typically in the range 1% to 2%.

In the ABR follow-up of babies referred by the screen not all will exhibit hearing loss. Figure 6.34 shows the outcome on 29 out of 500 at-risk babies that referred the ABR screen at 50 dB nHL in the Nottingham programme and were followed up at 46 weeks gestational age with assessment of ABR thresholds. Eight babies (28%) were identified as having a bilateral sensorineural hearing loss of greater than 50 dB HL. However, there were 13 babies (44%) that were subsequently normal on follow-up. Transient middle-ear pathology in the neonatal period is likely to be one of the main causes of normal outcome on follow-up. Those eight babies with severe to profound hearing loss on follow-up represent 1.6% of the sample at-risk population screened. Hearing aids have been fitted in five of these babies at a very early age. This incidence of severe to profound bilateral hearing loss is in good agreement with the published findings of 1% to 2% in the at-risk neonatal population.

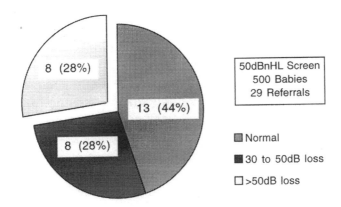

Figure 6.34. Outcome of follow-up ABR threshold measurements in 29 at-risk babies referred from the Nottingham Neonatal Hearing Screening Programme.

There are many reports that document values of sensitivity, specificity and false negative results for newborn hearing screening (Herrmann et al., 1995; Davis et al., 1997; Mason et al., 1998; Kennedy et al., 1998). Values of sensitivity, for example, are quoted from around 80% all the way up to 100%. However, it is important, when interpreting these results, to know whether they apply to the screening test itself or to the overall screening process. For example, a baby or infant with an acquired or progressive severe-to-profound hearing loss may pass the screen at the neonatal stage but subsequently may have the criterion level of loss. This baby could be classed as a false negative result (missed case of hearing loss) when analysis is based on the whole screening process, but will simply fall into the specificity numbers for just the screening test. There are also other potential causes of false negative results such as the frequency profile of the hearing loss and an incorrect interpretation of the screening test. Acceptable measures of the sensitivity and false negative rate for the screening process must include some follow-up of babies that pass the newborn hearing screen. The false negative rate of just the screening test can be investigated using no-stimulus runs.

Electrophysiological and objective measures in cochlear implantation

Cochlear implantation is an accepted approach to management of profoundly deafened children and adults who obtain little or no benefit from conventional amplification. The number of young children receiving cochlear implants is increasing worldwide as the benefits of early implantation become apparent. Electrophysiological and objective measures play a vital role in the management of these patients (Kileny, 1991; Shallop, 1997; Mason 2002a). Electrical stimulation of the cochlea, in addition to conventional acoustical stimulation, has led to the development of a whole range of electrophysiological and objective measures that can be implemented before implantation, at the time of surgery and afterwards. They have the capability to assess the degree of hearing loss, guide the selection of the ear and patient for implantation, monitor implant function, and provide valuable assistance with the tuning of the device in the difficult-to-test and very young children.

ERA before implantation

Electric response audiometry can be employed before implantation as a means of providing objective confirmation of a profound hearing loss and supporting the results of behavioural audiological assessment. In the Nottingham Paediatric Cochlear Implant Programme (NPCIP) the auditory brainstem response (ABR) is routinely employed using stimulus presentation through either conventional headphones or using the child's own hearing aid (Garnham et al., 2000; Mason 2002a). Aided ABRs are helpful to confirm the aided behavioural thresholds that form part of the audiological criteria for cochlear implantation. The ABR protocol in the NPCIP employs click stimuli and 1 kHz and 4 kHz tone-pips. It is not essential for all children to undergo ERA but those in most need tend to be the younger ones and complex cases and, for that reason, sedation is usually required. In the majority of children the test confirms the suspected profound bilateral hearing loss. Occasionally some significant residual hearing is identified which may necessitate a repeat audiological assessment to check the status of hearing before proceeding with implantation.

In a series of 70 young children from the NPCIP, the pre-implant ABR exhibited some residual response activity in 30 children (43%) and a short latency component in 18 children (25%). The click-evoked short latency component (SLC) was present in 15 (48%) of 31 congenitally deaf children but in only 2 (6%) of the children deafened after meningitis. The SLC has been described in more detail earlier in this chapter and in Mason et al. (1996). It is likely that the SLC arises from stimulation of sensory units of the vestibular system in the inner ear, when intense levels of stimulation are presented, with the recorded response originating primarily from the vestibular nuclei in the brainstem. The presence of the SLC is not a contraindication for proceeding with cochlear implantation. A similar component has also been observed on the EABR evoked by trans-tympanic electrical stimulation at the promontory.

Electrocochleography (ECochG) is available in the NPCIP test battery and is used in special cases. Typical indications for its use are inconsistency between the objective and behavioural audiological assessments, or the unexpected presence of evoked otoacoustic emissions which suggests the possibility of auditory neuropathy or retrocochlear pathology.

Electrical stimulation before implantation

The effectiveness of a cochlear implant depends not only on neuronal survival in the cochlea but on the ability for perception and cognition in central pathways and the cortex. The responsiveness of the peripheral auditory nerve to electrical stimulation can be assessed prior to cochlear implantation from recordings of the electrically evoked auditory brainstem response (EABR). The current spread from an electrical stimulus is not constrained by the mechanics of the middle ear and cochlea and it is therefore possible to apply a stimulus in the ear canal, at the promontory or on the round window. The closer the site is to the cochlea the more effective is the stimulus. Stimulation at the promontory in the middle ear has been extensively investigated being a good compromise between a minimally invasive approach and application of an effective stimulus (Mason et al., 1997). The EABR evoked by promontory stimulation (PromEABR) can be recorded in young children under general anaesthesia (Figure 6.35). There is evidence from animal work that the amplitude input/output (I/O) function of the EABR is correlated with neuronal survival (Hall, 1990).

In the NPCIP the PromEABR is targeted at complex cases where there is some doubt about the survival of the auditory nerve. It is a very valuable assessment tool to have available and if positive can guide a decision to proceed with implantation in difficult cases. Previously, the PromABR was recorded intra-operatively on all children, immediately before implantation,

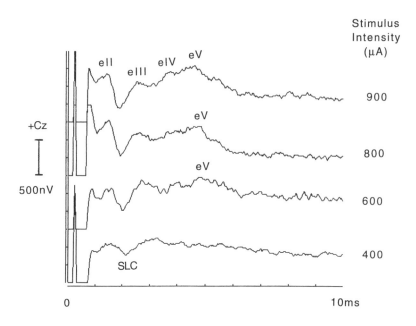

Figure 6.35. An intensity series of the electrically evoked auditory brainstem response (EABR) evoked by electrical stimulation at the promontory.

and the results were used to assist selection of the ear for implantation. However, a recent study of outcome measures (Nikolopoulos et al., 2000) did not provide any evidence to support the use of the technique in this way. Some children with an absent PromEABR still received significant benefit from a cochlear implant and it would therefore be inappropriate to use the technique to specifically exclude a child from undergoing cochlear implantation. In a study of 25 children (Mason et al., 1997), in 10 of the 50 ears tested (20%) it was not possible to identify a reliable response. Explanations for the absence of a response, in addition to the status of the auditory nerve, are lack of sensitivity of the test technique, difficult recording conditions and stimulus artefact. The latter make interpretation and identification of small responses challenging.

Intra-operative measurements

Several electrophysiological and objective measures can be employed at the time of implantation to assess the functioning of the cochlear implant and provide assistance with post-operative tuning of the device:

- back telemetry (BT);
- integrity testing (IT)
- electrically evoked stapedius reflex (ESR);
- electrical auditory brainstem response (EABR);
- electrical compound auditory nerve action potential (ECAP).

Many centres apply at least one or more of these intra-operative tests. In the NPCIP a protocol has been developed that encompasses many of these tests and provides a comprehensive evaluation of the implant. These results provide immediate reassurance to the surgeon and subsequently to the parents that the implanted receiver and electrode array are functioning normally and that the auditory nerve is being stimulated. Measurements obtained at this stage are also extremely valuable for the initial fitting and tuning session.

Back telemetry (BT)

All commercially available cochlear implant systems now have the capability to check the functioning of the internal implant and the integrity of the electrode array (for example, contact impedance of intra-cochlear electrodes) using a feature known as back telemetry (or reverse telemetry). This technique enables data, transmitted from the implant, to be picked up by the coil on the outside of the head. This direction of transmission is opposite to the way that the implant functions when stimulating.

Back telemetry is a valuable tool in the routine clinic, being simple and quick to implement across all electrodes on the array. In particular, measurement of contact impedance of intra-cochlear electrodes enables the detection of possible broken wires (high impedance) and shorting electrodes (very low impedance).

Integrity testing (IT)

The biphasic electrical pulse stimuli generated by the implant inside the cochlea can be recorded from surface electrodes on the scalp as a far-field potential. This is known as integrity testing (IT). It can be used to confirm the functioning of the implanted device and, where necessary, support the results of back telemetry. Signal averaging (typically 100 sweeps) is often employed and hence the term; averaged electrode voltages (AEV) is sometimes used. This is a relatively simple and quick investigation that can be carried out across all electrodes. The availability of IT and back telemetry at the time of surgery should eliminate the risk of implanting a faulty device.

Electrically evoked stapedius reflex (ESR)

The ESR is recorded intra-operatively from microscopic observation of the stapedius muscle/tendon before closure of the middle ear. The lowest stimulus level that causes contraction of the muscle (threshold) is measured on at least one electrode of the electrode array (for example, electrode 11 with the Nucleus Contour implant in the NPCIP protocol). Stimulation parameters are used that are similar to those that will be employed in the initial behavioural fitting session (for example, monopolar stimulation). The threshold of the ESR provides guidance as to the maximal levels of electrical stimulation that will be comfortable to the child at the initial fitting session.

Electrical auditory brainstem response (EABR)

A whole set of electrically evoked potentials can be recorded from the auditory pathway in much the same way as those generated by acoustical stimulation including the middle latency response (EMLR) and auditory cortical response (EACR). The origin of these response components is similar for both the acoustical and electrical modalities of stimulation. In young children, the electrical auditory brainstem response (EABR) and electrical compound action potential (ECAP) are valuable responses to record because they are stable and resistant to the effects of anaesthesia and sedation, similar to their counterparts in acoustical ERA.

The EABR can be evoked by a train of electrical biphasic pulses generated on a single channel of the electrode array by the implant and recorded from surface EEG scalp electrodes (Abbas and Brown, 1988; Mason, 2002b). The general morphology of the response is similar to the PromEABR but is normally larger with individual waves better defined. When compared to the acoustical ABR the EABR has shorter component latencies as shown in Figure 6.36. This arises primarily as a result of the mechanics of the cochlea being bypassed by the electrical stimulus.

The presence of a response confirms the functioning of the auditory nerve and brainstem pathways. Threshold of the intra-operative EABR can be used as a guide towards appropriate

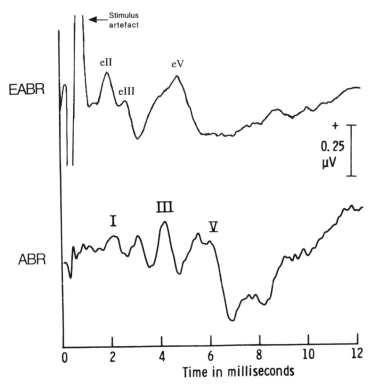

Figure 6.36. Typical waveforms for the acoustical ABR and the electrical ABR showing the different latency characteristics.

threshold levels of electrical stimulation for the first tuning session, providing appropriate correction factors are applied. A combination of the EABR (or ECAP) and ESRT can provide an objective indication of the appropriate dynamic range of electrical stimulation for a child.

Electrical compound action potential (ECAP)

Back telemetry techniques such as neural response telemetry (NRT) on the Nucleus Contour implant and neural response imaging (NRI) on the Advanced Bionics Clarion CII device provide us with the opportunity to record the ECAP, generated by the auditory nerve, from inside the cochlea. This is an exciting and valuable tool for the investigation of functioning of the peripheral auditory nerve and prediction of behavioural threshold levels (Hughes et al., 2000; Mason et al., 2001c). Testing is simple and relatively fast using custom-designed software and can easily be performed across all channels of the electrode array. Major attractions of the technique are: no external electrodes on the scalp, no additional evoked potential recording equipment, signals that are resistant to the effects of external electrical interference and patient movement. An intensity series of ECAP recordings recorded using NRT with the Nucleus Contour device is shown in Figure 6.37.

After implantation

The majority of electrophysiological and objective measures discussed previously can also be implemented after implantation. Back telemetry and IT investigations can confirm

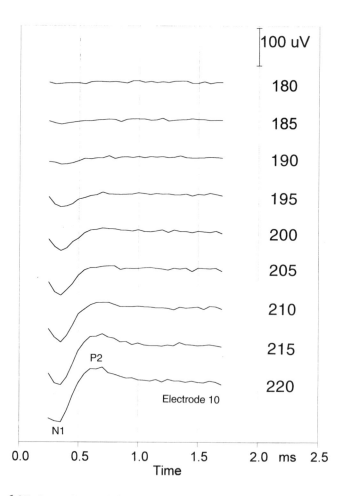

Figure 6.37. Recordings of the electrically evoked compound auditory nerve action potential (ECAP) with the Nucleus Contour cochlear implant using Neural Response Telemetry (NRT).

or exclude device malfunction (Mason, 2002a). It is important to remember that many children still have implants where back telemetry is not available and IT is therefore an essential objective test of implant function. In the NPCIP, all children have a routine IT investigation five years after implantation as part of the standard protocol (Garnham et al., 2000b) in addition to an on-demand basis.

The EABR and ECAP can also be employed post-operatively to monitor any unexpected changes in behavioural threshold levels of electrical stimulation and to assist with device fitting. It is very helpful to have the earlier intra-operative results available as these provide a reference data set that may enable any subtle change in the functioning of the implant to be detected.

Summary

Electric response audiometry, and in particular the auditory brainstem response, plays an essential role in the management of infants and young children when reliable behavioural assessment is not possible. The use of tone-pip stimuli to evoke the ABR has improved the frequency specificity of the objective estimations of hearing threshold. It is highly likely that steady state evoked potentials will contribute to ERA in the future. Cochlear implantation in young children and the introduction of newborn hearing screening in the UK are two areas of activity that are currently driving forward the development and application of ERA techniques.

References

Abbas P (1988) Electrophysiology of the auditory system. Clinical Physics and Physiological Measurement 9: 1–31.

Abbas P, Brown CJ (1988) Electrically evoked brainstem potentials in cochlear implant patients with multi-electrode stimulation. Hearing Research 36: 153–62.

Abramovich S (1990) Electric Response Audiometry in Clinical Practice. Edinburgh: Churchill Livingstone.

Achor LJ, Starr A (1980) Auditory brainstem responses in the cat. I. Intracranial and extracranial recordings. Electroencephalography and Clinical Neurophysiology 48: 154–73.

Alberti PW, Hyde M, Corbin H, Riko K, Abramovich S (1983) An evaluation of BERA for hearing screening in high-risk neonates. Laryngoscope 93: 1115–20.

Aoyagi M, Suzuki Y, Yokota M, Furuse H, Watanabe T, Ito T (1999) Reliability of 80 Hz amplitude-modulation following response detected by phase coherence. Audiology and Neuro-otology 4: 28–37.

Beagley HA, Kellogg SE (1968) A comparison of evoked response and subjective auditory thresholds. International Audiology 7: 420-1.

Bekesy G von (1947) The variation of phase along the basilar membrane with sinusoidal vibrations. Journal of the Acoustical Society of America 19: 452-62.

Bennett MJ (1975) The Auditory Response Cradle: a device for the objective assessment of auditory state in the neonate. Symposium of the Zoological Society 37: 291-305.

Berger H (1930) On the electroencephalogram of man. In Gloor P (ed.) Hans Berger on the Electroencephalogram of Man. Electroencephalography and Clinical Neurophysiology, Suppl. 28, 37, 1969.

Bickford RG, Galbraith RF, Jacobson JL (1963) The nature of average evoked potentials recorded from the human scalp. Electroencephalography and Clinical Neurophysiology 15: 720.

Brown DD (1982) The use of Middle Latency Response (MLR) for assessing low-frequency auditory thresholds. Journal of the Acoustical Society of America Suppl. 1, 71, S99.

Brownell WE (1986) Outer hair cell motility and cochlear frequency specificity. In Moore BCJ, Patterson RD (eds) Auditory Frequency Selectivity. New York: Plenum Press, pp. 109-20.

BS EN 60645-3 (1995) Audiometers Part 3. Auditory test signals of short duration for audiometric and neuro-otological purposes. London: British Standards Institution.

Chiappi KH, Gladstone KJ, Young RR (1979) Brainstem auditory evoked responses; studies of waveform variations in 50 normal human subjects. Archives of Audiology 36: 81-7.

Clark WA Jr (1958) Average Response Computer (ARC-1). Quarterly Progress Report No. 49 Research Laboratory of Electronics, Massachusetts Institute of Technology. Cambridge MA: MIT Press.

Coats AC, Martin JL (1977) Human auditory nerve action potentials and brainstem evoked responses. Archives of Otolaryngology 103: 605-22.

Cone-Wesson B (1995) Bone-conduction ABR tests. American Journal of Audiology 4: 14-19.

Davis A, Bamford J, Wilson I, Ramkalawan T, Forshaw M, Wright S (1997) A critical review of the role of neonatal hearing screening in the detection of congenital hearing impairment. Health Technology Assessment 1(10): 1-177.

Davis H (1976) Brainstem and other responses in electrical response audiometry. Annals of Otology 85: 3-14.

Davis H, Davis PA, Loomis AL, Harvey EN, Hobart G (1939) Electrical reactions of the human brain to auditory stimulation during sleep. Journal of Neurophysiology 2: 500-14.

Davis H, Hirsh SK (1976) The audiometric utility of brainstem responses to low-frequency sounds. Audiology 15: 181-95.

Davis H, Hirsh SK (1979) A slow brainstem response for low-frequency audiometry. Audiology 18: 445-61.

Davis H, Hirsh SK, Shelnutt J, Bowers C (1967) Further validation of evoked response audiometry (ERA). Journal of Speech and Hearing Research 10: 717-32.

Davis H, Hirsh SK, Turpin LL, Peacock ME (1985) Threshold sensitivity and frequency specificity in auditory brainstem response audiometry. Audiology 24: 54-70.

Davis PA (1939) Effects of acoustic stimuli on the waking human brain. Journal of Neurophysiology 2: 494–9.

Dawson GD (1951) A summation technique for detecting small signals in a large irregular background. Journal of Physiology 115: 2–3.

Don M, Elberling C, Waring M (1984) Objective detection of averaged auditory brainstem responses. Scandinavian Audiology 13: 219–28.

Douek EE, Gibson WPR, Humphries KM (1975) The crossed acoustic response. Revue de Laryngologie 96: 121–5.

Eggermont J (1982) The inadequacy of click-evoked auditory brainstem responses in audiological applications. Annals of the New York Academy of Sciences 388: 707–9.

Eggermont JJ, Stein L (1996) Maturation of the auditory system. Editors of the special issue: maturation of the auditory system. Ear and Hearing 17.

Finitzo-Hieber T, Friel-Patti S (1985) Conductive hearing loss and the ABR. In Jacobson JT (ed.) The Auditory Brainstem Response. San Diego, CA: College-Hill Press, pp. 113–32.

Fjermedal O, Laukli E (1989) Low-level 0.5 and 1 kHz auditory brainstem responses. Scandinavian Audiology 18: 177–83.

Folsom RC (1984) Frequency specificity of human auditory brainstem responses as revealed by pure-tone masking profiles. Journal of the Acoustical Society of America 75: 919–24.

Fria TJ, Sabo DL (1980) Auditory brainstem responses in children with otitis media and effusion. Annals of Otology, Rhinology, and Laryngology 68: 200–6.

Galambos R, Makeig S, Talamachoff PJ (1981) A 40 Hz auditory potential recorded from the human scalp. Proceedings of the National Academy of Science USA 78: 2643–7.

Garnham J, Cope Y, Durst C, McCormick B, Mason SM (2000a) Assessment of aided auditory brainstem response thresholds prior to cochlear implantation. British Journal of Audiology 34: 267–78.

Garnham J, Cope Y, Mason SM (2000b) Audit of five-year post-implantation routine integrity tests peformed on paediatric cochlear implantees. British Journal of Audiology 34: 285–92.

Geisler CD, Frishkopf LS, Rosenblith WA (1958) Extracranial responses to acoustic clicks in man. Science 128: 1210–11.

Gibson WPR (1978) Essentials of Clinical Electric Response Audiometry. London: Churchill Livingstone.

Glasscock ME, Jackson CG, Josey AF (1987) The ABR Handbook. London: Thieme Medical Publishers.

Gorga MP, Worthington DW, Reiland JK, Beuchaine KA, Goldgar DE (1985) Some comparisons between auditory brainstem response thresholds, latencies, and the pure tone audiogram. Ear and Hearing 6: 105–12.

Gravel J, Berg A, Bradley M, Cacace A, Campbell D, Dalzell L, DeCristofaro J, Greenberg E, Gross S, Orlando M, Pinheiro J, Regan J, Spivak L, Stevens F, Prieve B (2000) New York state universal newborn hearing screening demonstration project: effects of screening protocol on inpatient outcome measures. Ear and Hearing 21: 131–40.

Hall III JW (1992) Handbook of Auditory Evoked Potentials. Boston: Allyn & Bacon.

Hall RD (1990) Estimation of surviving spiral ganglion cells in the deaf rat using the electrically evoked auditory brainstem response. Hearing Research 45: 123–36.

Hashimoto I (1982) Auditory evoked potentials from the human midbrain: slow brain stem responses. Electroencephalography and Clinical Neurophysiology 53: 652–7.

Hawes MD, Greenberg HJ (1981) Slow brain stem responses (SN10) to tone pips in normally hearing newborns and adults. Audiology 20: 113–22.

Hecox K, Galambos R (1974) Brain stem auditory evoked responses in human infants and adults. Archives of Otolaryngology 99: 30–3.

Herrmann BS, Thornton AR, Joseph JM (1995) Automated infant hearing screening using the ABR: development and validation. American Journal of Audiology 4: 6–14.

Hood LJ (1998) Clinical Applications of the Auditory Brainstem Response. San Diego CA: Singular Publishing.

Hosford-Dunn H, Runge CA, Hillel A, Johnson SJ (1983) Auditory brain stem response testing in infants with collapsed ear canals. Ear and Hearing 4: 258–60.

Hughes ML, Brown CJ, Abbas PJ, Wolaver AA, Gervais JP (2000) Comparison of EAP thresholds with MAP levels in the Nucleus 24 cochlear implant: data from children. Ear and Hearing 21: 164–74.

Hyde ML (1985) The effect of cochlear lesions on the ABR. In Jacobson JT (ed.) The Auditory Brainstem Response. San Diego CA: College-Hill Press, pp. 133–46.

Hyde ML, Stephens SDG, Thornton ARD (1976) Stimulus repetition rate and the early brainstem responses. British Journal of Audiology 10: 41–6.

Hyde ML, Riko K, Malizia K (1990) Audiometric accuracy of the click ABR in infants at risk for hearing loss. Journal of the American Academy of Audiology 1: 59–66.

Jacobson JT (1985) The Auditory Brainstem Response. San Diego CA: College Hill Press.

Jewett DL, Williston JS (1971) Auditory-evoked far fields averaged from the scalp of humans. Brain 94: 681–96.

John MS, Picton TW (2000) Master: a Windows program for recording multiple auditory steady-state responses. Computer Methods and Programs in Biomedicine 61: 125–50.

Kato T, Shiraishi K, Eura Y, Shibata K, Sakata T, Morizono T, Soda T (1998) A neural response with 3-ms latency evoked by loud sound in profoundly deaf patients. Audiology and Neuro-otology 3: 253–64.

Keith WJ, Grenville KA (1987) Effects of audiometric configuration on the auditory brainstem response. Ear and Hearing 8: 49–55.

Kemp DT, Ryan S, Bray P (1990) A guide to the effective use of otoacoustic emissions. Ear and Hearing 11: 93–105.

Kennedy CR, Kimm L, Cafarelli Dees D, Campbell MJ, Thornton ARD (1998) Controlled trial of universal neonatal screening for early identification of permanent childhood hearing impairment. Lancet 352: 1957–64.

Kiang NY-S, Christ AH, French MA, Edwards AG (1963) Post-auricular electric response to acoustic stimuli in humans. Quarterly Progress Report of the Laboratory of Electronics, MIT 68: 218–25.

Kileny PR (1987) ALGO-1 automated infant hearing screener: preliminary results. Seminars in Hearing 8: 125.

Kileny PR (1991) Use of electrophysiologic measures in the management of children with cochlear implants: brainstem, middle latency, and cognitive (P300) responses. American Journal of Otology (Suppl) 12: 37–42.

Klein AJ (1983) Properties of the brain-stem response slow-wave component, I. Latency, amplitude and threshold sensitivity. Archives of Otolaryngology 109: 6-12.

Kramer SJ (1992) Frequency-specific auditory brainstem responses to bone-conducted stimuli. Audiology 31: 61-71.

Kraus N, Ozdamar O, Heydemann PT, Stein L, Reed N (1984) Auditory brainstem response in hydrocephalic patients. Electroencephalography and Clinical Neurophysiology 59: 310-31.

Kraus N, Ozdamar O, Hier D, Stein L (1982) Auditory middle latency responses (MLRs) in patients with cortical lesions. Electroencephalography and Clinical Neurophysiology 54: 275-87.

Lightfoot GR, Mason SM, Stevens JC (2002) Electric response audiometry and otoacoustic emissions : principles, techniques and clinical applications. Course notes, Harrogate, UK, 14-18 May 2001.

Lins OG, Picton PE, Picton TW, Champagne SC, Durieux-Smith A (1995) Auditory steady state responses to tones amplitude-modulated at 80-110Hz. Journal of the Acoustical Society of America 97: 3051-63.

Lutman ME, Davis AC, Fortnum HM, Wood S (1997) Field sensitivity of targeted neonatal hearing screening by transient otoacoustic emissions. Ear and Hearing 18: 265-76.

Mahoney TM (1985) Auditory brainstem response hearing aid applications. In Jacobson JT (ed.) The Auditory Brainstem Response. San Diego CA: College Hill Press, pp. 349-70.

Mason JDT, Mason SM, Gibbin KP (1995) Raised ABR threshold after suction aspiration of glue from the middle ear: three case studies. Journal of Laryngology and Otology 109: 726-8.

Mason SM (1984a) Effects of high-pass filtering on the detection of the auditory brainstem response. British Journal of Audiology 18: 155-61.

Mason SM (1984b) On-line computer scoring of the auditory brainstem response for estimation of hearing threshold. Audiology 23: 277-96.

Mason SM (1985) Objective waveform detection in electric response audiometry. PhD thesis, University of Nottingham.

Mason SM (1988) Automated system for screening hearing using the auditory brainstem response. British Journal of Audiology 22: 211-13.

Mason SM (1993) Electric response audiometry. In McCormick B (ed.) Paediatric Audiology 0-5 years. London: Whurr, pp. 187-249.

Mason SM (2002a) Electrophysiological and objective measures. In McCormick B (ed.) Cochlear Implants for Young Children. London: Whurr.

Mason SM (2002b) Electrical auditory brainstem response (EABR). In Cullington H (ed.) Cochlear Implants: Objective Measures. London: Whurr.

Mason SM, Cope Y, Garnham J, O'Donoghue GM, Gibbin KP (2001c) Intra-operative recordings of electrically evoked auditory nerve action potentials in young children by use of neural response telemetry with the Nucleus CI24M cochlear implant. British Journal of Audiology 35: 225-35.

Mason SM, Davis A, Wood S, Farnsworth A (1998) Field sensitivity of targeted neonatal hearing screening using the Nottingham ABR Screener. Ear and Hearing 19: 91-102.

Mason SM, Elliott C, Lightfoot GR, Parker D, Stapells D, Stevens JC, Sutton G, Vidler M (2001a) Auditory brainstem response testing in babies using tone pip stimulation: a recommended test protocol. Website: www.unhs.org.uk.

Mason SM, Elliott C, Lightfoot GR, Parker D, Stapells D, Stevens JC, Sutton G, Vidler M (2001b) Automated auditory brainstem response: information and guidelines for screening hearing in babies. Website: www.unhs.org.uk.

Mason SM, Field DL, Coles RAA (1990) Non-linearities of the click evoked ABR threshold in cochlear hearing loss. Presented at the Fourth International Evoked Potentials Symposium, Toronto, Canada, 30 September– 3 October.

Mason SM, Garnham CW, Hudson B (1996) Electric response audiometry in young children prior to cochlear implantation: a short latency component. Ear and Hearing 17: 537–43.

Mason SM, McCormick B, Wood S (1988) Auditory brainstem response in paediatric audiology. Archives of Disease in Childhood 63: 465–7.

Mason SM, O'Donoghue GM, Gibbin KP, Garnham CW, Jowett CA (1997) Perioperative electrical auditory brainstem response in candidates for pediatric cochlear implantation. American Journal of Otology 18: 466–71.

Mason SM, Singh CB, Brown PM (1980) Assessment of non-invasive electro-cochleography. Journal of Laryngology and Otology 94: 707–18.

Mokatoff B, Schulman-Galambos C, Galambos R (1977) Brain stem auditory evoked response in children. Archives of Otolaryngology 103: 38–43.

Moller AR (1999) Neural mechanisms of BAEP (review). Electroencephalography and Clinical Neurophysiology Supplement 49: 27–35.

Moller AR, Jannetta PJ (1984) Neural generators of the brainstem auditory evoked potential. In Nodar RH, Barber C (eds) Evoked Potentials II. Boston: Butterworth, pp. 137–44.

Moore BCJ (1989) Frequency selectivity, masking and the critical band. In Moore BCJ (ed.) An Introduction to the Psychology of Hearing. London: Academic Press, pp. 84–136.

Moore JK, Ponton CW, Eggermont JJ, Wu BJ-C, Huang JQ (1996) Perinatal maturation of the auditory brain stem response: changes in path length and conduction velocity. Ear and Hearing 17: 411–18.

Nikolopoulos TP, Mason SM, Gibbin KP, O'Donoghue GM (2000) The prognostic value of promontory electric auditory brainstem response in pediatric cochlear implantation. Ear and Hearing 21: 236–41.

Okitsu T (1984) Middle components of the auditory evoked response in young children. Scandinavian Audiology 13: 83–6.

Parving A, Salomon G, Elberling C, Larsen B, Lassen NA (1980) Middle components of the auditory evoked response in bilateral temporal lobe lesions. Scandinavian Audiology 9: 161–7.

Pickles JA (1988) An Introduction to the Physiology of Hearing. London: Academic Press.

Picton TW, Alain C, Woods DL, John MS, Scherg M, Valdes-Sosa P, Bosch-Bayard J, Trujillo NJ (1999) Intracerebral sources of human auditory-evoked potentials. Audiology and Neuro-otology 4: 64–79.

Picton TW, Champagne SC, Kellett AJC (1992) Human auditory evoked potentials recorded using maximum length sequences. Electroencephalography and Clinical Neurophysiology 84: 90–100.

Picton TW, Hillyard SA, Krausz HI, Galambos R (1974) Human auditory evoked potentials. I. Evaluation of components. Electroencephalography and Clinical Neurophysiology 36: 179–90.

Picton TW, Ouellette J, Hamel G, Smith AD (1979) Brainstem evoked potentials to tone pips in notched noise. Journal of Otolaryngology 10: 289–314.

Portmann M, Lebert G, Aran J-M (1967) Potentiels cochleares obtenus chez l'homme en dehors de toute intervention chirurgicale. Revue de Laryngologie 88: 157–64.

Ramkalawan TW, Davis AC (1992) The effects of hearing loss and age intervention on some language metrics in young hearing-impaired children. British Journal of Audiology 26: 97–107.

Rance G, Dowell RC, Rickards FW, Beer DE, Clark GM (1998) Steady-state evoked potential and behavioural hearing thresholds in a group of children with absent click-evoked auditory brainstem response. Ear and Hearing 19: 48–60.

Rance G, Beer DE, Cone-Wesson B, Shepherd RK, Dowell RC, King AM, Rickards FW, Clarke GM (1999) Clinical findings for a group of infants and young children with auditory neuropathy. Ear and Hearing 20: 238–52.

Reid A, Thornton ARD (1983) The effects of contralateral masking upon the brainstem electric responses. British Journal of Audiology 17: 155–62.

Sahley TL, Nodar RH, Musiek FE (1997) Efferent Auditory System: Structure and Function. San Diego CA: Singular.

Salamy A, McKean CM (1976) Postnatal development of human brainstem potentials during the first year of life. Electroencephalography and Clinical Neurophysiology 40: 418–26.

Seeley RR, Stephens TD, Tate P (1992) Anatomy and Physiology. St Louis MI: Mosby Year Book.

Shallop J K (1997) Objective measurements and the audiological management of cochlear implant patients. In Alford BR, Jerger J, Jenkins HA (eds) Electrophysiological Evaluation in Otolaryngology. Advances in Otorhinolaryngology. Basel: Karger 53: 85–111.

Simmons FB, Russ FN (1974) Automated newborn hearing screening, The Crib-O-Gram. Archives of Otolaryngology 100: 1–7.

Sininger YS, Abdala C (1996) Hearing threshold as measured by auditory brain stem response in human neonates. Ear and Hearing 17: 395–401.

Sininger YS, Hyde M, Luo P (2001) Statistical algorithms for automated detection of ABR: newborn hearing screening and tone burst diagnostic applications. Presented at the Seventeenth Biennial Symposium of the International Evoked Response Audiometry Study Group, Vancouver, Canada, 22–27 July.

Sininger YS, Masuda A (1990) Effect of click polarity on ABR threshold. Ear and Hearing 11: 206–9.

Sininger YS, Starr A (2001) Auditory Neuropathy: A New Perspective on Hearing Disorders. San Diego CA: Singular.

Sohmer H, Feinmesser M (1967) Cochlear action potentials recorded from the external ear in man. Annals of Otology, Rhinology and Laryngology 76: 427–35.

Stapells DR, Oates P (1997) Estimation of the pure tone audiogram by the audiitory brainstem response: a review. Audiology and Neuro-otology 2: 257–80.

Stapells DR, Picton TW, Perez-Abalo M, Read D, Smith A (1985) Frequency specificity in evoked potential audiometry. In Jacobson JT (ed.) The Auditory Brainstem Response. San Diego CA: College Hill Press, pp. 147–80.

Stapells DR, Galambos R, Costello JA, Makeig S (1988) Inconsistency of auditory middle latency and steady-state responses in infants. Electroencephalography and Clinical Neurophysiology 71: 289–95.

Starr A, Picton TW, Sininger YS, Hood LJ, Berlin CI (1996) Auditory neuropathy. Brain 119: 741–53.

Stevens JC, Baldwin M, Elliott C, Lightfoot GR, Mason SM, Parker D, Stapells D, Sutton G, Vidler M (2001a) Bone conduction auditory brainstem response testing in babies: a recommended protocol. Website: www.unhs.org.uk.

Stevens JC, Elliott C, Lightfoot G, Mason SM, Parker D, Stapells D, Sutton G, Vidler M (2001b) Click auditory brainstem response testing in babies – a recommended test protocol. Website: www.unhs.org.uk.

Stevens JC, Webb HD, Hutchinson J, Connell J, Smith MF, Buffin JT (1990) Click evoked otoacoustic emissions in neonatal screening. Ear and Hearing 11: 128-33.

Stockard JJ, Rossiter MA (1977) Clinical and pathologic correlates of brain stem auditory response abnormalities. Neurology 27: 316-25.

Stockard JJ, Stockard JE, Sharbrough FW (1977) Detection and localization of occult lesions with brainstem auditory responses. Proceedings of the Mayo Clinic 52: 761-9.

Sutton G, Baldwin M, Gravel J, Thornton R (2001) Tympanometry in neonates and infants under four months: a recommended test protocol. Website: www.unhs.org.uk.

Thornton ARD (1987) Electrophysiological measures of hearing function in hearing disorders. British Medical Bulletin 43: 926-39.

Thornton ARD, Coleman MJ (1975) The adaptation of cochlear and brainstem auditory evoked potentials in humans. Electroencephalography and Clinical Neurophysiology 39: 399-406.

Thornton AR, Hermann BS, Berick JM (1985) Automated neonatal hearing screening using the auditory brainstem response. Paper presented at the Ninth Biennial Symposium of the International Electric Response Audiometry Study Group, Erlangen, Germany.

Van der Drift JFC, Brocaar MP, Van Zanten GA (1987) The relation between the pure tone audiogram and the click auditory brainstem response threshold in cochlear hearing loss. Audiology 26: 1-10.

Wood S, Mason S, Farnsworth A, Davis A, Curnock DA, Lutman ME (1998) Anomalous screening outcomes from click-evoked otoacoustic emissions and auditory brainstem response tests. British Journal of Audiology 32: 399-410.

Yang EY, Stuart A, Mencher GT, Mencher LS, Vincer MJ (1993) Auditory brain stem responses to air and bone-conducted clicks in the audiological assessment of at-risk infants. Ear and Hearing 14: 175-82.

Yoshinaga-Itano C (1999) Benefits of early intervention for children with hearing loss. Otolaryngologic Clinics of North America 32: 1089-102.

Chapter 7
Otoacoustic emissions

Christian J. Durst, Jackie Moon

Introduction

Since the initial documentation of otoacoustic emissions by Kemp (1978) the study of these phenomena has contributed to our knowledge of the mechanisms of the auditory system, and otoacoustic emission testing has become a valued part of the audiological test battery. Commercial test equipment is widely available and its use is common during audiological evaluations. The most widespread use of emissions has so far been in assessment of peripheral auditory function. However, study of suppression effects may lead to insights into more central hearing pathways.

Emission testing does not require a behavioural response from the subject; thus it is best described as a physiological rather than a behavioural test, and it can have certain advantages in testing paediatric populations. Emissions are likely to play a key role in screening programmes, particularly with the planned introduction of universal neonatal screening.

As will be discussed later, it is widely accepted that otoacoustic emissions are generated within the cochlea. Due to the pathways involved their successful detection in a subject depends on the status of the middle ear and ear canal, as well as cochlear function.

This chapter focuses on OAE results obtained in human subjects and more specifically, where appropriate, on results from the paediatric population. Observations from a wealth of animal studies are included as appropriate.

Recording of OAEs

Otoacoustic emissions are detectable as acoustic energy present in the ear canal, either spontaneously, or as the result of external stimulation. These signals can be sampled or recorded using a probe assembly that is usually sealed in the ear canal. The probe will usually contain at least two transducers. One is a sensitive microphone used to record the emission response. The other is used to deliver the eliciting acoustic stimulus to the ear in the case of evoked otoacoustic emissions. The actual sound pressure level of the emission is usually very small in comparison to background noise. Therefore a combination of techniques are used to improve the signal-to-noise ratio. A schematic of a typical set up is given in Figure 7.1. A subject undergoing the test is shown in Figure 7.2.

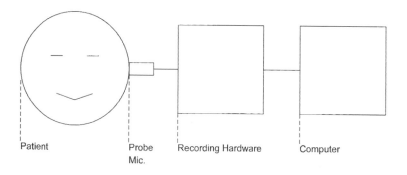

Patient   Probe   Recording Hardware   Computer
                     Mic.

Figure 7.1. Schematic set-up for OAE testing.

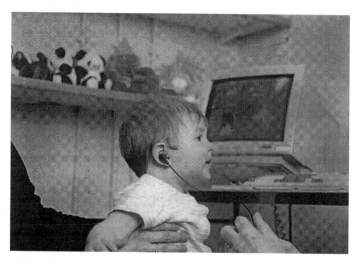

Figure 7.2. Subject undergoing OAE testing.

In most commercial equipment the signal is amplified and passed on to a computer-based processing system. A large number of stimulus presentations or 'sweeps' can be combined to allow averaging. This works on the principle that features of the response occur at invariant latencies following stimulus onset. Noise will occur at random times. Thus averaging tends to lessen the effects of background noise. Artefact rejection excludes sweeps where the signal level is deemed too high to be an emission. Frequency areas not of interest and likely to contain only noise are excluded using frequency filtering. Time windowing is used to exclude information from latencies not of interest – for click evoked emissions the very early latencies may be dominated by artefacts such as ringing of the stimulus. The methods used are analogous to those used in evoked response testing such as the auditory brainstem response (ABR). Sometimes these parameters can be altered in real time during recording, or applied retrospectively to the information stored in computer memory.

In most cases the OAEs of interest demonstrate non-linear behaviour. The recording equipment should therefore be as linear or high fidelity as possible in order to reduce the possibility of equipment artefacts being mistaken for an emission response.

A common technique in commercial equipment is to store alternate sweeps in separate computer buffers. This allows the correlation between the two buffers to be analysed. A high degree of correlation indicates that the response is highly repeatable and therefore unlikely to be due to random noise. Random noise will tend to produce a low level of correlation.

Analysis in the frequency domain using the fast fourier transform is also often employed. This can aid in identifying an emission at a specific frequency, or in the case of a wide-band response, provide information over chosen ranges of frequencies.

Systems that provide the ability to examine a wide range of parameters, including information in the frequency domain – the power spectrum of the response, as well as the time domain – the waveform of the response, are the most desirable for the experienced clinician. Single measure systems such as overall waveform correlation may 'fail' responses that are present but marginal (Kapadia and Lutman, 1997) or 'pass' emissions that are present but only at limited frequencies, which may be important in an individual case. Overall waveform measures are useful but it is the authors' opinion that they are best used in conjunction with observation of less processed data such as time-domain waveform.

A computer-based system will also allow data from tests to be stored (usually to a computer hard drive). Files can then be recalled for later re-analysis and comparisons over time can be made.

Summary

- Recording of OAEs requires a probe with stimulus transducer and sensitive microphone. The system must be highly linear.
- Signal-to-noise ratio is improved by repeated sweeps, time windowing, frequency filtering and artefact rejection.
- Computer-based systems can allow statistical analysis of the response.

Classification and characteristics of OAEs

The term otoacoustic emission refers to a range of phenomena that can be classified into several groups. The broadest grouping is those that occur spontaneously without an external stimulus; spontaneous OAEs, and those that are produced as a result of an applied stimulus; evoked OAEs. Evoked OAEs are most commonly classified by the type of precipitating stimulus, giving rise to:

- transiently evoked OAEs (TEOAEs) – produced in response to brief duration acoustic stimuli such as clicks and tone bursts;
- distortion product OAEs (DPOAEs) – produced in response to multiple pure-tone stimuli;.
- stimulus frequency OAEs (SFOAEs) – produced at frequencies similar to a pure-tone stimulus.

An additional class of OAEs comes from animal studies. Electrical stimulation of the cochlea can lead to the production of acoustic energy in the ear canal, giving rise to the further class of electrically evoked OAEs.

The principal characteristics of the OAE classes are given in Table 7.1.

Table 7.1. Characteristics of otoacoustic emission types

OAE	Stimulus	Form (in terms of ear canal signal)	Prevalence (in audiologically normal ears)
SOAE (Spontaneous)	None	Peaks in ear canal frequency spectrum above noise level.	Many ears.
TEOAE (Transient Evoked)	Transient – e.g. broad-band click Frequencies correspond to stimulus frequency.	Wide-band response above noise level.	Close to all ears.
DPOAE (Distortion Product)	Two tone complex	Narrow-band response above noise level. Frequency algebraically related to stimulus frequencies.	Close to all ears.
SFOAE (Stimulus Frequency)	Pure tone (usually swept in frequency)	Non-linear peaks and troughs in phase or magnitude of ear canal phase and magnitude.	Vast majority of ears.

Spontaneous otoacoustic emissions

In the absence of external stimuli it is possible for the ear to emit acoustic energy. This can be recorded by a sensitive microphone placed in the ear canal. The signal is then amplified and passed to a computer system for analysis. Commonly, a fast fourier transform is used to analyse the spectrum of the signal. Filtering and averaging techniques are employed to further improve the signal-to-noise ratio. Sometimes this is facilitated by introducing a low-level transient stimulus into the ear canal, with which the spontaneous emission becomes synchronized. (If this is employed it is important to discard responses from latencies that could be TEOAEs.) The spontaneous emission takes the form of peaks in the ear canal power spectrum, at discrete frequency bands, above the noise floor of the recording (Figure 7.3).

Spontaneous emissions have been separated into two groups. High-level emissions are less common and can be associated with sensorineural hearing loss. These are often at the frequencies of the hearing loss or its boundaries and can have absolute levels as high as 50 dB SPL (Glanville, Coles and Sullivan, 1971; Yamamoto et al., 1987). The rest of this section will refer to low-level spontaneous OAEs (SOAEs) unless stated otherwise.

Low-level emissions are more common, present in approximately 30% to 60% of the population with normal

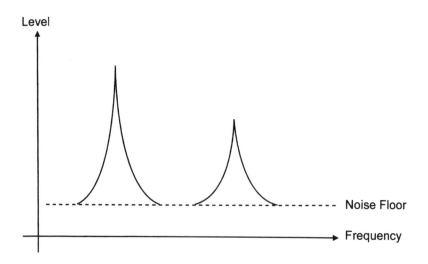

Figure 7.3. Schematic of SOAE.

hearing sensitivity (Zurek, 1981; Strickland, Burns and Tubis, 1985; Bonfils, 1989). These estimates vary widely but do not seem to be directly related to the sensitivity or noise floor of the recording apparatus (Probst, Lonsbury-Martin and Martin, 1991). However Penner and Zhang (1997) found that the recording techniques could alter the apparent prevalence of SOAEs. The frequency resolution employed and the number of spectral averages taken influenced SOAE detectability.

A number of studies have shown that spontaneous OAEs are more prevalent in female rather than male ears (Zurek, 1981; Probst et al., 1986; Lonsbury-Martin et al., 1990). It remains unclear as to why this is the case. Cope and Lutman (1993) proposed an effect of ear canal volume, positing that as female ears are typically smaller, the acoustic energy being delivered to a smaller air volume will tend to produce a more detectable sound level. Probst, Lonsbury-Martin and Martin (1991) speculate that anatomical differences in the cochlea may contribute.

Population and twin studies have demonstrated evidence for a genetic component to the characteristics of SOAEs (for example, Russell and Bilger, 1992). Differences in SOAES between Asiatic, Afro-Caribbean and Caucasian subjects were shown by Whitehead et al. (1993).

Various authors have documented SOAEs occurring across the frequency range 0.5 to 6 kHz. The vast majority of studies indicate that the greatest number of SOAEs are found between 1 and 2 kHz. Kemp (1980) showed the reverse transfer function of the middle ear to be most efficient at these frequencies, suggesting the presence of a middle-ear effect.

The frequency structure of SOAEs in an ear does not appear to be random. Where multiple emissions are present in an ear there is evidence for a preferred minimum frequency spacing, constant on a logarithmic scale and approximately equal to a musical interval of one semitone (Braun, 1997). Braun (1997) also showed multiple emission spacing to have a peak in prevalence for intervals of 1 to 2 critical bands. The critical band is a measure of the frequency resolution of the auditory system (see Moore, 1989). There is also a tendency for emission frequencies present in one ear of an individual to be present also in the contralateral ear (Braun, 1998). Braun (1998) suggested that this reflected the involvement of the efferent system and higher centres in the auditory system.

A high degree of stability over time is generally observed in the frequencies present in an individual's SOAE. However Kohler and Fritz (1992) found significant changes in the emissions of a large proportion of ears after a long time interval (mean: 68 months). They suggested that this might be due to age-related changes. Penner (1996) documented the emergence and disappearance of intense OAEs in a subject, possibly due to noise exposure. Strickland et al. (1985) noted that the frequency change over time in SOAEs was related to the absolute emission frequency, and Dallmayr (1987) calculated that this corresponded to an equal spacing along the cochlear partition. In other words, the variability could be accounted for by a shift in site of emission origin on the cochlear partition within consistent limits.

The amplitude of SOAEs is usually within the region between –10 dB and 20 dB SPL (Probst et al., 1991; Probst and Harris, 1997). The amplitude of SOAEs shows less stability compared to frequency, at least over intervals greater than several hours (Dallmayr, 1987).

The presence of a SOAE at a given frequency is associated with greater hearing sensitivity at this frequency, compared with adjacent regions (Zwicker and Schloth, 1984; Long and Tubis, 1988). Probst et al. (1987) concluded that where SOAEs are found, hearing threshold at that frequency will not exceed 15 dB HL.

It should be recognized that the absence of a SOAE does not necessarily indicate the presence of any pathology, as a large proportion of ears can demonstrate normal hearing sensitivity, and the absence of recordable spontaneous activity. Whether future advances in recording techniques or other fields will allow us to conclude that all normal ears show some spontaneous activity remains to be seen. In the meantime it is suggested that although SOAE measurements may be useful in monitoring cochlear status in some subjects during, for example, the administration of ototoxic drugs, evoked OAEs currently provide a more useful investigative tool in providing information regarding subjects' hearing sensitivity.

Summary

- Spontaneous OAEs take the form of one or more narrow-band signals above the noise floor of the ear canal.
- They are present in the majority of normal ears.

- Amplitudes of −10 to 20 dB SPL are common and SOAEs have been observed over the frequency range 0.5 kHz to 9 kHz.
- The pattern in a particular ear is stable over time.
- Audiologically normal ears can exhibit none, one, or several narrow-band SOAEs.

Transient evoked OAEs (TEOAEs)

Transient OAEs are produced in response to a brief duration acoustic stimulus. This is commonly a click, or a tone-pip (Figure 7.4). Click stimuli are broad-band and thus (with appropriate analysis) can yield information simultaneously across a wide range of frequencies. Tone-pips are more frequency specific and can limit the information to a given frequency range if desired. Recording equipment and procedure are as described above. Commonly a high-pass filter, artefact rejection and timelocked averaging are used to increase the signal-to-noise ratio. This is essentially analogous to the recording of auditory evoked potentials.

The click-evoked OAE (CEOAE) takes the form of a linear component over latencies of approximately 0 to 5 ms. This is attributable to the response of the probe transducers, ear canal and middle ear, along with a passive response from the cochlea,

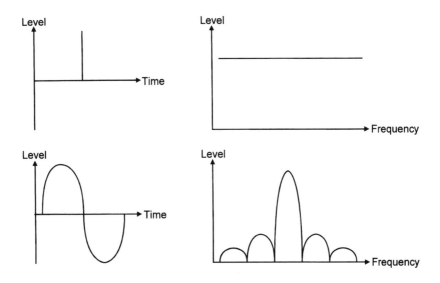

Figure 7.4. Click and tone-pip characteristics.

to the impulse stimulus. A non-linear component follows this, observable up to latencies of 100 ms (Wit and Ritsma, 1980). The non-linear component is seen to saturate at higher stimulus levels (Kemp, 1978; Grandori, 1985). It is the non-linear component that is deemed of greatest interest as the characteristics of this reflect the function of the cochlea. Commonly, in the literature, the term CEOAE (or TEOAE) refers to the non-linear portion of the response.

Two principal methods of extracting the non-linear component can be employed (Figure 7.5). One is to record the response at two stimulus levels. The amplitude of the higher level response is scaled (linearly) by the difference in stimulus levels and the waveforms subtracted (for example, Probst et al., 1986). This will eliminate any component that increases linearly with stimulus level and will yield the non-linear component. Alternatively, a 'stimulus package' can be designed that manipulates the response to automatically eliminate linear components. One such package employed in commercial equipment is a non-linear click train (for example, Kemp et al., 1986). This consists of a train of four clicks. The initial three are

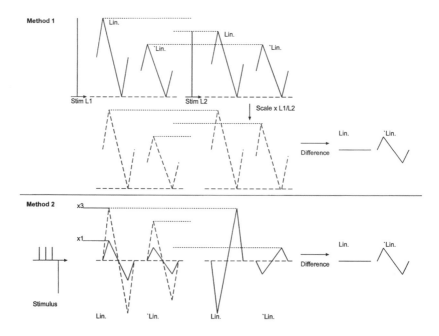

Figure 7.5. Extraction of non-linear components.

of similar polarity and amplitude. The final click is of reversed polarity and three times the amplitude. The summed response to this will include three linear responses of one polarity, and one linear response of opposite polarity at three times the amplitude. Therefore the linear portion is cancelled, yielding the non-linear emission.

A typical response waveform (with the non-linear component isolated) is given in Figure 7.6). The waveform typically shows oscillatory characteristics at different latencies.

The non-linear response is dispersive with regard to frequency (Kemp, 1978; Grandori, 1985) (Figure 7.7). High

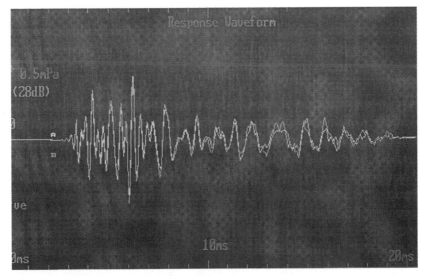

Figure 7.6. Non-linear TEOAE in time domain.

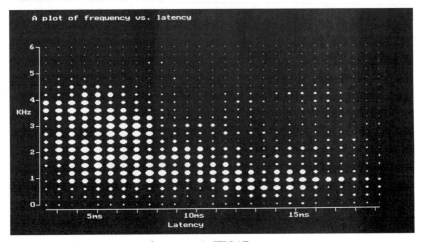

Figure 7.7. Latency versus frequency in TEOAE.

frequency energy in the response occurs at lower latencies compared to lower frequency energy. It has been proposed that this reflects the time taken for the travelling wave produced by the stimulus on the basilar membrane to reach the site of response origin, and the time taken for this to be transmitted back along the cochlea. The pattern coincides with the tonotopic organization of the cochlea.

Useful information can be derived through frequency analysis of the response, usually achieved through a fast fourier transform. An example of a typical spectrum is given in Figure 7.8. A typical response will take the form of peaks and troughs in energy above the resultant background noise level after averaging. The power spectrum of the response depends in part on the eliciting stimulus. Where the stimulus is broad-band (for example, a click), most ears demonstrate a characteristic pattern of discrete, or dominant, frequencies (see, for example, Kemp, 1981; Probst et al., 1986; Bray, 1989). These dominant frequencies will also be present in response to narrower band stimuli as long as the stimulus contains sufficient energy at the dominant frequencies.

The pattern of dominant frequencies is highly stable over time barring changes in cochlea and/or middle-ear function. Johnsen and Elberling (1982) found little or no change in responses over a five-week interval. Antonelli and Grandori (1986) demonstrated similar findings but over a four-year period. The author's ear has been used in biological calibration checks of OAE equipment over several years on a weekly basis and has not demonstrated any significant changes. There do,

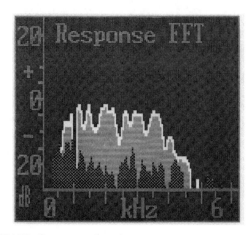

Figure 7.8. TEOAE in frequency domain.

however, appear to be maturational and ageing effects on OAE spectra. These will be discussed below.

Emission energy and dominant frequencies are commonly within the frequency range 0.5 kHz to 4 kHz for CEOAEs (Kemp, 1981; Probst et al., 1986). In an analogy with SOAEs, the greatest emission energy is usually in the region 1 kHz to 2 kHz, again possibly reflecting the maximum efficiency region of the middle ear reverse transfer function.

As higher frequency energy in the emission response tends to occur at earlier latencies there are technical difficulties with recording higher frequencies from the TEOAE response. Even slight amounts of stimulus ringing can contaminate very early latencies and thus higher frequency energy in the response. For practical purposes (including transducer limitations) most commercial equipment cannot provide much useful information on emission energy above approximately 4 kHz to 5 kHz.

For TEOAEs evoked by other stimuli (such as tone bursts) the spectrum of the response is dependent on the spectrum of the eliciting stimulus. For tone bursts maximum emission energy will occur at or near the peak energy of the stimulus (Elberling et al., 1985; Norton and Neely, 1987). Elberling et al. (1985) and Probst et al. (1986) showed that the form of the CEOAE is well predicted by the summation of a number of tone burst responses (sufficient to cover a wide frequency range similar to the click).

The absolute amplitude of the TEOAE response is dependent on stimulus level as well as the middle-ear response, recording system response and of course the characteristics of the cochlea under test. The response sound pressure level is almost always below 20 dB SPL. As mentioned above, responses show saturation as higher stimulus levels are observed.

Otoacoustic emissions can be detected for levels lower than psychoacoustic threshold (Kemp 1978; Probst et al., 1986). Kemp (1978) reported that emission waveform changed with stimulus level, although identifiable 'key' features of the response were always present. As will be discussed later, a general rule can be applied such that, where hearing levels are normal or near normal, TEOAEs are detectable. Where significant hearing loss is present they are not. This applies (generally) regardless of stimulus level used. Thus the minimum stimulus level required to elicit an OAE - the detection threshold - is not held to offer highly useful clinical information. In most commercial equipment the stimulus is presented at high levels, for example 60 dB SPL to 80 dB SPL, to ensure a high degree of saturation non-linearity and thus a higher signal-to-noise ratio of the emission portion of interest.

The majority of studies into the prevalence of TEOAEs suggests that they can be detected in almost all ears with normal audiometric thresholds, for example:

- Kemp (1978): 100%;
- Probst et al. (1986) 96%;
- Avan et al. (1991) 100%;
- Kapadia and Lutman (1997) 99.2%.

This finding appears to be consistent even when different response criteria and recording conditions are used. A study by Dijk and Wit (1987) reported a much lower prevalence of 40% but it has since been suggested that this may have been due to technical limitations of the equipment used (e.g. Probst et al., 1991).

In the case of tone-burst OAEs the prevalence depends partly on the stimulus frequency. Probst et al. (1986) reported a greater number of subjects showing responses for 1.5 kHz tone bursts than for 0.5 kHz tone bursts. Wit and Ritsma (1980) showed that higher tone-burst frequencies led to smaller emission responses.

Summary

- TEOAEs are produced in response to brief duration stimuli such as clicks and tone bursts.
- Energy is present in the form of distinct peaks and troughs at various frequencies.
- Scaling or cancellation methods are used to derive the non-linear portion of the response.
- They are present in almost all normal ears.
- Amplitudes of <20 dB SPL are reported and a frequency range of 0.5–4 kHz is common.
- The pattern of responses in an ear is highly stable over time.

Distortion product OAEs

Non-linearity in terms of response amplitude growth was discussed in the section on TEOAEs. Another form of non-linearity is exhibited by the ear when it is stimulated with two (or more) tones. Inter-modulation distortion can occur, resulting in distortion products occurring at predictable frequencies, which can be recorded at the ear canal. The presence of distortion products in the human ear has been known for many years (Helmholtz, for example, reported them in the nineteenth century). Distortion products can be detectable by subjects and have been extensively researched psychoacoustically (where they are often referred to as combination tones).

If the two eliciting (or primary) tones have frequencies f1 and f2 (f2 being the higher) then tones can be generated with frequencies of pf1 + qf2, where p and q are integers. Commonly in DPOAE literature, the primaries are referred to as 'f1 and f2' in terms of frequency and 'L1 and L2' in terms of level. The highest amplitude distortion product and consequently the most studied, in the human ear, is usually 2f1-f2, though others such as 2f2-f1 can be detected. A schematic is shown in Figure 7.9.

Distortion product otoacoustic emission recording is similar to that described for other types of evoked OAEs. Linearity and ultra-low distortion are required properties of the recording system. Multiple tones can be delivered to the ear canal either by multiple transducers or a single transducer driven with an appropriate signal. If the latter method is used linearity of the transducer under these conditions must be verified.

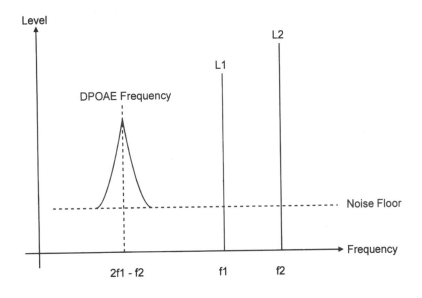

Figure 7.9. Schematic of DPOAE.

Studies are again suggestive that DPOAEs are a feature of virtually all normally hearing ears (for example, Kemp, 1986; Lonsbury-Martin et al., 1990).

Distortion product amplitude is highly dependent on the eliciting stimulus. There is considerable inter-subject variability, although results in a single subject are typically stable over time. A complex relationship exists between distortion product response and both primary frequencies and amplitudes. Not only are the absolute values of the overall primary amplitude and frequency important, their relative values (for example L2 – L1 and f2/f1) also play a crucial role. To date research has not indicated definitive ideal values for these parameters, partly as they may vary depending on which characteristics are of interest when examining DPOAEs. Generalizations for the parameters in the clinical use of DPOAEs as indicators of hearing sensitivity are, however, possible.

It is possible to examine the peak amplitude of a DPOAE as a function of f2/f1 ratio. An f2 to f1 ratio of approximately 1.2 maximizes the response (see, for example, Kemp and Brown, 1983; Harris et al., 1989; Lasky, 1998). Some studies have reported a tendency for DPOAE amplitude to peak at lower f2/f1 ratio as overall frequency increases (Lonsbury-Martin et al., 1987; Lasky, 1998) but the deviation from 1.2 appears only slight.

The level difference in the primaries is also important. Lasky (1998) suggests that positive L1 – L2 differences are favourable (where L1 > L2). Level differences in the order of 6 dB to 15 dB for clinically used stimuli are favourable (see, for example, Hauser and Probst, 1990).

Beattie and Jones (1998) suggested that the absolute levels of L1 and L2 influence the optimum level difference for eliciting responses. Higher overall levels showed a zero level difference to be favourable. Moderate levels favoured 5 dB to 10 dB differences. Low stimulus levels did not indicate any particular level difference to be favourable but it was much less likely that DPOAEs were detectable anyway under these conditions.

Distortion product otoacoustic emissions have been reported for a wide range of frequencies, for example 0.5 kHz to 8 kHz (Smurzynski and Kim, 1992). The ability for DPOAEs to provide information over higher frequencies suggests that a combination of TEOAE and DPOAE testing is highly effective where detailed information over a broad frequency range is required, given the limitations of TEOAEs at higher frequencies.

As mentioned above, DPOAE amplitude is highly dependent on the eliciting stimuli. Maximal amplitude, however, is typically in the order of 60 dB below the primaries (Kemp et al., 1986; Lonsbury-Martin et al., 1990). Cases of higher amplitude emissions have been noted where DPOAE frequency is at or close to a subject's SOAE (Wier et al., 1988). Evidence from animal studies (for example, Whitehead, Lonsbury-Martin and Martin, 1992) suggest that two types of DPOAEs can be elicited: a high-amplitude type elicited by levels at or in excess of 60–70 dB SPL, and a low-amplitude type that is more vulnerable than the higher amplitude to physiological manipulations that degrade cochlear function. Lonsbury Martin et al. (1987) found that in post-mortem studies high level emissions, produced in response to stimuli >70 dB SPL, degraded much more slowly than those elicited by lower level stimuli. This is suggestive of different generator mechanisms, and indicates that for tests of cochlear status low level, physiologically vulnerable emissions are the most useful. Bonfils and Avan (1992) suggested that caution is required in interpreting distortion products in humans for stimuli in excess of approximately 50 dB SPL, for these reasons.

The latency of DPOAEs has been studied by examination of the phase relationship of the response to the primaries. The latency appears to be dependent on the $f2/f1$ ratio (Kemp, 1986). Increasing $f2/f1$ ratio gave rise to a range of latencies from 2 ms to 8 ms. Latency also depends on overall stimulus frequency. Higher frequencies give rise to lower latencies as the site of stimulus response and generator site become more basal along the cochlear partition (Probst and Harris, 1997).

Three principal methods of studying DPOAE responses have been described (Figure 7.10). One is to set the relative level and relative frequency of the stimulus tone pair. The overall absolute stimulus frequency is then varied and DPOAE amplitude above noise floor is examined. This is often referred to as the 'distortion product audiogram'. Commonly, parameters are set in order to produce maximum response amplitude; the $2f1-f2$ frequency is examined, a frequency ratio of ~1.2 and a level difference of ~10 dB, with an overall stimulus level of ~50 to 60 dB SPL is used. This is the method most widely employed in commercial clinical equipment. Stimulus frequencies can be chosen to correspond to audiogram frequencies or swept across a chosen frequency range at a pre-determined resolution.

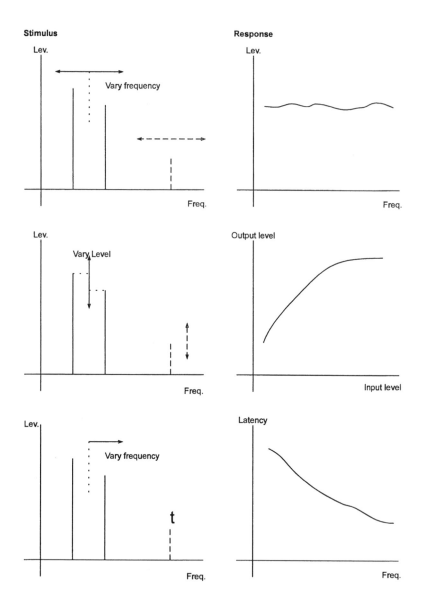

Figure 7.10. Methods of DPOAE testing.

Repeated sweeps are used to improve the signal-to-noise ratio and can give a statistical indicator in terms of level above the noise floor of the reliability of the response.

Another technique is to examine DPOAE detection threshold or produce in/out functions for stimulus and response. With this method f1 and f2 are fixed both in relative and overall absolute frequency terms, and L1 and L2 are varied either separately or together. Again, it is common to use fixed parameters that maximize the DPOAE response. Lonsbury-Martin et al. (1990) demonstrated a detection threshold of approximately 35 to 45 dB SPL for a response 3 dB above the noise floor over the frequency range 0.5 to 8 kHz. Where response frequency coincides with an SOAE frequency, much lower thresholds have been reported of the order of 5 dB SPL (for example, Wier et al., 1988). Detection threshold will also depend on the sensitivity and overall noise floor of the recording conditions. Characteristics of the I/O function can be dependent upon the stimulus parameters used. Lonsbury-Martin et al. (1990) showed shallower growth functions for lower overall frequencies (1 to 2 kHz) compared to higher frequencies (3 to 8 kHz). Typical growth functions have a monotonic gradient tending to unity until overall stimulus levels of 60 to 70 dB SPL are reached, where saturation occurs (Probst, Lonsbury-Martin and Martin, 1991). However deviations from this pattern occur in a significant number of ears. Flat or near flat, and non-monotonic growth functions have been reported (for example, Lonsbury Martin et al, 1990; Prieve et al., 1997).

Thirdly latency as a function of stimulus frequency can be investigated. A monotonic decrease in latency is expected as stimulus and generator site become more basal with increasing stimulus frequency. Deviations from this pattern are likely to be caused by the lack of emission energy and therefore may suggest a degree of cochlear degradation.

Summary

- Distortion product otoacoustic emissions are produced in response to two or more primary tones and take the form of narrow-band energy at frequencies algebraically related to the primaries. The highest amplitude DPOAE in humans is 2f1 – f2.
- A frequency ratio of f2 to f1 of ~1.2 and a level difference of L1-L2 of ~10 dB tends to favour maximum response amplitude of the 2f1-f2 product.
- They are present in almost all normal ears.
- They can be elicited over the frequency range 0.5 to 8 kHz.
- The pattern of responses in an ear is stable over time.

Stimulus frequency OAEs

Stimulus frequency OAEs are a steady-state response produced at frequencies of the eliciting tonal stimulus (Figure 7.11). They are recordable as additional energy present along with the stimulus tone in the ear canal. They are probably the least studied of the major OAE classes. This is probably partly to be due to the technical difficulties inherent in recording them as the stimulus and response are not separated either by frequency (cf. DPOAEs) or time (cf. TEOAEs).

The eliciting stimulus is typically a pure tone that is swept in frequency at a rate of several Hz per second. Vector summation (taking into account the phase of the signal and response) is carried out. This requires the use of specialized equipment such as a lock-in amplifier. Both the phase and magnitude of the ear canal signal can be examined as a function of stimulus frequency. Linear effects of ear canal resonances can be cancelled by scaling techniques. Non-linear maxima and minima

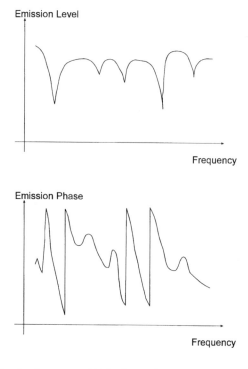

Figure 7.11. Stimulus frequency OAE schematic.

in the magnitude recorded indicate the presence of SFOAEs. In similarity with other classes of OAEs the pattern produced is unique to the ear under test.

Evidence has been presented that SFOAEs are generated at particular sites along the cochlear partition (Kemp and Chum, 1980; Zwicker and Schloth, 1984). Phase interactions between the responses generated at these sites and the stimulus tone are thought to give rise to the pattern of minima and maxima observed.

The frequency spacing of maxima and minima increases with increasing stimulus frequency (Zwicker and Schloth, 1984; Lonsbury-Martin et al., 1990) and seem to show a similarity to psychoacoustic critical bandwidth measures (Zwicker and Schloth, 1984; Dallmayr, 1987). Phase measurements have indicated that SFOAEs have latencies in the region of 10–12 ms (Kemp and Chum, 1980; Kemp and Brown, 1983). Stimulus frequency OAE amplitudes between –20 and +10 dB SPL are typical (Kemp and Chum, 1980; Dallmayr, 1987). As with other OAEs, saturation effects are apparent with increasing stimulus levels (Zwicker and Schloth, 1984; Probst, Lonsbury-Martin and Martin, 1991).

Stimulus frequency OAEs appear to be present in the vast majority of normally hearing ears – 93% to 94% according to Probst, Lonsbury-Martin and Martin, 1991 – although it is possible that this figure may actually be higher given the inherent technical difficulties in recording SFOAEs.

Summary

- Stimulus frequency OAEs are elicited by pure-tone stimuli and take the form of additional acoustic energy present in the ear canal at the same frequency as the stimulus.
- They are present in the majority of normal ears.
- Amplitudes of –10 to +20 dB SPL are reported.

Evidence for site of origin/mechanism

There was much initial scepticism regarding the proposal that a physiological mechanism within the cochlea was responsible for OAE production. It was assumed by many that OAEs originated artefactually, from the recording apparatus, from the middle ear, or from neural activity.

Recording artefacts such as ear-canal resonances, or 'ringing' of transient stimuli (and passive mechanical responses), would demonstrate linear behaviour – for a given increase in stimulus level, a similar increase in response level should be observed. As has been described above, OAEs demonstrate non-linear features.

Middle-ear muscle activity can also be ruled out as otoacoustic emissions can be produced at stimulus levels well below those required to initiate this muscle activity. Moreover, the administration of muscle relaxing drugs does not abolish OAE responses (Evans, Wilson and Boerwe, 1981 demonstrated this in the guinea pig). General anaesthetic and muscle relaxant administration in humans also does not abolish OAE responses (Probst and Beck, 1987). Other OAE characteristics such as long latencies, saturation and frequency dispersion cannot be explained in terms of the known vibratory properties of the middle-ear system (Probst, Lonsbury-Martin and Martin, 1991).

Neural responses can be shown to adapt at high stimulation rates – a phenomenon not shown by OAEs (for example, Kemp, 1978). In addition OAEs can be elicited at stimulus levels below psychoacoustic detection thresholds, again countering the proposal of a neural origin for OAEs (for example, Kemp, 1978; Bonfils, Bertrand and Uziel, 1988).

A cochlear origin for OAEs is supported by the finding that insults to the cochlea such as excessive acoustic stimulation and ototoxic drugs can degrade or abolish emission responses. Administration of salicylate has been shown to both produce reversible sensorineural hearing loss and degrade SOAEs and DPOAEs (Wier et al., 1988) as well as TEOAEs (Johnsen and Elberling, 1982).

Sound exposures that produce temporary threshold shifts also reduce OAEs and these show complex recovery patterns similar to psychoacoustic threshold recovery (for example, Norton et al., 1989). Animal studies have shown that prolonged exposure inducing permanent hearing loss also degrades OAE responses. Hypoxia and anoxia also degrade OAE responses.

Spontaneous OAEs and TEOAEs are absent at frequencies where there is hearing loss greater than 25 to 35 dB HL, but can be present in the same ear for frequencies where there is better sensitivity. Suppression effects on OAE responses also show fine frequency tuning very similar in nature to cochlear frequency selectivity (Clark et al., 1984).

Having accepted that OAEs are cochlear in origin, the next question to ask is why they occur at all. Bekesy demonstrated the frequency tuning of the passive cochlear, showing that stimulation by a tone of given frequency caused maximum mechanical activity at a particular point on the basilar membrane. The frequency resolution shown in these experiments can be modelled adequately using passive mechanics. Subsequent research into psychophysical frequency selectivity, neural tuning curves and physiological research of healthy cochleae has demonstrated much finer frequency resolution; so fine that no passive mechanical model of the cochlea to date can entirely replicate this resolution. Models where an active source of mechanical energy is allowed can achieve the required resolution. The requirement for a cochlear energy source was posited as early as the 1940s by Gold. The addition of an active energy source immediately introduces the possibility of energy transference back to the ear canal. The presence of an energy source also accounts for non-linearity and helps to explain the observation that emissions at a given frequency with greater energy than the input stimulus can occur, as well as SOAEs.

A growing body of evidence supports the outer hair cell (OHC) as the site of origin of this active process, and therefore OAEs. Innervation of the cochlea is not only afferent: efferent fibres from the crossed olivocochlear bundle predominantly terminate on OHCs. Stimulation of this efferent system has been shown to reduce DPOAEs in animals. Puel and Rebillard (1990) demonstrated that section of this efferent system abolished this effect.

Outer hair cells demonstrate electromotility. Electrical stimulation of isolated hair cells *in vitro* can produce reversible shape changes (Ashmore and Brownell, 1986). Depending on the polarity of stimulation, active reductions or increases over a 'resting' length are brought about. This distinguishes them from muscle cells in which only contracting phases produce force. A further distinction is that OHC electromotility can be observed at high frequencies, well into the audio frequency range where OAEs are found (Evans, 1988; Evans et al., 1989). Such rapid rates are not observed for muscle cells.

Electromotility also displays non-linearity, necessary to account for some OAE phenomena such as DPOAEs. Under certain stimulus conditions, *in vitro* and with high stimulation frequencies, OHC elongation saturates and shortening dominates (Evans, 1988; Evans et al., 1989). It is likely that these conditions also exist *in vivo* (Brownell, 1996). The arrangement of the OHCs and supporting cells in the organ of Corti is commensurate with allowing the forces created by the OHC to be transmitted to the cochlear partition and thus provide a positive mechanical feedback that can amplify responses close to threshold (Brownell, 1996). The non-linearity generated could be transmitted back to the ear canal as energy at the stimulus frequency – a SOAE. There is inherent instability in high gain systems. The presence of three rows of OHCs in humans may reflect a compromise between the required stability and overloading the basilar membrane with excess mass (Brownell, 1996).

It is beyond the scope of this chapter to illustrate the detailed theoretical mechanisms of OAE production. The reader is referred to the reference list.

Summary

- Evidence suggests that OAEs are generated within the cochlear, with OHCs playing an integral role.
- The efferent innervation of OHCs is shown to be important to the generation of OAEs.
- The electromotility displayed by OHCs is consistent with providing the additional energy and hence non-linearities associated with OAE phenomena.

Age-related differences in OAEs

A number of findings in relation to age effects are discussed below for the various classes of OAEs. To date SFOAEs have only been widely studied in younger adults and do not address age effects. On the whole the characteristics of OAEs found in adults are largely mirrored in the findings from children, infants and neonates. Differences are generally relatively subtle changes in OAE frequency content and amplitude.

Spontaneous OAEs

Some studies have reported a lower prevalence of SOAEs in infants (for example, Bargones and Burns, 1988). However the likelihood of less favourable recording conditions as a factor in this can not be discounted. Other studies have occasionally found a higher prevalence in infant ears (Bonfils, Uziel and Narcy, 1989), or similar prevalence in infant ears (for example, Burns et al., 1992). Ageing effects have also been noted. Bonfils (1989) reported no OAEs in ears >70 years, and reduced prevalence in ears between 50 and 69 years. Lonsbury-Martin et al. (1991) showed that the number of SOAE frequencies present in ears decreased with increasing age.

Transient evoked OAEs

Prevalence rates similar to those for adults have been recorded in neonatal populations; for example, Elberling et al. (1985) – 100%; Stevens et al. (1987) – 100%; Dolhen et al. (1991) – 95%. For graduates of neonatal intensive care units, many of whom have low gestational ages, lower incidences are reported; for example, Stevens et al. (1987) – 81%, Stevens et al. (1990) – 82%. Stevens et al. (1990) proposed that this may be due to a number of factors; a higher incidence of sensorineural hearing loss in this population, middle-ear disorder and difficulty in obtaining good probe coupling in small/unusually shaped external auditory meati.

Neonates have higher amplitude TEOAEs compared to adults and older children (Norton, 1993, 1994). Johnsen, Parbo and Elberling (1989) compared TEOAE amplitude at birth to age four years in the same subject group. Less energy was found as the subjects became older. Spektor et al. (1991) found that TEOAE levels in children (four to 10 years) was higher than in an adult group. Norton and Widen (1990) discovered significant differences in TEOAE amplitude across an age range of 17 days to 30 years.

Prieve et al. (1997) showed that higher amplitudes overall are demonstrated by subjects less than one year old in terms of TEOAE input/output functions. A progressive decrease in amplitude for ages up to and above 17 years was shown. They proposed developmental changes in the external auditory meatus and middle-ear system are factors.

Differences in OAE frequency spectra have also been noted. Johnsen et al. (1989) found less high-frequency energy in OAEs in subjects age four years compared to neonates, and that the dominant regions in the spectrum shifted to lower frequencies as age increased. Kemp, Ryan and Bray (1990) reported OAEs in neonates covering a greater frequency range than in adults. Similar findings were demonstrated by Uziel and Piron (1991).

The reasons for these differences are still unclear. As mentioned above, developmental changes in the external and middle ear are possible factors. Developmental changes in the cochlea are less likely as studies have suggested that cochleae at 40 conceptual weeks are largely mature (see, for example, Abdala 1996; Gorga et al., 1989), although this cannot be entirely ruled out. Other possibilities put forward include 'wear and tear' on the cochlea due to typical environmental noise or toxin exposure.

Distortion product OAEs

The findings in DPOAEs are complicated by the fact that there are a greater number of stimulus parameters to consider. Some studies have suggested that DPOAEs in neonates are qualitatively similar to those in adults, but amplitude is different for some frequency regions (see, for example, Smurzynski et al., 1993; Lasky et al., 1992). The frequency region of the effect and its sign differs between studies. Bergman et al. (1995) reported higher DPOAE amplitude in neonates compared to adults over mid to high frequency ranges. Prieve et al. (1997) report a frequency-dependent effect on DPOAE amplitude (as examined by in/out functions), with children <1 year having greater amplitude than children of one to three years who, in turn, showed greater amplitude compared to adults. The effect was not dependent on stimulus level. Lasky (1998) reported frequency-dependent amplitude differences in neonates compared to adults, with higher amplitudes at certain frequency regions.

The available data suggest that, overall, DPOAE amplitude tends to decrease with increasing age to adulthood, at least over some frequency ranges.

Lasky (1998) reported some differences between in/out functions, with neonates showing saturation at lower primary levels compared to adults. However qualitatively overall in/out functions were similar to those seen in adults.

Summary

- Otoacoustic emissions display age-related effects.
- The type of effect varies slightly for different OAE classes and between studies, but a general trend of greater emission energy for lower ages can be identified.
- Otoacoustic emission responses seem to degrade with increasing age beyond young adulthood.

Otoacoustic emissions in hearing loss

Conductive hearing loss

The middle-ear system plays an important role in acoustic emissions. The middle-ear system is required not only to transmit the stimulus successfully (where used) to the inner ear, but also to perform the reverse role of transmitting energy from the cochlea back to the ear canal. As would be expected, the literature suggests that degradation in middle-ear function can degrade or abolish otoacoustic emissions. Kemp (1978), Decreton, Hanssens and De Sloovere (1991) and Koike and Wetmore (1999) demonstrated that in cases where middle-ear compliance was low, emissions could not be recorded. Experimentally induced positive and negative middle-ear pressures have been shown to degrade emission responses, with greater effects for lower frequencies (Robinson and Haughton, 1991; Veuillet, Collet and Morgon, 1992; Naeve et al., 1993; and Kemp, Ryan and Bray, 1990). Compensation of abnormal middle-ear pressure by introducing pressure change in the ear canal has been shown to increase emission amplitude (Trine, Hirsch and Margolis, 1993), and reduce middle-ear pressure effects on TEOAE spectra (Marshall, Heller and Westhusin, 1997). Significant changes in TEOAE spectra for relatively small amounts of negative middle-ear pressure have been demonstrated and TEOAE reliability has been shown to be compromised by negative middle-ear pressures of as little as –60 to –75 daPa (Marshall, Heller and Westhusin, 1997).

The evidence suggests that diagnostic interpretation of OAEs requires tympanometric data. This has some bearing on situations where neonates or very young infants are being tested. Standard low frequency probe tone tympanometry can give misleading results in the very young ear (Marchant et al., 1986; Holte et al., 1991). A degree of correspondence between high-frequency tympanometry and TEOAE findings has been reported by McKinley, Grose and Roush (1997). A strong relationship between tympanometry with a 678 Hz probe tone and OAE findings was reported by Sutton, Gleadle and Rowe (1996) in neonates.

In the authors' clinic some examples have been found where TEOAEs were identifiable even in ears with flat (type D) tympanograms. It would therefore be unwise to use the presence of OAEs as an indicator of entirely normal middle-ear function.

The presence of grommets or ventilation tubes can also affect OAEs. Cullington et al. (1998) were able to record OAEs in only 32% of children following grommet insertion, although the vast majority had normal hearing sensitivity demonstrated through behavioural testing at follow-up. Koike and Wetmore (1999) were able to demonstrate OAEs in 60% of cases with patent grommets. Otoacoustic emission recordings performed shortly after surgery could be affected by threshold shifts due to the noise of suctioning or mechanical trauma. However possible effects of a grommet on the reverse transmission of energy from the cochlea cannot be entirely discounted.

Summary

- Relatively minor middle-ear pathology can degrade or abolish OAEs.
- Independent assessment of middle-ear status is required for diagnostic interpretation of OAE results.

Sensorineural hearing loss

Given the cochlear origin of OAEs, it is reasonable to assume that cases where hearing loss is due to damage to the cochlea, OAEs recorded from that ear will be degraded or absent. This is indeed demonstrated in the literature, and is generally true for all classes of emissions. Due to the difficulties in recording SFOAEs, their properties in hearing impaired ears have been less studied. Different recording and classification techniques between researchers, as well as inter-subject variability, make it difficult to identify an exact level or configuration of hearing loss that will cause a specific degradation of OAEs. However examination of the literature indicates a general trend for increasing hearing loss to increase the likelihood of degradation or absence of an emission. There is also a trend for frequency specificity across the emission types, i.e. greater hearing loss at a given frequency reduces the likelihood of detecting emission energy at this frequency. This however is much less well defined than the trend for increasing degree of hearing loss.

As a general rule, the presence of an OAE indicates the presence of normal or near normal hearing sensitivity for at least some frequency regions.

Otoacoustic emissions depend primarily on cochlear function. It is therefore important to bear in mind that cases of retrocochlear hearing loss could be expected to exhibit OAEs. Ferguson et al. (1996) were able to detect OAEs in 53% of ears with confirmed retrocochlear lesions (CPA tumours). It is likely in the remainder of cases that a cochlear component to the hearing loss was present, possibly caused by interruption of the vascular supply or cochlear innervation. The detection of OAEs in the presence of reliable data indicating hearing loss must therefore raise the suspicion of retrocochlear pathology. Conversely, the absence of OAEs in the presence of hearing loss cannot be used to rule out a retrocochlear component.

A further point of importance is that, although OAE testing can identify the presence of hearing loss, it does not quantify the degree of loss. Thus mild to profound hearing losses could exhibit similar results on an OAE test.

Spontaneous OAEs

Examples of ears where there is significant hearing loss, in the presence of detectable SOAEs have been documented (Zurek, 1981; Probst et al., 1987). Only high-level emissions have been documented at frequencies where there are losses greater than 30 dB HL (for example, Glanville et al., 1971). In general, as discussed above, normal hearing sensitivity is predicted for frequencies where low-level SOAEs are detectable. However, as SOAEs are only present in a high proportion of, rather then nearly all, ears classed as normal their absence does not necessarily indicate any pathology.

It is rare for a spontaneous emission to be associated with troublesome tinnitus. Zurek (1981), Penner and Burns (1987) and Bonfils (1989) could not find any general associations of tinnitus with SOAEs, and observed a lack of correlation between tinnitus pitch match and SOAE frequency. There is evidence that at least some cases of tinnitus may have correlation with SOAEs: Penner (1988) reported the case of a subject in which suppression of the SOAEs reduced the audibility of the tinnitus. Administration of aspirin in sufficient quantity to reduce SOAE amplitude can also reduce tinnitus perception (Penner and Coles, 1992). Penner (1990) estimated that only approximately 4% of troublesome tinnitus is related to SOAEs. However Ceranic, Prasher and Luxon (1998) showed that tinnitus sufferers demonstrated greater variability in the frequency structure of SOAEs compared to a control group.

Transient evoked OAEs

Kemp (1978) found that TEOAEs were absent in cases of sensorineural hearing loss >30 dB HL. Rutten (1980) demonstrated that, in ears with high-frequency losses, emissions could be detected, but the dominant frequencies in the OAE spectra related to frequencies where thresholds were 15 dB HL or better. Where mean thresholds across 0.5, 1 2 and 4 kHz are greater than around 35 dB HL, OAEs are not detectable (Kemp et al., 1986; Cope and Lutman, 1993). Lutman (1989) demonstrated that, in virtually all cases where the best two average of audiometric thresholds was less than 25 dB HL, an emission was nearly always present. Kapadia and Lutman (1997) showed from a large dataset (n = 397) that 99.2% with normal thresholds (≤20 dB HL across audiometric frequencies to 4 kHz) had detectable OAEs as defined by a cross-correlation method. Furthermore, expert observer analysis of the remainder of waveforms yielded evidence that an OAE was probably present in these cases.

The detection threshold for the OAE stimulus itself has also been examined. Stevens and Ip (1988) showed that, for a click stimulus, a threshold of 18 dB nHL or better was required for OAE detection. Bonfils and Uziel (1989) were not able to record OAEs where click threshold was 35 dB nHL or worse. Hauser, Probst and Lohle (1991) indicated that where an OAE was present threshold for at least one frequency was better than 30 dB HL.

Several conclusions are possible from the data:

- the detection of an OAE depends on the method of OAE classification, recording conditions and technique, and definition criteria for the hearing loss;
- a cut-off level of hearing loss exists above which an OAE will not be detectable;
- Virtually all audiometrically normal ears will demonstrate detectable OAEs.

The spectra of the click-evoked OAE does not predict the audiometric configuration well. This may be partly due to the wide inter-subject variability. Collet et al. (1991) demonstrated that better hearing at higher frequencies in a subject increased the likelihood of high frequency components in the OAE. However the absence of OAE energy at a given frequency cannot be used to infer audiometric threshold at that point (Probst et al., 1987; Cope and Lutman, 1993). The absence does not predict that hearing threshold at that point is greater than normal or near normal.

More recent research by Vinck et al. (1998) has shown promise for greater predictive power in terms of degree and configuration of hearing loss using TEOAEs. Using multivariate analysis techniques of both click-evoked and tone-burst OAEs, predictions of thresholds over audiometric frequencies 0.5 to 4 kHz were accurate to within approximately 10 dB for losses up to 60 dB HL in a patient population. The authors acknowledge that the process is much more time consuming than standard TEOAE testing and thus of limited applicability in the paediatric population. Their findings are contrary to the majority of the literature, but the study is relatively unique in using both tone-burst and click-evoked OAEs.

Distortion product OAEs

Kemp et al. (1986) reported results in patients with high frequency losses that suggested DPOAE amplitude is diminished in regions where there was hearing loss. Kimberley and Nelson (1989) reported very good agreement between degradation in DPOAE amplitude and auditory threshold. Harris (1990) using DPOAE in/out functions reported that thresholds of 15 dB HL or better were always associated with detectable OAEs, and thresholds in excess of 50 dB HL were associated with absent or attenuated OAEs. Despite these overall good reported agreements, there is still considerable variability in findings in pathological ears. Probst and Harris (1997), considering the evidence from a range of researchers, conclude that DPOAE testing cannot replace conventional tests of hearing sensitivity. The evidence suggests a similar conclusion to that for TEOAEs: the presence of a DPOAE is indicative of normal or near normal hearing sensitivity for the frequencies under consideration, there is a cut-off point in terms of hearing threshold above which OAEs are abolished. The absence of a DPOAE for the frequencies considered should raise the suspicion of a degree of hearing loss.

Summary

- For cochlear hearing losses greater loss has greater likelihood of abolishing or degrading OAE responses. As a rule of thumb, dependent on the recording parameters used, the presence of an OAE indicates normal or close to normal cochlear sensitivity.
- A trend for frequency specificity is observed. The absence of OAE energy at a given frequency raises a degree of suspicion regarding the hearing sensitivity at that frequency.

Suppression effects

Suppression is a phenomenon widely studied in the field of psychoacoustics and neural responses to sound stimuli. Here suppression describes an effect where the introduction of a second stimulus to an original stimulus reduces the activity level (or audibility) resulting as compared with the activity level when the original stimulus is presented alone. In the case of OAEs, most researchers use suppression to refer to effects where the introduction of an acoustic stimulus (in addition to the eliciting stimulus where required) reduces the amplitude of OAEs. Suppression effects on measures of OAE latency have also been described (Figure 7.12). Suppression stimuli can be presented to the test ear (ipsilateral suppression), to the opposite ear (contralateral suppression), or binaurally. Where

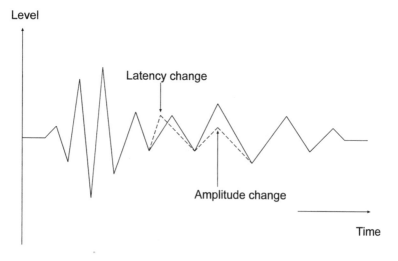

Figure 7.12. Suppression effects.

suppression stimuli are presented contralaterally, it is important to be aware of possible acoustic crosstalk to the test ear, and in all cases possible middle-ear reflex effects must be considered.

Suppression is thought to be mediated by the efferent neural pathways, with involvement of the olivocochlear system. Therefore examination of suppression effects can lead to inferences regarding the status of these central hearing pathways.

Again there is less evidence from studies involving SFOAEs, and the majority of studies focus on TEOAEs.

Probst, Lonsbury-Martin and Martin (1991) conclude that suppression effects on SOAEs follow the well-documented characteristics of psychophysical suppression as measured through tuning curves. The most efficient suppression effects are from acoustic stimuli of slightly higher frequency than the SOAE (Dallmayr, 1987). More rapid growth in suppression effect with suppressor stimulus level is seen for stimulus frequencies lower than the SOAE under observation (Rabinowitz and Widin, 1984). The suppressed SOAE generally reappears with a latency of approximately 5.5 ms and grows exponentially to return to its original value (Schloth and Zwicker, 1983). More intense suppression stimuli produce effects similar to those seen in temporary threshold shift studies (Probst, Lonsbury-Martin and Martin, 1991).

In the case of TEOAEs, similar suppression effects as seen in SOAEs have been documented by several researchers (for example, Wit and Ritsma, 1980; Schloth, 1982). Masking effects on TEOAE responses similar to psychophysical phenomena have been demonstrated (for example, Zwicker et al., 1987). Similar suppression findings are also reported for DPOAEs (for example, Brown and Kemp, 1984).

A complex pattern of supression effects occurs depending on parameters such as site of suppressor stimulation (ipsi/contra/binaural), suppressor level and duration, eliciting stimulus level, type of suppressor (for example, tone/broad-band noise), and temporal separation of suppressor and click onset. On the whole, suppressor parameters with greater overall suppressor energy tend to favour increased suppression effects.

In the case of TEOAEs, binaural suppressors show greater effects than ipsilateral suppressors, which in turn show more effect than contralateral suppressors (Berlin et al., 1995).

Hood et al. (1993) and Collet et al. (1990) have reported on the effect of contralateral acoustic stimulation on TEOAEs. Small but consistent reductions in response amplitude of around 1–2 dB were noted. Hood et al. (1996) note that the magnitude of supression effects both on latency and amplitude are variable between subjects but that all normally hearing subjects demonstrate some suppression. Increasing the level of contralateral suppressor increases suppression amplitude and broadens the latency range over which suppression occurs. Other latency changes are also described. The addition of a contralateral suppressor causes peaks and/or zero crossings in the OAE waveform to occur earlier than if no suppressor is used. This is referred to as a 'negative time delay'. Increasing suppressor levels causes earlier latencies to become involved. Hood et al. (1993) report that these suppression effects show good test-retest reliability. Maximal suppression effects occur for response latencies of 8 ms to 18 ms, and some subjects only show suppression effects over narrow latency ranges.

Starr et al. (1996) have presented cases where subjects with auditory neuropathy demonstrate little effect of suppressors on OAE responses. It is envisaged that further study of suppression effects could lead to the development of clinic tests that aid the differentiation of peripheral and central auditory disorder.

Summary

- Suppression in OAEs is manifest as changes in the phase or level of OAE components.
- Suppression is mediated by higher auditory pathways, as demonstrated by contralateral suppression.

Application of OAE testing in the paediatric clinic

The lower prevalence of SOAEs compared to other OAE classes, and the inherent technical difficulties (and lack of commercial equipment) with recording SFOAEs leads to the conclusion that TEOAEs and DPOAEs are the most applicable to the testing of a paediatric population, at least for the present. The advantage of TEOAEs in simultaneously providing information over a wide frequency range can not be overlooked, and this is the most widely clinically employed OAE test.

Given the lack of absolutely clear-cut relationships of OAEs to hearing sensitivity, it is important that the clinician has a full understanding of the scientific underpinning of the test regime adopted, including an awareness of its potential pitfalls.

In diagnostic applications, for the reasons outlined above, OAE results should always be interpreted in the light of other results from the chosen test battery. For example the absence of OAEs in the presence of raised sound-field or air conduction behavioural thresholds and normal middle-ear function is indicative of a cochlear hearing loss. However if tympanometric or other data indicates a conductive element no information regarding cochlear status can be inferred from the absence of an OAE.

It is advantageous to obtain tympanometric data prior to OAE testing. Where middle-ear function is compromised the value of even attempting OAE testing is debatable.

It is desirable to carry out testing in an area with minimal background noise. However, soundproofing to audiometric standard is not required. A quiet office room will usually suffice. Rhoades et al. (1998) reported the effects of background noise on TEOAEs. Parameters including wave reproducibility were significantly affected only once room noise began to exceed 50 dB A to 55 dB A. In the paediatric population the noise sources are usually principally from the child i.e. breathing, movement and vocalizations.

The stiller and quieter the subject, the better, and it is advantageous for the child to be asleep. In the authors' clinic if a child is asleep when brought into the clinic, otoacoustic emission testing may be carried out before other tests. Patience is often required in allowing the child to settle down. Many younger children will often sleep if left alone with their parents in a quiet room for some time, allowing a window of opportunity for testing.

The coupling of the probe to the ear is very important. Most equipment uses disposable probe tips of varying sizes. A poor fit can introduce background noise and/or promote stimulus ringing. In some commercial equipment there is a facility to monitor the quality of the probe fit. If the fit is unsatisfactory readjustment may be required. The absence of a measurable probe signal indicates that the probe tip is against the ear canal wall, or is blocked with wax, or there is another malfunction of the equipment.

Some commercial systems allow a degree of intervention by the operator during testing. This can be to alter the rejection levels for noise or to pause recording if, for example, the child becomes active or noisy. With experience the clinician can monitor the recording and adjust parameters as required to minimize the test time required, or obtain a useable test result in the presence of adverse recording conditions.

Some TEOAE test equipment offers screening paradigms that can be more robust to noise (Rhoades et al., 1998) and reduce test time. This is often at the expense of obtaining some information, for example reducing the frequency range tested, by manipulating the time windowing of the response, so allowing more stimulus presentation per unit time. Alternatively, or in addition, more extreme low cut filtering can be used, to reduce background noise effects but this can reduce energy from low frequency emissions. The clinician must determine if such adjustments are necessary, and then interpret the response accordingly.

The range of possible application of OAEs is very wide. There are a numerous scenarios where OAE testing is particularly useful. The most common in the authors' clinic is in the testing of children with a low developmental age, or with other problems that prevent reliable determination of behavioural threshold data. Sometimes in these cases it is possible to obtain repeatable but suprathreshold response levels from behavioural observation. Coupled with good OAE results this provides good evidence of a normally functional hearing pathway. Some aspects of higher auditory function can also be investigated without behavioural responses using for example, acoustic reflex testing.

Otoacoustic emission testing can also help in cases of suspected non-organic hearing loss. Where there is suspicion of a non-organic component, and there is normal middle-ear function, otoacoustic emission testing can help to resolve this. Caution should be exercised, however, as the presence of an OAE cannot rule out retrocochlear pathology. It is also possible that a mild loss sufficient to abolish an OAE is being exaggerated.

In the author's clinic it is considered desirable to routinely follow-up patients in most cases where hearing status indication is predominantly given by OAE testing alone. This is considered necessary due to the variable degree of frequency specificity exhibited by OAEs and their possible detection in milder hearing impairments. This does not detract from the usefulness of positive OAE results in reassuring patients/parents and in helping to determine an appropriate interval for follow-up, when the child may be mature enough to allow reliable behavioural testing to be carried out. In the case of negative OAE results and the absence of good behavioural data, further testing, such as an auditory brainstem response test, is indicated.

With hearing aid users and cochlear implant candidates OAEs can be used as a first-line screening test (coupled with diagnostic imaging and other tests as required) to help confirm the absence of retrocochlear pathology. As mentioned above, with further development, tests of suppression effects may further aid the differentiation of cochlear and retrocochlear disorders.

Interpretation

In common with other audiological tests often defined as 'objective', there is a degree of subjectivity in interpreting the results of an OAE test. However the availability of correlation scores or statistical analysis of the noise floor can reduce the degree of subjectivity. It is of course highly important that the clinician takes into account all factors in interpreting OAE results: not just waveform appearance, recording conditions and machine scoring but also other test results, case history and so on. It is vitally important that the clinician be able to incorporate OAE results into the wider clinical picture before any management decisions are reached.

Characteristics of 'good' OAE responses are given below:

1. Emission energy is present with levels significantly above the noise floor.
2. Emission energy is present over a wide frequency range (not necessarily for SOAEs).
3. Applicable replicate measures show a high degree of correlation.
4. The stimulus has been stable throughout testing.
5. Recording conditions have not been too noisy.

An absent or 'poor' response is indicated by the opposite of points 1 to 3 above. However, in this case, if conditions 4 and 5 are not met, the lack of an emission response may be simply due to poor recording conditions, perhaps indicating the test should be repeated.

Transient evoked OAEs

With computer-based recording it is possible to obtain replicate measures by storing alternate responses in separate computer buffers. The degree of cross correlation between buffers can be analysed. Higher levels of cross correlation indicate repeatable responses, or 'genuine' emissions. Background noise is predominantly random in nature and not timelocked to the stimulus. Therefore this shows a low degree of correlation. Cross correlation can be obtained either on the entirety of the accepted data, or carried out after the response has been filtered into different frequency bands. Signal-to-noise ratio is also usually available. Again, the better (higher) this is, the greater the likelihood that a true emission response has been detected. Some commercial equipment allows the stability of the stimulus to be monitored throughout a test. A high degree of stability is desirable. Where stability has been too variable a repeat test is indicated. In general a 'good' emission response requires high stimulus stability, and high signal-to-noise ratio coupled with high cross correlation scores. Examination of the waveforms from each buffer is also important. These should ideally show a high degree of similarity across all latencies. Waveforms showing high correlation only over very early latencies should be treated with some suspicion as stimulus artefacts may influence these latencies. Examples of a 'good' and absent TEOAE are given in Figures 7.13 and 7.14.

A positive OAE response across a broad frequency range is indicative of normal or near normal hearing sensitivity. A completely absent response suggests hearing impairment of mild or greater degree. A partial response with OAE energy only at a limited frequency range should raise the suspicion of degree of hearing loss at some frequencies.

Distortion product OAEs

Interpretation of DPOAE findings is obviously dependent on the test paradigm adopted. The most widely applied paradigm in DPOAE testing is the DP audiogram method (see above). Interpretation is analogous to that for TEOAEs. This method uses repeated stimulus sweeps to determine the level of any DPOAE above the noise floor. Statistical analysis is usually available to determine how likely the signal is to be 'genuine' or due to chance in terms of its amplitude above the noise floor. As with

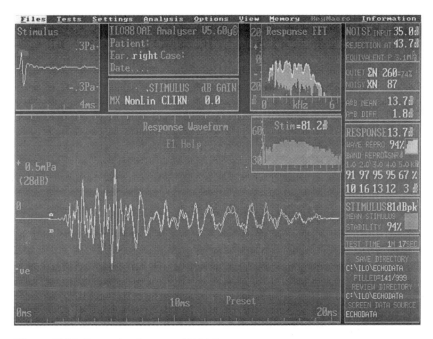

Figure 7.13. Example of present TEOAE.

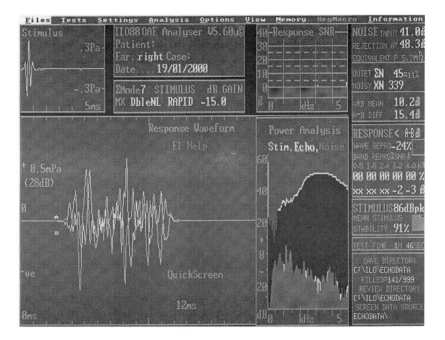

Figure 7.14. Example of absent TEOAE.

TEOAEs good responses across a wide frequency range are consistent with normal or near normal hearing sensitivity. Completely absent responses suggest hearing impairment. Partial responses for limited frequency ranges must raise suspicion of a degree of hearing loss at some frequencies.

Definitive comments on interpretation of the other DPOAE paradigms are more difficult as they are less studied and less routinely employed. Stimulus/response in/out functions that differ from those described above should raise suspicion, particularly where no emission is detected until stimulus levels are high (~60–70 dB SPL). Latency functions departing from monotonicity are also suspicious as this suggests that latency could not be determined, possibly due to absence of OAE energy at the point in question.

Summary

- Otoacoustic emission testing can be useful in a wide range of clinical scenarios.
- Absent OAEs must raise suspicion of a degree of hearing loss. Other audiological tests are required to determine the nature and extent of any possible loss.
- Interpretation in light of the 'wider clinical picture' is necessary.

Neonatal screening

A screening programme can be defined as a procedure that effectively identifies a subset of the population with a high probability of having the condition that the screen is designed to identify. The set is then referred on for further diagnostic testing. The condition in question must be of significant importance to warrant the expense of a screening programme. The identification of a subset of the population avoids the prohibitive cost of applying diagnostic testing to the entire population. The effectiveness of a screening test is measured through two principle parameters: *sensitivity* – indicated by the percentage with the condition that correctly fail the test; and *specificity* – indicated by the percentage without the condition that correctly pass the test. The closer these are to 100%, the 'better', or more effective, the screening test. However increasing sensitivity (correctly finding more of those with the condition) usually comes at the expense of decreasing specificity and thus failing more of the population who don't have the condition and increasing the workload on the diagnostic test services.

The issue of screening the paediatric population for hearing loss has been widely debated. As this chapter is being written it is almost without doubt that a universal neonatal screening programme will eventually be adopted on a nationwide basis. Current estimates suggest the prevalence of significant congenital hearing impairment to be approximately 1 per 1,000 live births, yielding an estimated 840 born per year in the UK (Bamford and Davis, 1998).

Correlations exist between earlier diagnosis and better outcomes (reviewed in Davis et al., 1997). So far there is less available evidence to suggest that extremely early diagnosis produces even better outcomes, but there can be little doubt that late diagnosis and intervention leads to more negative outcomes, and a greater negative impact on the family and child. It therefore follows that the goal of a screening programme is to accurately identify the greatest possible number of hearing impaired children, at the earliest age possible, with the least possible cost. The NDCS 'quality standards in paediatric audiology' document (1994) sets a target for the early identification of permanent congenital hearing impairment (40% by age six months; 80% by age 12 months).

Current practice in the UK for most regions involves a universal Health Visitor Distraction Test (HVDT), carried out at around seven to eight months of age. There are somewhat varied reports of its effectiveness in the literature (Bamford and Davis, 1998; Wood, Davis and McCormick, 1997). With appropriate high-quality implementation, the test can yield good sensitivity (Davis and Wood, 1992) but poorer performance has been demonstrated in some regions (Sutton and Scanlon, 1999). Even with the best performance figures the HVDT will have obvious difficulties in meeting the NDCS target for the six-month age group.

In some regions the HVDT is combined with a targeted neonatal screening programme (Wood, Davis and McCormick, 1997). This selects neonates to undergo screening on the basis of risk factors such as family history and requirement for a neonatal intensive care unit stay. An alternative strategy sometimes employed is focused community/professional surveillance programmes, often referred to as 'vigilance', such as described by Scanlon and Bamford (1990).

The report of Davis et al. (1997) considered a number of options, including those above, which could possibly meet the NDCS target, and included analysis of the cost-benefit ratio. Their conclusion was that a universal neonatal screen is required as a core component of any programme to meet these goals. This would involve the vast majority of neonates undergoing the test before being discharged from hospital.

There are several key features desirable for a neonatal hearing screening test:

- high sensitivity and specificity, requiring a well defined cut-off point dividing normal and abnormal results;
- applicability to the entire population in question;
- required test time is short;
- minimally invasive and thus well tolerated by subjects;
- affordable both in terms of equipment costs and staffing costs
- the level of expertise required to administer the test should not be inordinate.

A comparison of the OAE types indicates that the CEOAE is the most suitable for large scale screening programmes. Stimulus frequency OAEs can be eliminated on the basis of the technical difficulties and time-consuming recording process. Spontaneous OAEs can be absent in too high a proportion of 'normal' ears. Distortion product OAEs would provide more frequency specific information, but this is at the cost of extra time to cover a wide frequency range. The CEOAE provides information simultaneously over a wide frequency range and as discussed above there exists a cut-off hearing threshold level above which responses are absent or identifiably degraded (approximately 30 dB HL). The CEOAE is also amenable to refinements in test paradigms that can reduce the required test time. For instance, if information from longer latency areas is considered less important for screening purposes, a more rapid click repetition rate can be employed. Frequency regions deemed less important for screening (for example, lower frequencies) can be filtered out resulting in lessened effects of background noise. In fact, click repetition rates can be increased even to the point of overlapping latencies of interest through the use of maximum length sequences (Thornton, Folkard and Chambers, 1994). With this technique the response waveform can be extracted (deconvolved) from the stimulus waveform where they are overlapping in time. The feasibility of applying this in neonates has been documented by Rasmussen et al. (1998).

The utility of the CEOAE as a screening tool has been well documented in terms of sensitivity, specificity, and so forth (Stevens et al., 1990; Cope and Lutman, 1993; Aidan, Avan and Bonfils, 1999). Aggregate machine-based cross correlation scores can be used (Cope and Lutman, 1993), removing the need for high level expert interpretation at the screening stage. Commercial screening equipment is available that can use this or related methods to provide an overall 'test score' that can be compared against a criterion of pass or fail. Buller and Lutman (1998) showed that artificial neural networks can also be used as an effective means of deciding on the presence or absence of OAE responses. At the screening level, then, highly expert knowledge of OAEs is not required as machine automation can effectively determine passed or failed tests.

In summary, CEOAEs meet the requirements of a neonatal screening test. Bamford and Davis (1998) suggest a universal screening procedure with TEOAEs forming a 'first line' screen for the majority of babies.

As a final point it is worth noting that there cannot be an instantaneous shift to universal neonatal screening. This would lead to the cohort of children already born but below the health visitor test age missing any form of screening, which is clearly unacceptable. Conversely the cost of running the two programmes in parallel for a transition period is likely to be prohibitive. At the time of writing this issue is not fully resolved.

Summary

- Current screening practice typically involves universal screening based on the health visitor distraction test at age 6-9 months.
- It is widely accepted that changing practice to a universal neonatal screen is required.
- Otoacoustic emissions and in particular CEOAEs are highly likely to play a key role in this.

Summary

Otoacoustic emission testing in its varied forms has been shown to be of high utility and effectiveness. The addition of OAE capabilities to the diagnostic clinic situation can be extremely useful in adding an objective, and usually rapid, test of cochlear function. As with any test, it is essential their results are interpreted in the light of the entire clinical picture. That OAEs will play a high-profile role in neonatal screening programmes is beyond doubt. Further advances in the study of suppression effects are likely to lead to the development of clinical tests of more central auditory function. They will also play an ongoing role in the study of the development of the auditory system.

Acknowledgement

Figures 7.6, 7.7, 7.8, 7.13 and 7.14 were produced using the Otodynamics ILO88 OAE Analyser software, version 5.6, (c) 1997 Otodynamics Limited.

References

Abdala C (1996) DPOAE amplitude as a function of f2/f1 frequency in humans. J Acoust Soc Am 100: 3726-40.

Aidan D, Avan P, Bonfils P (1999) Auditory screening in neonates by means of transient evoked otoacoustic emissions: a report of 2,842 recordings. Ann Otol Rhinol Laryngol 108: 525-31.

Antonelli A, Grandori F (1986) Long term stability, influence of the head position and modelling considerations for evoked otoacoustic emissions. Scand Audiol Suppl 25: 97-108.

Ashmore JF, Brownell WE (1986) Kilohertz movements induced by electrical stimulation in outer hair cells isolated from the guinea pig cochlea. J Physiol 377: 41.

Avan P, Bonfils P, Loth D, Narcy P, Trotoux J (1991) Quantitative assessment of human cochlear function by evoked otoacoustic emissions. Hear Res 52: 99-112.

Bamford J, Davis AC (1998) Neonatal hearing screening: a step towards better services for children and families. Br J Audiol 32: 1-6.

Bargones JY, Burns EM (1988) Suppression tuning for spontaneous otoacoustic emissions in infants and adults. J Acoust Soc Am 83: 1809-16.

Beattie RC, Jones RL (1998) Effects of relative levels of primary tones on distortion product otoacoustic emissions in normal hearing. Audiology 37: 187-97.

Bergman BM, Gorga MP, Neely ST, Kaminski JR, Beauchaine KL, Peters J (1995) Preliminary description of transient evoked and distortion product otoacoustic emissions from graduates of an intensive care nursery. J Am Acad Audiol 6: 150-62.

Berlin CI, Hood LJ, Hurley A, Wen H, Kemp DT (1995) Binaural noise suppresses linear click-evoked otoacoustic emissions more than ipsilateral or contralateral noise. Hear Res 59: 112-30.

Bonfils P (1989) Spontaneous otoacoustic emissions: clinical interest. Laryngoscope 99:752-6.

Bonfils P, Avan P (1992) Hearing Diagnostic Model Evaluation using Distortion Product Otoacoustic Emissions. Presented to Third International Symposium on Cochlear Mechanics and Otoacoustic Emissions, Rome.

Bonfils P, Bertrand Y, Uziel A (1988) Evoked otoacoustic emissions: normative data and presbyacucis. Audiology 27: 27-35.

Bonfils P, Uziel A (1989) Clinical applications of evoked acoustic emissions: results in normally hearing and hearing impaired subjects. Ann Otol Rhinol Laryngol 98: 326-31.

Bonfils P, Uziel A, Narcy P (1989) The properties of spontaneous and evoked emissions in neonates and children. A preliminary report. Arch Otorhinolaryngol 26: 249-51.

Braun M (1997) Frequency spacing of multiple spontaneous otoacoustic emissions shows relation to critical bands: a large scale cumulative study. Hear Res 114: 197-203.

Braun M (1998) Accurate binaural mirroring of spontaneous otoacoustic emissions suggest influence of time-locking in medial efferents. Hear Res 118: 129-38.

Bray P (1989) Click evoked otoacoustic emissions and the development of a clinical otoacoustic hearing test instrument. Doctoral thesis, University of London.

Brown AM, Kemp DT (1984) Suppressibility of the 2f1-f2 stimulated acoustic emissions in gerbil and man. Hear Res 13: 29-37.

Brownell WE (1996) Outer hair cell electromotility and otoacoustic emissions. In Berlin C (ed) Hair Cells and Hearing Aids. San Diego: Singular Publishing Co.

Buller G, Lutman ME (1998) Automatic classification of transiently evoked otoacoustic emissions using an artificial neural network. Br J Audiol 32: 235-47.

Burns E, Hoberg Arehart K, Campbell SL (1992) Prevalence of spontaneous otoacoustic emission in neonates. J Acoust Soc Am 91: 1571-5.

Ceranic BJ, Prasher DK, Luxon LM (1998) Presence of tinnitus indicated by variable spontaneous otoacoustic emissions. Audiol Neuro-otol 3(5): 332-44.

Clark WW, Kim DO, Zurek PM, Bohne BZ (1984) Spontaneous otoacoustic emissions in chinchilla ear canals: correlation with histopathology and supression by external tones. Hear Res 16: 299-314.

Collet L, Kemp DT, Veuillet E, Duclaux R, Moulin A, Morgon A (1990) Effect of contralateral auditory stimuli on active cochlear micro-mechanical properties in human subjects. Hear Res 43: 251-62.

Collet L, Veuillet E, Chanal JM, Morgon A (1991) Evoked otoacoustic emissions: correlations between spectrum analysis and audiogram. Audiol 30: 164-72.

Cope Y, Lutman ME (1993) Oto-acoustic emissions. In McCormick B (ed.) Paediatric Audiology 0-5 Years. 2 edn. London: Whurr, pp. 250-90.

Cullington HE, Kumar BU, Flood LM (1998) Feasibility of otoacoustic emissions as a hearing screen following grommet insertion. Br J Audiol 32: 57-62.

Dallmayr C (1987) Stationary and dynamic properties of simultaneous evoked otoacoustic emissions (SEOAE). Acustica 63: 243-55.

Davis A, Wood S (1992) The epidemiology of childhood hearing impairment: factors relevant to planning services. Br J Audiol 26: 77-90.

Davis A, Bamford B, Wilson J, Ramkalawan T, Forshaw M, Wright S (1997) A critical review of neonatal screening in the detection of congenital hearing impairment. Health Technol Assessment 1: 10.

Decreton SJRC, Hanssens K, De Sloovere M (1991) Evoked otoacoustic emissions in infant hearing screening. Int J Paed Otorhinolaryngol 21: 235-47.

Dijk van P, Wit HP (1987) The occurrence of click-evoked otoacoustic emissions (Kemp echoes) in normal hearing ears. Scand Audiol 16: 62–4.

Dolhen P, Hennaux C, Chantry P, Hennenbert D (1991) The occurrence of evoked otoacoustic emissions in a normal adult population and neonates. Scand Audiol 20: 203–4.

Elberling C, Parbo J, Johnsen NJ, Bagi P (1985) Evoked otoacoustic emissions: clinical applications. Acta Otolaryngol Suppl 421: 77–85.

Evans BN (1988) Asymmetries in outer hair cell electro-mechanical responses. Abstracts of the Midwinter Meeting of the Association for Research in Otolaryngology 11: 29.

Evans B, Dallos P, Hallworth R (1989) Asymmetries in motile responses of hair cells in simulated in vivo conditions. In Wilson JP, Kemp DT (eds) Cochlear Mechanisms Structure Function and Models. New York: Plenum Press, pp. 205–6.

Evans EF, Wilson JP, Borerwe TA (1981) Animal models of tinnitus. In Tinnitus, CIBA foundation symposium. London: Pitman, pp. 300–2.

Ferguson MA, Smith PA, Lutman ME, Mason S, Coles RRA, Gibbin KP (1996) Efficiency of tests used to screen for cerebello-pontine angle tumours: a prospective study. Br J Audiol 30: 159–76.

Glanville JD, Coles RRA, Sullivan BM (1971) A family with high-tonal objective tinnitus. J Laryngol Otol 85: 1–10.

Gorga MP, Kaminski J, Beauchaine K, Jestead W, Neely S (1989) Auditory brainstem responses from children three months to three years of age: normal patterns of response. J Speech Hear Res 32: 281–8.

Grandori F (1985) Nonlinear phenomena in click and tone burst evoked otoacoustic emissions. Audiology 24: 71–80.

Harris FP (1990) Distortion product otoacoustic emissions in humans with high frequency sensorineural hearing loss. J Speech Hear Res 33: 594–600.

Harris FP, Lonsbury-Martin BL, Stagner BB, Coats AC, Martin GK (1989) Acoustic distortion products in humans: systematic changes in amplitude as a function of f2/f1 ratio. J Acoust Soc Am 85: 220–9.

Hauser R, Probst R (1990) The influence of systematic primary tone level variation L2-L1 on the acoustic distortion product emission 2f1-f2 in normal human ears. J Acoust Soc Am 89: 280–6.

Hauser R, Probst R, Lohle R (1991) Click and tone burst evoked otoacoustic emissions in normally hearing ears and ears with high frequency sensorineural hearing loss. Eur Arch Oto-Rhino-Laryngol 248: 345–52.

Holte L, Margolis R, Cavanagh R (1991) Developmental changes in multifrequency tympanograms. Audiology 30: 1–24.

Hood LJ, Hurley A, Wen H, Berlin C I, Jackson DF (1993) A new view of contralateral suppression of transient evoked otoacoustic emissions. Abstracts of the sixteenth midwinter research meeting. Association for Research in Otolaryngology 18: 123.

Hood LJ, Berlin CI, Hurley A, Wen H (1996) Suppression of otoacoustic emissions in normal hearing individuals. In Berlin C (ed) Hair Cells and Hearing Aids. San Diego, CA: Singular Publishing Co.

Johnsen NJ, Elberling C (1982) Evoked acoustic emissions from the human ear II. Normative data in young adults and influence of posture. Scand Audiol 11: 69–77.

Johnsen NJ, Parbo J, Eleberling C (1989) Evoked acoustic emissions from the human ear. V. Developmental changes. Scand. Audiol. 18: 5962–75.

Kapadia S, Lutman ME (1997) Are normal hearing thresholds a sufficient condition for click-evoked otoacoustic emissions? J Acoust Soc Am 101: 3566-76.

Kemp DT (1978) Stimulated acoustic emissions from within the human auditory system. J Acoust Soc Am 64: 1386-91.

Kemp DT (1980) Towards a model for the origin of cochlear echoes. Hear Res 2: 533-48.

Kemp DT (1981) Physiologically active cochlear micromechanics – one source of tinnitus. In Tinnitus. CIBA Foundation Symposium. London: Pitman, pp. 300-2.

Kemp DT (1986) Otoacoustic emissions , travelling waves and cochlear mechanisms. Hear Res 22: 95-104.

Kemp DT, Bray P, Alexander L, Brown AM (1986) Acoustic emission cochleography - practical aspects. Scand Audiol Suppl 25: 71-95.

Kemp DT, Brown AM (1983) An integrated view of cochlear mechanical non-linearities observable from the ear canal. In E de Boer and MA Viergever (eds) Mechanics of Hearing. The Hague: Martinus Nijhoff.

Kemp DT, Chum RA (1980) Properties of the generator of stimulated acoustic emissions. Hear Res 2: 213-32.

Kemp DT, Ryan S, Bray P (1990) A guide to the effective use of otoacoustic emissions. Ear Hear 11: 93-105.

Kimberley BP, Nelson DA (1989) Distortion product emissions and sensorineural hearing loss. J Otolaryngol 18: 365-9.

Kohler W, Fritz W (1992) A long term observation of spontaneous otoacoustic emissions (SOAEs). Scand Audiol 21: 55-8.

Koike KJ, Wetmore SJ (1999) Interactive effects of the middle ear pathology and the associated hearing loss on transient-evoked otoacoustic emissions. Otolaryngol Head Neck Surg 121: 238-44.

Lasky RE (1998a) Distortion product otoacoustic emissions in human newborns. I. Frequency effects. J Acoust Soc Am 103: 981-91.

Lasky RE (1998b) Distortion product otoacoustic emissions in human newborns. II. Level effects. J Acoust Soc Am 103: 992-1000.

Lasky RE, Perlman J, Helcox KE (1992) Distortion product otoacoustic emissions input/output functions as a function of frequency in human adults. J Am Acad Audiol 5: 183-94.

Long GR, Tubis A, Jones K (1988) Modification of spontaneous and evoked otoacoustic emissions and associated psychoacoustic microstructure by aspirin consumption. J Acoust Soc Am 84: 1343-53.

Lonsbury-Martin BL, Cutler WM, Martin GK (1991) Evidence for the influence of ageing on distortion-product otoacoustic emissions in humans. J Acoust Soc Am.

Lonsbury-Martin BL, Harris FP, Stagner BB, Hawkins MD, Martin GK (1990) Distortion product emissions in humans: I Basic properties in normally hearing subjects. Ann Otol Rhinol Laryngol Suppl 147: 3-14.

Lonsbury-Martin BL, Harris FP, Stagner BB, Hawkins MD, Martin GK (1990) Distortion product emissions in humans: II Relations to acoustic immitance and stimulus frequency and spontaneous otoacoustic emissions in normally hearing subjects. Ann Otol Rhinol. Laryngol Suppl 147: 15-29.

Lonsbury-Martin BL, Matin GK, Probst R, Coats AC (1987) Acoustic distortion products in the rabbit ear canal. I Basic features and physiological vulnerability. Hear Res 28: 173-89.

Lutman ME (1989) Evoked otoacoustic emissions in adults: implications for screening. Audiology in Practice 6(3): 6-8.

Marchant CD, McMillan PM, Shurin PA, Johnson CE, Turczyk VA, Feinstein JC, Panek SM (1986) Objective diagnosis of otitis media in early infancy by tympanometry and ipsilateral acoustic reflex thresholds. J Pediatr 109: 590–5.

Marshall L, Heller LM, Westhusin LJ (1997) Effect of negative middle-ear pressure on transient-evoked otoacoustic emissions. Ear Hear 18: 218–26.

McKinley AM, Grose JH, Roush J (1997) Multifrequency tympanometry and evoked otoacoustic emissions in neonates during the first 24 hours of life. J Am Acad Audiol 8: 218–23.

Moore BCJ (1989) An Introduction to the Psychology of Hearing. London: Academic Press.

Naeve SL, Margolis RH, Levine SC, Fournier EM (1993) Effect of ear canal pressure on evoked otoacoustic emission. J Acoust Soc Am 91: 2091–5.

NDCS (1994) Quality Standards in Paediatric Audiology. Vol 1. London: NDCS.

Norton SJ (1993) Application of transient evoked otoacoustic emissions to pediatric populations. Ear Hear 16: 515–20.

Norton SJ (1994) Emerging role of otoacoustic emissions in neonatal hearing screening. Am J Otol Suppl 15: 4–12.

Norton SJ, Mott JB, Champlin CA (1989) Behaviour of spontaneous otoacoustic emissions following intense acoustic stimulation. Hear Res 38: 243–58.

Norton SJ, Neely ST (1987) Tone-burst evoked otoacoustic emissions from normal-hearing subjects. J Acoust Soc Am 81: 1860–72.

Norton SJ, Widen JE (1990) Evoked otoacoustic emissions in normal-hearing infants and children: emerging data and issues. Ear Hear 11: 121–7.

Penner MJ (1988) Audible and annoying spontaneous otoacoustic emissions. Arch Otolaryngol Head Neck Surg 114: 150–3.

Penner MJ (1990) An estimate of the prevalence of tinnitus caused by spontaneous otoacoustic emissions. Arch Otolaryngol Head Neck Surg 116: 418–23.

Penner MJ (1996) The emergence and disappearance of one subject's spontaneous otoacoustic emissions. Ear and Hearing 17: 116–19.

Penner MJ, Burns EM (1987) The dissociation of SOAEs and tinnitus. J Speech Hear Res 30: 396–403.

Penner MJ, Coles RRA (1992) Indications for aspirin as a palliative for tinnitus caused by SOAEs: a case study. Br J Audiol 26: 91–6.

Penner MJ, Zhang T (1997) Prevalence of spontaneous otoacoustic emissions in adults revisited. Hear Res 103: 28–34.

Prieve BA, Fitzgerald TS, Schulte LE, Kemp DT (1997a) Basic characteristics of click-evoked otoacoustic emissions in infants and children. J Acoust Soc Am 102: 2860–70.

Prieve BA, Fitzgerald TS, Schulte LE, Kemp DT (1997b) Basic characteristics of distortion product otoacoustic emissions in infants and children. J Acoust Soc Am 102: 2871–8.

Probst R, Beck D (1987) Influence of general anaesthesia on spontaneous otoacoustic emissions. Assoc Res Otolaryngol Abstr 10: 17.

Probst R, Coats AC, Martin GK, Lonsbury-Martin BL (1986) Otoacoustic emissions in ears with hearing loss. Am J Otolaryngol 8: 73–81.

Probst R, Harris FP (1997) Otoacoustic emissions. Adv Otorhinolaryng 53: 182–204.

Probst R, Lonsbury-Martin BL, Martin GK (1991) A review of otoacoustic emissions. J Acoust Soc Am 2027–67.

Probst R, Lonsbury-Martin BL, Martin GK, Coats AC (1987) Spontaneous, click-and toneburst-evoked otoacoustic emissions from normal ears. Hear Res 21: 261–75.

Puel GL, Rebillard G (1990) Effect of contralateral sound stimulation on the distortion product 2f1-f2: evidence that the medial efferent system is involved. J Acoust Soc Am 87: 1630-5.

Rabinowitz WM, Widin GP (1984) Interaction of spontaneous otoacoustic emissions and external sounds. J Acoust Soc Am 76: 1713-20.

Rasmussen AN, Osterhammel PA, Johannesen PT, Borgkvist B (1998) Neonatal hearing screening using otoacoustic emissions elicited by maximum length sequences. Br J Audiol 32: 355-66.

Rhoades K, McPherson B, Smyth V, Kei J, Baglioni A (1998) Effects of background noise on click-evoked otoacoustic emissions. Ear Hear 19: 450-62.

Robinson PM, Haughton PM (1991) Modification of evoked otoacoustic emissions by changes in pressure in the external ear. Br J Audiol 25: 131-3.

Russell AF, Bilger RC (1992) A twin study of spontaneous otoacoustic emissions. J Acoust Soc Am 92: 2409.

Rutten WLC (1980) Evoked acoustic emissions from within normal and abnormal ears: comparison with audiometric and electrocochleographic findings. Hear Res 2: 263-71.

Scanlon PE, Bamford JM (1990) Identification of hearing loss: screening and surveillance methods. Arch Dis Child 65: 479-85.

Schloth E, Zwicker E (1983) Mechanical and acoustical influences on spontaneous oto-acoustic emissions. Hear Res 11: 285-93.

Smurzynski J, Kim DO (1992) Distortion-product and click evoked otoacoustic emissions of normally hearing adults. Hear Res 58: 227-40.

Smurzynski J, Jung MD, Lafrieniere D, Kim DO, Kamath V, Rowe J, Holman MC, Leonard G (1993) Distortion product and click evoked otoacoustic emissions of preterm and full term infants. Ear Hear 14: 258-74.

Spektor Z, Leonard G, Kim DO, Jung MD, Smurzynski J (1991) Otoacoustic emission in normal and hearing impaired children and normal adults. Laryngoscope 101: 965-76.

Starr A, Picton TW, Sininger Y, Hood LJ, Berlin CI (1996) Auditory neuropathy. Brain 119: 741-53.

Stevens JC, Ip CB (1988) Click evoked otoacoustic emissions in normal and hearing impaired adults. Br J Audiol 22: 45-9.

Stevens JC, Webb HD, Smith ME, Buffin JT, Ruddy H (1987) A comparison of otoacoustic emissions and brain stem electric response audiometry in the normal newborn and babies admitted to a special care baby unit. Clin Phys Physiolog Meas 8: 95-104.

Stevens JC, Webb HD, Smith ME, Buffin JT (1990) The effect of stimulus level on click evoked oto-acoustic emissions and brainstem responses in neonates under intensive care. Br J Audiol 24: 293-300.

Strickland AE, Burns EM, Tubis A (1985) Incidence of spontaneous otoacoustic emissions in children and infants. J Acoust Soc Am 78: 931-5.

Sutton GJ, Scanlon PE (1999) Health visitor screening versus vigilance: outcomes of programmes for detecting permanent childhood hearing loss in West Berkshire. Br J Audiol 3: 145-56.

Sutton GJ, Gleadle P, Rowe SJ (1996) Tympanometry and otoacoustic emissions in a cohort of special care neonates. Br J Audiol 30: 9-18.

Thornton ARD, Folkard TJ, Chambers JD (1994) Technical aspects of recording evoked otoacoustic emissions using maximum length sequences. Scand Audiol 24: 83-90.

Trine MB, Hirsch JE, Margolis R (1993) The effect of middle ear pressure on transient evoked otoacoustic emissions. Ear Hear 14: 401-7.

Uziel A, Piron JP (1991) Evoked otoacoustic emissions from normal newborns and babies admitted to an intensive care baby unit. Acta Otolaryngol Suppl 482: 85-91.

Veuillet E, Collet L, Morgon A (1992) Differential effects of ear canal pressure and contralateral acoustic stimulation on evoked otoacoustic emissions in humans. Hear Res 61: 47-55.

Vinck BM, Van Cauwenberge PB, Corthals P, De Vel E (1998) Multivariate analysis of otoacoustic emissions and estimation of hearing thresholds: transient evoked otoacoustic emissions. Audiol 37: 315-34.

Whitehead ML, Lonsbury-Martin BL, Martin GK (1992) Evidence for two discrete sources of 2f1-f2 distortion product otoacoustic emissions in rabbit: I. Differential dependence on stimulus parameter. J Acoust Soc Am 91:1587-606.

Whitehead ML, Kamal N, Lonsbury-Martin BL, Martin GK (1993) Spontaneous otoacoustic emissions in different racial groups. Scand Audiol 22: 3-10.

Wier CC, Pasanen EG, McFadden D (1988) Partial dissociation of spontaneous otoacoustic emissions and distortion products during aspirin use in humans. J Acoust Soc Am 84: 230-7.

Wit HP, Ritsma RJ (1980) Evoked acoustical responses from the human ear: some experimental results. Hear Res 2: 253-61.

Wood S, Davis AC, McCormick B (1997) Changing performance of the Health Visitor Distraction Test when targeted neonatal screening is introduced into a health district. Br J Audiol 31: 55-61.

Yamamoto E, Takagi A, Hirono Y, Yagi N (1987) A case of spontaneous otoacoustic emission. Arch Otolaryngol Head Neck Surg 113: 1316-18.

Zurek PM (1981) Spontaneous narrowband acoustic signals emitted by human ears. J Acoust Soc Am 69: 514-23.

Zwicker E, Schloth E (1984) Interrelation of different otoacoustic emissions. J Acoust Soc Am 75: 1148-54.

Zwicker E, Stecker M, Hind J (1987) Relations between masking, otoacoustic emissions, and evoked potentials. Acustica 64: 102-9.

Chapter 8
Analysis of the middle ear

CLAIRE L BENTON, JACQUELINE E BROUGH,
MICHELLE C DODD

Introduction

The assessment of middle-ear function is of great diagnostic relevance and, since the early 1970s, has become one of the most common clinical procedures performed in paediatric audiology.

The first documented attempt at using acoustic admittance measurements as a diagnostic tool was reported by Lucae (1867). Interest in determining the acoustic impedance of the human middle ear continued in the early 1900s, mainly as a result of developing telephone technology. The first account of measurements undertaken on human ears was by West (1928). This was, however, of more technical than diagnostic interest – it was published in the *Post Office Electrical Engineers Journal*. The 'pneumophone' developed in the mid-1930s by Van Dishoek (Sutherland and Campbell, 1990) allowed the pressure in the external ear canal to be varied. The middle-ear pressure was determined subjectively by the patient reporting when the probe tone was at its loudest. Metz (1946) is reported to be the first person to initiate the use of these measures in clinical audiological applications in the differentiation of conductive and sensorineural hearing loss. In 1934 he developed the equipment that forms the basis of present day systems. Clinical application was made more straightforward by Terkildsen and Scott-Neilson (1960) developing the electroacoustic bridge. This was easy to operate and could be made airtight thus enabling tympanometry to be carried out. Madsen Electronics, a Danish audiometer company then manufactured and marketed the bridge. The first clinical procedure for tympanometry was published by Terkildsen and Thomsen (1959). The use of middle-ear assessment techniques then sparked widespread interest throughout the world and the procedure became a routine part of diagnostic clinical audiological evaluations.

Teele and Teele (1984) developed the acoustic otoscope in an attempt to overcome the sometimes problematic airtight seal essential for acoustic admittance measurements to be completed. The origin of the theory behind acoustic reflectometry however can also be attributed to Lucae's early work on quarter wavelength cancellation.

Marchbanks and Martin (1984) developed a new technique, tympanic membrane displacement (TMD). This technique involves the measurement of very small volume displacements of the tympanic membrane. Clinical applications of TMD are still being researched at present.

Principles

A description of the terminology used to describe attributes of tympanometry is given in the appendix.

The complex ratio between sound pressure and velocity determines the characteristic impedance of the medium through which sound waves are propagated and provides a measure of how the flow of sound is opposed within that medium.

For effective acoustic transmission to occur within the middle ear, the system should ideally offer high admittance and low impedance to the flow of sound. The term acoustic impedance was derived from electronics, an analogy drawn from the impedance to electrical flow within an alternating current circuit. As previously defined it provides a measure of the total opposition to sound flow within the middle-ear system.

The vast majority of middle-ear function assessment techniques, although often referred to as 'impedance tests', in fact use the measurement of acoustic admittance rather than impedance to determine the total opposition to sound flow at the lateral surface of the tympanic membrane of the test ear.

In a normally functioning middle ear, the relatively large tympanic membrane offers little resistance to the propagation of sound waves from the air-filled outer ear to the air-filled middle ear. The primary resistance to sound flow within the middle ear occurs as a result of the coupling of the stapes footplate at the oval window. The transmission of sound waves at the smaller oval window to the hair cells in the endolymph filled inner ear would, theoretically, result in much of the incoming sound being reflected. The characteristic impedance of endolymph is higher than that of air and the middle-ear apparatus acts as an impedance transformer enabling effective energy transfer across the air-endolymph boundary.

Acoustic impedance is affected by the mass, elasticity and frictional properties of the middle ear. These include the mass of the middle-ear ossicles, the stiffness of the ossicular ligaments and muscles, the stiffness of the tympanic membrane as well as the stiffness of the air within the middle-ear space. The compression and expansion of air in the middle-ear space, as the tympanic membrane vibrates in sympathy with sound pressure waves in the external canal, causes mass and frictional changes which also affect the acoustic impedance.

These factors influence the way in which sounds of different frequency are transmitted. Frictional changes reduce efficiency across the whole auditory spectrum. Alteration of mass elements is rare but affects transmission of sound at higher frequencies. Changes in elasticity are more common and affect low frequencies.

Determination of middle-ear pressure by means of measuring the admittance of the tympanic membrane is of great clinical use. There are also measures of reflectivity and displacement of the tympanic membrane that provide valuable clinical information. The equipment and procedures associated with these techniques will be described later.

Tympanometry

Middle-ear disease is one of the most common medical complaints to effect young children. Approximately 50% of all children will experience at least one episode of acute otitis media by their first birthday, with one-third of all children experiencing three or more episodes prior to their third birthday (Harsten et al., 1993). It is known that children who have early otitis media are at higher risk of persistent problems, with the complication of middle-ear effusion. The effects of a hearing loss caused by repeated or prolonged episodes of otitis media with effusion have been well documented (Bluestone and Klein, 1995). Diagnosis of the condition and follow-up management are, therefore, very important. Tympanometry provides a quick, objective method of obtaining information about the status of the middle ear and should be included routinely in a child's audiological assessment.

Equipment used for tympanometry

There are a variety of systems available that, as mentioned before, mostly look at the admittance of the middle-ear system. The commonest method, albeit the most limited, of evaluating the magnitude of middle-ear admittance is vector tympanometry. The basic principle of this test involves introducing an acoustic signal and measuring the sound pressure level of this in the ear canal. The acoustic signal internationally recommended and typically used in paediatric testing is a 226 Hz pure tone generated from a miniature loudspeaker housed in a probe unit. Some setups allow multiple probe tone frequencies to be used.

Figure 8.1 illustrates the main components of a tympanometer. The end of the probe unit is surrounded by a soft tip, available in various sizes to enable an airtight seal to be achieved when the probe is placed into the external ear canal. The sound pressure level of the probe tone is measured by a microphone in the probe unit, which measures the sound pressure level at the

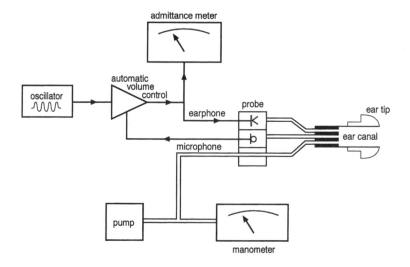

Figure 8.1. Middle-ear measurement system block diagram.

opening of the auditory meatus. The sound pressure level as measured at the probe tip is directly proportional to the acoustic impedance offered by the ear at the point of measure and is inversely proportional to the acoustic admittance – the higher the probe tone SPL, the higher the impedance, the lower the admittance. There is an air pressure sub-system to provide a means of introducing and adjusting the ear-canal pressure via an air pump and a manometer to monitor air-pressure changes within the ear canal. In a normally functioning middle ear, the admittance will be at its greatest when the pressure on either side of the tympanic membrane is equal. If the pressure is adjusted on either side of the tympanic membrane, there will be a decrease in admittance.

Under measurement plane conditions, the acoustic admittance actually measured includes contributions of the ear canal, tympanic membrane, in fact the whole middle-ear system including the coupling of the ossicular chain to the inner ear. Introducing a substantial positive or negative ear-canal pressure effectively stiffens the tympanic membrane and middle-ear transmission system. If the pressure is sufficient, the acoustic admittance at the probe tip is approximately equivalent to the acoustic admittance offered just by the volume of air within the ear canal. Subtracting the value of the acoustic admittance attributable to the air in the outer ear from the total acoustic admittance at ambient ear-canal pressure in a normally functioning middle ear then gives an estimate of the acoustic admittance at the lateral surface of the tympanic membrane referred to as the peak compensated static acoustic admittance of the ear under test at the tympanic membrane. Peak compensated measures are clinically the most commonly used although tympanometry can be undertaken under compensated or plane measurement conditions. Using the plane measure-ment condition may be preferable, however, when using a manual system with a plotter, as this provides a visible means of determining ear-canal volume. This gives valuable information regarding the probe tip placement within the ear canal. If the probe is placed against the meatal wall, the ear canal volume will be low and the probe can be moved accordingly to achieve the correct position. If this occurred with compensated tympanometry, a misleading flat trace could be obtained.

The vector tympanogram obtained represents a single component, the acoustic admittance. For the majority of middle-ear measurement systems admittance is expressed as just one component of admittance, compliance. This approximates well to admittance for the low-frequency probe tone routinely used.

Another sub-system is involved in the measurement of ipsilateral and contralateral stapedial reflexes. For ipsilateral reflex testing, a second probe tone needs to be introduced as well as a means of recording the decrease in acoustic admittance, which occurs with elicitation of the reflex. Contralateral testing involves presentation of the acoustic signal in the opposite 'stimulus ear' to the probe and are usually presented via a conventional supra-aural headphone or an insert earphone placed in the external ear canal. The change in acoustic admittance is measured in the opposite 'probe ear'.

Test variables

There are several parameter options available when carrying out tympanometry, both between different manufacturers' tympanometers and with any one tympanometer. Different options may be more suitable for the paediatric population than for adults.

Rate of pressure change

The recommended rate of pressure change is 50 decaPascals per second (daPa/s) (British Society of Audiology, 1992). However, with young children a faster rate of change may be desirable in order to reduce the time of the test. Most automatic tympanometers use a variable rate of pressure change of 600/200 daPa/s when in screening mode. With manual tympanometers the rate of pressure change is decided by the operator and therefore is more adaptable. The primary effect of the rate is on the peak static admittance, that is peak static admittance decreases as rate increases. Therefore, those who are used to interpreting tympanograms at the slower rate will noticed a shift to the left in the peak when using a screening option using a faster rate. The magnitude of the decrease in peak admittance varies between individuals, but should not affect the use of the normal values in interpretation.

Direction of pressure change

Tympanometers have the option of using different directions of pressure change, from negative pressure to positive or vice versa. The direction of pressure change will have an effect on the shape of the tympanogram with there being a higher chance of notching with a negative to positive direction. The peak static admittance is also affected by the direction of pressure change. A negative-to-positive sweep will give a more positive peak static admittance than a positive to negative sweep. Therefore, if using a classification scheme for the interpretation of tympanograms, for example Jerger's (Jerger, 1970), it is important to match the classification to the direction of sweep.

A recommended reference pressure is 200 daPa (British Society of Audiology, 1992). This is where the indicated admittance is that of the air-filled space between the tip of the probe and the tympanic membrane and there is no influence from the middle ear. It is recommended that tympanometry should commence at this reference pressure and therefore use a positive-to-negative direction of pressure change. This direction is also recommended for neonatal tympanometry as a collapsed ear canal is more common with a negative-to-positive direction.

Probe tone frequency

The standard probe tone frequency used is 226 Hz and, until recently, this was the only option available on most tympanometers, especially those used as a screening tool. However, there is growing evidence that the information that can be gained from using higher frequency probe tones is proving useful in several populations. Most commonly encountered middle-ear pathologies such as otitis media, Eustachian tube dysfunction (with tympanic membrane retraction) or otosclerosis, increase middle-ear stiffness. These can be adequately detected by a low frequency probe tone and acoustic compliance (the reciprocal of stiffness). The usefulness of a 226 Hz probe tone in children below the age of seven months is open to question. Neonatal tympanograms with a 226 Hz probe tone characteristically produce a W-shape and have been known to give results which resemble 'normal' tympanograms in the presence of middle-ear effusion. It is commonly assumed that this is due to the hypermobility of the neonate's ear canal wall. The resting ear canal diameter changes in response to pneumatic stimulation (Holte, Margolis and Cavanaugh Jr, 1991). This change decreases with age, as the bony portion of the ear canal develops. However, this is not the sole factor responsible for producing atypical tympanogram shapes. This also occurs due to the different physiology of the neonatal middle ear. The mass and resistive components of the tympanic membrane and middle ear are more pronounced for neonates, giving a more positive reactance. With advancing age this changes to a stiffness-controlled system with negative reactance. These changes can be shown by the increase in admittance phase angle in the first few months of life. The increase in the mass component of the neonatal middle ear produces a lower resonant frequency for the system than that for an adult or older child. A higher probe-tone frequency is, therefore, more sensitive to the characteristics of the neonatal middle ear.

A probe tone of 660 Hz or 678 Hz has been shown to be more accurate than a lower probe tone frequency at predicting middle-ear effusion in neonates (Shurin, Pelton and Finkelstein, 1977; Marchant et al., 1986; Sutton, Gleadle and Rowe, 1996). Considering multiple components of the high-frequency tympanograms, susceptance (B), conductance (G) as well as the usual admittance (Y), gives more information to aid the interpretation. These variables will be discussed in more detail later in this chapter.

Test procedure

The child should be examined for any contraindications for tympanometry, such as discharging ears or recent tenderness. They should be sat sideways on their parent or carer's knee if very young or nervous. If the child is disturbed the parent or carer should hold the child comfortably against their chest to reduce the chance of movement: this also serves to reassure the child. The procedure should be explained clearly to the parent, explaining that it is best if the child is still. An appropriately sized ear tip should be placed at the entrance of the ear canal (Figure 8.2). A good seal is required and is helped by pulling the pinna gently back, in order to straighten the ear canal. Automatic tympanometers will start as soon as a hermetic seal is achieved. It can be useful to involve older children more by showing them the equipment and explaining what will happen in order to allay any anxiety. As described above, the pressure sweep should be started at 200 daPa and it is often helpful to extend the lower limit to –400 daPa or –600 daPa to obtain a more accurate tympanogram.

Erroneous results can occur with poor test technique. Not positioning the ear tip in the external ear canal and manipulating

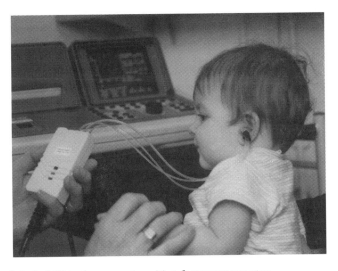

Figure 8.2. A child in the correct position for tympanometry.

the pinna accordingly can cause the probe to rest against the canal wall, a tympanogram with suspiciously low ear-canal volume should be repeated. Wax blocking the probe can also prevent accurate results. False peaks can occur in the tympanogram if the child moves or is particularly noisy. If the child is very restless or continuously crying the tympanogram will be inconclusive. Again, tympanograms with unusual shapes should always be repeated.

Interpretation of results

When interpreting a tympanogram, it is important that the result is not considered in isolation but as part of the test battery. By taking into account all of the audiological test results and the patient's history, it is less likely that an incorrect diagnosis will be reached, which could otherwise result in the mismanagement of the patient.

Various attempts have been made to classify tympanometric patterns, obtained using a 226 Hz probe tone (Brooks, 1969; Jerger, 1970). Such classifications are certainly useful, but not essential for the understanding of tympanometry and tympanometric patterns and are not generally used in reporting results. The classifications are only applicable to single component tympanometry and are not suitable for use with the more complex tympanometric patterns obtained using multifrequency, multicomponent tympanometry.

Normal tympanogram - classified as 'Type A'

Middle-ear pressure: –100 to +50 daPa.
Middle-ear compliance: 0.3 to 1.5 ml.

A normal tympanogram (Figure 8.3a) is usually suggestive of normal or, essentially normal middle ear and Eustachian tube function, for the probe tone used. Normal tympanograms can be obtained from those children with normal hearing sensitivity or a sensorineural hearing loss.

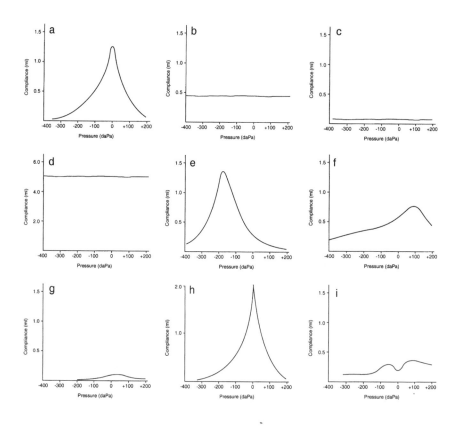

Figure 8.3. (a) A normal tympanogram. (b) A flat tympanogram with normal middle-ear volume. (c) A flat tympanogram with a low middle-ear volume. (d) A tympanogram consistent with a high middle-ear volume. (e) A tympanogram exhibiting negative middle-ear pressure. (f) A tympanogram exhibiting positive middle-ear pressure. (g) A tympanogram exhibiting reduced middle-ear compliance. (h) A tympanogram exhibiting elevated middle-ear compliance. (i) A double-peaked neonatal tympanogram.

Flattened tympanogram – classified as 'Type B'

A flattened tympanogram is probably the most common type encountered in the paediatric population. In children, a flat trace with normal ear-canal volume is usually suggestive of the presence of middle-ear effusion, where the middle-ear space is filled with fluid, as opposed to air, and the Eustachian tube is failing to function (Figure 8.3b). Children presenting with middle-ear effusion may also have an associated conductive hearing loss.

If a flat trace is obtained at a particularly high or low middle-ear volume then interpretation of the tympanogram is quite different. For example, if a volume of almost zero is obtained, this can be suggestive of some occluding wax in the ear canal (Figure 8.3c). Alternatively, the probe may be blocked with wax or debris, or it may have been positioned against the ear canal wall during testing. If, following a visual check and repositioning the probe, a reliable tympanogram is still unobtainable, otoscopic examination will ascertain if it is the presence of wax that is producing the low volume.

In children with patent grommets *in situ,* a large ear canal volume (for example, 4 ml) will be evident (Figure 8.3d). For those children with grommets, tympanometry is a simple way of checking if the grommet is patent, blocked or if it has been extruded from the tympanic membrane. Should the grommet be blocked and *in situ,* then a flattened trace showing normal ear canal volume might be obtained. Otoscopic examination and the patient's history will distinguish this trace from one obtained in the presence of middle-ear effusion.

If the grommet has been extruded, a variety of tympanograms may be obtained, depending upon the status of the middle ear and the tympanic membrane. For example, if the tympanic membrane has healed following the grommet extrusion and the middle ear is now clear from effusion, a normal tympanogram would be obtained. If, however, the middle-ear effusion has returned, then a flat trace with normal middle-ear volume would be seen.

It may be that following the grommet extrusion, the tympanic membrane has failed to heal. If the eardrum is perforated due to this or following, for example, repeated attacks of otitis media, this would result in a flat tympanogram exhibiting a large middle-ear volume (Figure 8.3d), as the volume of the middle-ear space is being measured, in addition to that of the ear canal. Otoscopic examination and a thorough patient history would distinguish a perforated tympanic membrane from a patent grommet *in situ*.

Tympanogram showing negative middle-ear pressure – classified as 'Type C'

Middle-ear pressure: less than –100 daPa.
Middle-ear compliance: 0.3 to 1.5 ml.

Negative middle-ear pressure is an indicator of dysfunction of the Eustachian tube (Figure 8.3e). In such cases, on otoscopic examination, the tympanic membrane would appear retracted.

Tympanogram showing positive middle-ear pressure

Middle-ear pressure: greater than +50 daPa.
Middle-ear compliance: 0.3 to 1.5 ml.

Links have been established between positive middle-ear pressure and the presence of acute middle-ear pathology (Figure 8.3f).

Tympanogram showing reduced middle-ear compliance

Middle-ear pressure: –100 daPa to +50 daPa.
Middle-ear compliance: approximately 0.5 to 0.66 of normal compliance values.

Flattened tympanograms exhibiting low compliance and normal middle-ear pressure (Figure 8.3g) are associated with stiffening of the tympanic membrane, resulting in its reduced mobility, and also with ossicular fixation – for example in patients with otosclerosis.

Tympanogram showing elevated middle-ear compliance

Middle-ear pressure: –100 daPa to +50 daPa.
Middle-ear compliance: greater than 1.5 ml.

Sharply peaked tympanograms are usually indicative of a hypermobile tympanic membrane, caused by scarring and thinning, possibly as a result of frequent ear infections, healed perforations of the tympanic membrane or a history of middle-ear effusion (Figure 8.3h). Elevated middle-ear compliance can, however, also be found in patients with ossicular discontinuity, although tympanic membrane hypermobility is more likely.

Interpretation of neonatal tympanograms

Recent developments in the literature have focused on the use and interpretation of tympanometry in the neonatal population. Tympanograms obtained from this group have been found to differ quite significantly from those recorded in older children and in adults. A tentative classification scheme for neonatal tympanograms has been suggested by Sutton, Gleadle and Rowe (1996). The authors however admit that further work is needed in this area before such a scheme could be validated.

Great care must be taken when interpreting a neonatal tympanogram. As previously mentioned, use of the standard 226 Hz probe often results in a double-peaked ('notched' or 'W-shaped') tympanogram (Figure 8.3i), as opposed to the single-peaked pattern seen in older children and adults. Both double-peaked and normal tympanograms have been found in neonates with known middle-ear effusion (Paradise, Smith and Bluestone, 1976; Marchant et al., 1986; Hunter and Margolis, 1992). In cases where a flat tympanogram is obtained, with a low ear-canal volume, this is usually a sign of debris in the ear canal, rather than the presence of middle-ear effusion. Most studies agree that the usefulness of the standard 226 Hz probe is therefore questionable for diagnostic use with the neonatal group (Paradise, Smith and Bluestone, 1976).

It was stated earlier in this chapter that various studies have investigated the use of multifrequency, multicomponent tympanometry for the detection of middle-ear effusion in neonates (Hirsch, Margolis and Rykken, 1992; Holte, Margolis and Cavanaugh Jr, 1991; McKinley, Grose and Roush, 1997; Sutton, Gleadle and Rowe, 1996). In particular, the use of high-frequency probe tones (typically 660 Hz) has been discussed as an alternative to the standard 226 Hz probe tone (Keefe and Levi, 1996, Meyer, Jardine and Deverson, 1997). Sutton, Gleadle and Rowe (1996) reported a strong association between tympanometric patterns obtained using a 660 Hz probe tone and the presence/absence of otoacoustic emissions in a neonatal group. It is well documented that detection of an otoacoustic emission is affected by the presence of middle-ear effusion. Classification of tympanometric patterns obtained using multifrequency, multicomponent tympanometry is still unfortunately presently in its infancy, with the tympanometric patterns obtained being very complex – often double or multiple peaks. Vanhuyse, Creten and Van Camp (1975) proposed a system for classification of multicomponent tympanograms obtained from older children and adults, based on the number of extrema or peaks in the tympanogram. Unfortunately the classification scheme is unsuitable for the interpretation of a neonatal tympanogram or those obtained from younger children, as the tympanometric patterns are known to differ in these groups. Additional data is therefore required from neonates and younger children with known middle-ear problems before a classification scheme can be established to distinguish normal tympanometric patterns from those associated with middle-ear disorders in these groups (Hunter and Margolis, 1992).

The acoustic reflex

The acoustic reflex is the name of the reflex arc that encompasses the eighth cranial nerve, brainstem and seventh cranial nerve. Its presence confirms the integrity of all parts of this pathway. The reflex is evoked by sound and results in the contraction of the stapedius muscle. An intense sound presented to one ear causes the innervation of the eighth cranial nerve that continues up to the synapse with the ventral cochlear nucleus in the brainstem. The ventral cochlear nucleus has several pathways (seventh cranial nerve) which terminate in the ipsilateral and contralateral stapedius muscles (Figure 8.4). There is a three-neuron ipsilateral pathway, a four-neuron ipsilateral pathway and two four-neuron contralateral pathways, one through each superior olivary complex. The bilaterality of the reflex pathway means that a sound presented to one ear causes contraction of the stapedius muscle in both ears. The reflex can therefore be measured in the stimulated ear (ipsilateral reflex) or the non-stimulated ear (contralateral reflex). The contraction of the stapedius muscle causes stiffening of the ossicular chain and consequently there is a decrease in admittance. Thus, its occurrence can be measured with a tympanometer. The reflex is abolished by pathologies at any point on the pathway. Therefore, cochlear damage, eighth

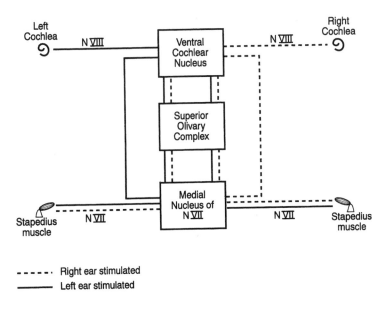

Figure 8.4. Schematic diagram of the acoustic reflex pathway.

nerve tumours, brainstem lesions to the superior olive level, facial nerve paralysis, myasthenia gravis and conductive lesions (except a fractured crura) cause a disappearance of the acoustic reflex.

The main use of the acoustic reflex is the measurement of its threshold. The threshold of the reflex decreases with an increase in bandwidth of the stimulus. The interpretation of the acoustic reflex thresholds together with the results from the behavioural testing can indicate whether there is a conductive loss, a sensorineural loss, or a sensorineural loss with abnormal loudness growth.

An intact tympanic membrane is essential for the measurement of acoustic reflexes, therefore they are carried out after tympanometry. As the reflex causes a relatively small change in admittance they must be measured at the point of peak static admittance where the greatest response will be seen. Most screening tympanometers carry out a screening ipsilateral reflex measurement at one or more frequencies once tympanometry is completed. Although measures of contralateral acoustic reflexes are considered more robust than ipsilateral measurements, from a practical point of view ipsilateral measures are more achievable with young children. However, ipsilateral reflexes can be contaminated by artefacts. This is caused by the interaction of the probe tone and stimulating tone. This can be subtractive where intermodulation between the probe tone and stimulation produces products that cause the removal of energy from the probe tone, the artefact will grow with an increase in stimulus level. The interaction may conversely be additive where there is a reaction between probe tone, stimulus and the ear canal walls. This occurs at high stimulation levels when the canal walls become non-linear producing sub-harmonics at the probe tone frequency. This can cause the artefact to be mistaken for a true response. Some equipment setups attempt to overcome this problem by presenting the stimulus in rapid pulses. A probe tone frequency of 660 Hz or higher is contaminated less by artefacts.

As the acoustic reflex arc is known to be functional from birth, it is possible for an acoustic reflex to be elicited in neonates, as well as in infants and older children (Vincent and Gerber, 1987). However, when testing a neonate, a higher frequency probe tone is recommended, as with tympanometry. Detection of the neonatal acoustic reflex is improved when using a 660 Hz probe tone, as opposed to the more standard 220 Hz or 226 Hz probe tone, routinely used with older children and adults (Margolis, 1993; Sprague, Wiley and Goldstein, 1985, Weatherby and Bennett, 1980).

The use of acoustic reflexes, both threshold and decay measures, for indicating a retrocochlear lesion or locating the site of the lesion has now been generally superceded by advanced imaging techniques due to their superior specificity and sensitivity.

Interpretation of results

In a normal ear – one free from any middle-ear disorder and hearing loss – the acoustic reflex threshold (ART) is usually found to lie between 80–85 dB HL (if using pure-tone stimuli, 250 Hz –4 kHz) and 60 dB HL – 65 dB HL (if using broad-band noise stimuli). It is important, however, to consider acoustic reflex testing along with other audiological test results. Absence of an acoustic reflex may occur for a number of reasons. In some patients, for example, the stapedius muscle itself may be absent. However, if it is possible to elicit a reflex, this is usually an indication that no significant middle-ear disorder exists.

Conductive hearing loss

For those children with a conductive hearing loss, the results of acoustic reflex testing depend upon the degree of hearing loss and whether it is a unilateral or bilateral loss. In the case of a unilateral conductive loss, if the ear being acoustically stimulated during testing is the affected ear, then the contralateral ART will be raised, often beyond the limitations of the equipment. Generally, if the auditory threshold is 35 dB HL or less, then the ART will be raised, but measurable. However, if the auditory threshold is greater than 35 dB HL, the contralateral acoustic reflex is usually absent. When the unaffected ear is stimulated, the contraction of the stapedius muscle cannot be detected and the contralateral acoustic reflex will therefore be obscured. The ipsilateral reflex will, however, only be absent on the side of the affected ear. In the case of a bilateral conductive hearing loss, even if only mild in nature, both the ipsilateral and contralateral acoustic reflexes will be absent bilaterally.

Sensorineural hearing loss

In children with sensorineural hearing losses, the results of acoustic reflex testing are, as with conductive losses, dependent upon the degree of the hearing loss and whether the loss is unilateral or bilateral. Acoustic reflex thresholds have been found to be elevated in those with a sensorineural hearing loss, and closer to the measured auditory threshold than in the normally hearing population. The degree of threshold elevation increases the greater the severity of the hearing loss. Acoustic stimulation using broad-band stimuli results in a greater elevation in the ART measured than when pure-tone stimuli are used, as the degree of hearing loss worsens. Patients with hearing losses greater than 80 dB HL tend not to have measurable reflexes. Whereas, those with hearing losses of 50 dB HL or less may have normal or essentially normal ARTs. Metz (1952) stated that when the ART and auditory threshold were found to differ by less than 60 dB, recruitment (abnormal loudness growth) was probable in the stimulated ear.

Non-organic hearing loss

Measurement of the ART is a useful tool in helping to distinguish those with a non-organic hearing loss from those with a true hearing loss. If the measured ART is found to be lower than the behavioural auditory threshold, then a non-organic hearing loss should be suspected.

Acoustic reflex decay (ARD)

When the stapedius muscle contracts in response to an auditory stimulus, it should remain contracted for the duration of the stimulus. However, if this normal pattern of response is absent, in that the stapedius muscle fails to maintain its contraction, this can be indicative of eighth nerve pathology (such as a tumour) or a cochlear disorder. The duration of the stapedius muscle contraction is measured in response to continuous high-level acoustic stimulation, usually 10 dB HL above the reflex threshold, with a stimulus duration of usually 10 s. The decay is measured as the percentage reduction in admittance during the 10 s. Greater than 50% decay in 5 s is an indication of a retrocochlear pathology.

Acoustic reflex testing can unfortunately produce a high false positive rate for eighth nerve pathologies and therefore, the results of all investigations should be considered before reaching a conclusive diagnosis.

Acoustic reflectometry

Acoustic reflectometry is based on the principle of a sound wave travelling in a closed tube that is completely reflected when it strikes the closed end of the tube. Reflected sound waves from the middle-ear cancel the original probe sound waves at a distance of one-quarter wavelength from the tympanic membrane. This can give an estimation of the length of the ear canal and an indication of the presence of middle-ear fluid. The greater the amount of sound reflected the greater the possibility of middle-ear fluid being present as this indicates that the tympanic membrane is more 'solid'. The results are reported in reflectance units, from 0.0 to 9.0. If the shape of the reflection is plotted then the results can also be described in terms of the spectral gradient, or curve angle. For ease of interpretation some manufacturer's separate the results into 'levels' ($1 \geq 95$, $2 = 70$ to 95, $3 = 60$ to 69, $4 = 49$ to 59, $5 \leq 49$).

Unlike tympanometry, acoustic reflectometry does not require an airtight seal of the ear canal. Neither is it affected by the child crying, so little co-operation is required. However, acoustic reflectometry is less reliable when there is negative middle-ear pressure, especially in cases where, on otoscopy, there has been evidence of fluid with air bubbles behind the tympanic membrane. False positive results have occurred when there are abnormalities of the tympanic membrane such as tympanosclerosis and extreme scarring. Acoustic reflectometry is proving to be a useful tool for clinicians when time is short and where only a diagnosis of the presence or absence of middle-ear effusion is required. Tympanometry, however, gives a more detailed insight into the function of the middle ear and when carried out effectively also takes very little time. In most cases in the audiological assessment of a child, tympanometry is preferable.

Equipment for acoustic reflectometry

The equipment used for this technique consists of a probe that emits a burst of sound sweeping from 2 kHz to 5 kHz in 1 s. A microphone in the probe measures the sound pressure level at the meatus. Summation of the incident and reflected sound wave occurs and if the tympanic membrane is functioning normally reflection should be minimal and the sound pressure level should be around 80 dB SPL. Rigidity of the tympanic membrane will result in measurable reflection of incident sound energy. The frequency at which the ear canal length is equivalent to one-quarter of the wavelength of the reflected signal. Cancellation will occur with the incident signal, the wavelength of this being half the reflected signal. The frequency at which the cancellation occurs can be used to calculate the ear canal length. At the quarter wavelength frequency, the degree of cancellation can also be determined.

Interpretation of results

The readout from the instrument gives a measure of reflectivity, expressed in terms of reflectance units (RU). Although normative data have not yet been obtained, recommended 'cut points' (the lowest number, as shown on the readout, thought to indicate the presence of effusion) of 4, 5 and 6 RU have been quoted in the literature (Babonis et al., 1994; Douniadakis et al., 1993; Kemaloglu et al., 1999). As the number of reflectance units increases, the greater the likelihood of the presence of middle-ear effusion. Babonis et al. (1994) found that children presenting with reduced middle-ear compliance on tympanometry tended to have reflectometry results greater than 6 RU.

Another parameter used in acoustic reflectometry is the spectral gradient angle (SGA). The SGA, as given on the readout of the instrument, corresponds to a level that the manufacturers associate with the likelihood of the presence/absence of middle-ear effusion. It has been reported that when the SGA was classified as level five, 88% of children (age range six months to 14 years) were found to have middle-ear effusion (Barnett et al., 1998). However, all younger children (under two years of age) with a SGA of less than 49 were found to have middle-ear effusion. According to the manufacturer's classification, an SGA corresponding to level one or level two means that the child is probably free of middle-ear effusion. A result classified as level three, four or five means that middle-ear effusion is probably present (Block et al., 1999). Comparisons were also made of the SGA measured and the results of children's audiological assessment. This revealed that children presenting with hearing difficulties often had a small SGA. Although acoustic reflectometry has been proved a clinically useful tool in predicting the presence of effusion in infants and older children, its use in the neonatal population is yet to be established.

Tests of Eustachian tube function

Eustachian tube dysfunction is known to be one of the causal factors of otitis media with effusion. The infant Eustachian tube differs anatomically from that of adults in that it has a shorter length and a smaller angle of inclination. This may impede its ventilation and clearance function. Once the Eustachian tube becomes blocked, air pressure in the middle ear decreases at the rate of approximately 50 daPa/hour if the tube remains closed. As the air pressure becomes increasingly negative, fluid is drawn out of the cells lining the middle ear.

There are several methods of measuring Eustachian tube function. An assumption that underlies tympanometry is that the acoustic admittance measured at the probe tip is maximal when the air pressure on both sides of the tympanic membrane is equal. Therefore, the air pressure at the tympanogram peak is an approximation of middle-ear resting pressure, and consequently provides a means of evaluating the ventilatory function of the Eustachian tube. Normal middle-ear pressure implies that the Eustachian tube must be functioning to maintain the equilibrium between ambient air pressure and middle-ear pressure. Where there is Eustachian tube dysfunction the tympanogram shows a shift in peak static admittance to the left indicating negative middle-ear pressure. A tympanogram that fluctuates in time with the patient's breathing can be an indication of a patulous Eustachian tube.

Tympanometry can also be used to assess Eustachian tube function by carrying out the simple Toynbee test. Patients are instructed to swallow whilst holding their nose closed. Tympanometry is carried out before and after the manoeuvre. If negative middle-ear pressure develops during the closed nose swallowing the Eustachian tube function can be considered to be normal. Tympanometry is also required for the nine-step inflation-deflation test. The test investigates the Eustachian tube's ability to equilibrate both induced positive and negative middle-ear pressure. Active opening of the Eustachian tube is induced by the patient being instructed to swallow at several points through out the test and is assessed by recording tympanograms at intervals. The tympanic membrane must be intact for this test to be carried out, although it can be modified if there is a perforation. In this case the passive opening and closing pressures can be recorded by observation of the tympanometer's pressure gauge (Bluestone and Cantekin, 1981).

The tests just described mainly rely upon creating an artificial pressure gradient across the Eustachian tube. Sonotubometry detects Eustachian tube opening under physiological conditions. Sonotubometry involves introducing a tone into the nasal cavity via a miniature transducer, whilst placing a microphone in the ipsilateral ear canal. If the probe tone used is below the attenuation value of the head then the microphone will not detect the signal. If the Eustachian tube opens, usually through a swallow, attenuation is decreased and the probe tone is detected. This method means the function of the Eustachian tube can be assessed with a perforated tympanic membrane.

Specific tests of Eustachian tube function are not routinely carried out in paediatric assessment. Tympanometry provides sufficient information for the clinician to make intelligent inferences about the state of the Eustachian tube.

Tympanic membrane displacement

Tympanic membrane displacement (TMD) provides an indirect measurement of intra-cochlear fluid pressure and was first described by Marchbanks and Martin (1984). Small displacements of the tympanic membrane caused by the contraction of the stapedius muscle during the acoustic reflex are observed. The cochlear aqueduct must be patent for the measurements to be possible, there must also be an intact acoustic reflex with normal middle-ear pressure. The cochlear aqueduct connects the cerebrospinal and peri-lymphatic fluids. Therefore, peri-lymphatic pressure is a direct reflection of intra-cranial pressure. Raised peri-lymphatic pressure displaces the resting position of the stapes footplate laterally. The tympanic membrane moves in an inward direction on stapedial contraction in this situation. Low peri-lymphatic pressure causes an outward movement of the tympanic membrane due to the stapes footplate being displaced medially. The TMD technique elicits an acoustic reflex with a 1 kHz ipsilateral stimulus and then measures the small changes in volume of the external auditory canal caused by the displacement of the tympanic membrane. The displacement is quantified by two parameters, both expressed in nanolitres (nl). Vi is the maximum inward displacement and Vm is the mean displacement of the tympanic membrane measured from the time at which Vi is reached until the acoustic stimulus stops. This method provides a non-invasive method of assessing intra-cranial pressure and has been used to monitor patients after ventricular shunt operations. Raised intra-cranial pressure can have otological symptoms such has tinnitus, vertigo and sometimes hearing loss. Tympanic membrane displacement can help to provide a differential diagnosis between a neurological disorder and a peripheral labyrinthine disorder caused by raised intra-cranial pressure. At present TMD is only routinely used in some clinics: its use, however, is becoming more widespread as an alternative to the more invasive methods of assessing intra-cranial pressure.

Equipment for tympanic membrane displacement (TMD)

The probe for this technique is connected to an external cavity containing a low-frequency pressure microphone and a reference diaphragm. Movement of the tympanic membrane produces pressure changes that are detected by the low frequency microphone. The signal from the microphone drives the feedback control mechanism that moves the diaphragm to equalize the pressure. The volume displacement of the diaphragm is equivalent to the volume displacement of the tympanic membrane. The technique enables tympanic membrane displacements of down to 1 nanolitre to be measured. The signal voltage of the diaphragm (TDH 39) provides a measure of TMD. The frequency response of the system is 0 Hz to 140 Hz. For sonotubometry, a miniature loudspeaker with an inflatable cuff generates a continuous pure tone, usually 7 kHz. The TMD probe used is the same as described earlier. When the Eustachian tube opens sound is transmitted via the nasopharynx and the Eustachian tube to the middle and external ear. The TMD probe detects this sound.

Interpretation of results

As mentioned previously intra-cranial pressure can be assessed using the TMD technique, for example in children with shunted hydrocephalus (Samuel, Burge and Marchbanks, 1998). It has been reported that when intra-cranial pressure is elevated, Vm values in the region of -200 nl and lower are typical, corresponding to an inward displacement of the tympanic membrane. When the intra-cranial pressure is low and the tympanic membrane is displaced outwards, Vm values of $+200$ nl and greater are seen. Vm values between -200 nl and $+200$ nl are found when the intra-cranial pressure is classed as normal.

Calibration

Daily checks as well as more detailed calibration on a yearly basis are recommended for equipment. There are calibration procedures available developed by the British Standards Institution (BS EN 61027, 1993).

The evaluation of the function of all the equipment components must be completed to ensure that this corresponds to the appropriate manufacturer's standard. These standards are provided with the equipment and give data to enable correct calibration.

Calibration involves ensuring the probe unit is functioning as specified – the probe tone frequency is accurate at the appropriate level and free of distortion and noise. This is completed by connecting the probe using an airtight seal to a 2cc (HA1) coupler. The airtight seal in this centre's set-up was achieved by making an impression material cuff into which the probe is placed. The coupler is then connected to a microphone and sound level meter. The sound level meter monitors the acoustic signal in the coupler (Figure 8.5).

The specific output level of the probe signal can then be determined and compared to the manufacturer's data for that particular piece of equipment using the BSI standard.

The accuracy of the probe tone frequency also has to be checked and this is achieved using a digital frequency counter. The output of the sound level meter is directed to the frequency counter and a digital display of the frequency measured for the probe tone used is provided.

The probe tone should also be evaluated to ensure that the level of any harmonic distortion and noise is much lower than the level of the probe tone. This is more realistic than expecting the signal to be completely pure as there is usually always some harmonic distortion and noise present. The probe signal from the coupler is directed via the sound level meter to a distortion analyser that monitors the signal levels for discrete frequency regions – in other words, each successive harmonic.

Calibration of the middle-ear measurement system to ensure that measured compliance values are accurate is achieved by using cylindrical calibration cavities of known and specified

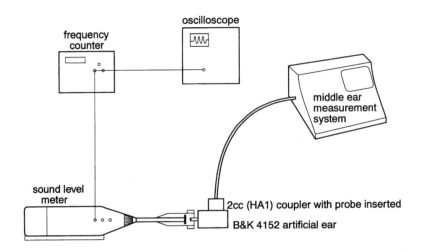

Figure 8.5. General set-up for calibration of a middle-ear measurement system.

volumes. Manufacturers provide preset calibration values for test cavities, taking into account the important effect of ambient temperature and barometric pressure, for equipment.

The acoustic admittance measured should be equal to the volume of the fixed cavity used over the pressure range used. This check is routinely carried out daily and if any inequality is discovered this can be corrected either manually by use of trimpots or through software commands for computerized equipment.

The air pressure system's manometer accuracy is also of great importance and has to be compared to manufacturers and the BSI standard. This is achieved using an external manometer such as a U-tube marked with graduations of known value and less than those in which the instrument is to be calibrated. The probe unit is attached to this via a small tube and the pressure setting on the equipment is then varied over the range clinically used. The corresponding value on the U-tube manometer is recorded and compared to specifications.

Due to the variation in tympanogram characteristics with the rate of change in air pressure, the pump speed, usually expressed in decaPascals per second has to be checked. This can be achieved on some systems by measuring the auxiliary output voltage, the size of which corresponds to the pump pressure output.

The tympanogram is usually recorded on a printer or plotter. If a plotter is used, the volume displayed can be checked on a daily basis using the calibration cavities. It has to be ensured that the volume of the cavity as well as the pressure change on the manometer corresponds to that plotted.

For calibration of the contralateral acoustic reflex measurement signals, the standards and equipment used are generally the same as for audiometers (BS EN 60645-1, 1995) with some exceptions which are detailed in the appropriate standards. The standards used provide information regarding frequency accuracy, output levels, attenuator linearity, harmonic distortion and other required specifications. If an insert earphone is used then reference to the appropriate manufacturer's standard is recommended. This also applies to ipsilateral stimuli, the procedure involves coupling of the probe to a 2cc (HA1) coupler in the same way as described earlier for calibration of the pure-tone signal used in the measurement of acoustic admittance.

To cover the calibration of reflectometers and TMD setups is beyond the scope of this text. It is therefore advised that the associated manufacturer's guidelines be consulted.

Conclusion

It has been shown that the assessment of middle-ear function in the paediatric population can assist in a differential diagnosis and therefore help decide the management for each case. With the advent of neonatal screening it will become increasingly important to be able accurately to assess the middle-ear function of this age group. The area of multifrequency tympanometry and the interpretation of complex tympanograms will become of greater importance.

Appendix

Terminology

Acoustic admittance (Ya)

The ease with which the tympanic membrane and middle-ear system accepts a flow of acoustic energy. In reality, it is the sum of the admittance of the tympanic membrane, the middle ear and the enclosed ear canal volume. Admittance is measured in acoustic mhos.

Acoustic conductance (Ga)

A component of acoustic admittance. Conductance is the component that dissipates acoustic energy.

Acoustic immittance

A general term referring to acoustic admittance, to acoustic impedance or, to both.

Acoustic impedance (Za)

The opposition that the middle-ear system presents to the flow of acoustic energy. Acoustic impedance is the reciprocal of acoustic admittance. It is measured in acoustic ohms.

Acoustic reactance (Xa)

A component of acoustic impedance. Reactance is the component that stores acoustic energy.

Acoustic resistance (Ra)

A component of acoustic impedance. Resistance is the component that dissipates acoustic energy.

Acoustic stapedial reflex

The contraction of the stapedius muscle due to intense acoustic stimulation, which results in changes in the immittance of the middle ear.

Acoustic stapedial reflex decay

The relaxation of the stapedius muscle, as measured by a change in immittance, during the presentation of an extended acoustic signal.

Acoustic stapedial reflex threshold

The lowest intensity of acoustic stimulation required to elicit the contraction of the stapedius muscle.

Acoustic susceptance (Ba)

A component of acoustic admittance. Susceptance is the component that stores acoustic energy.

Ambient compensated static acoustic immittance

The compensated static acoustic immittance measured when the external auditory meatal pressure is at atmospheric pressure.

Compensated static acoustic immittance

The static acoustic immittance measured when the acoustic immittance of the external auditory meatus has been taken into account. It therefore represents the static acoustic immittance at the lateral surface of the tympanic membrane.

Compensated tympanometry

When the acoustic immittance is measured, having taken into account the acoustic immittance of the ear canal. The measurements are effectively made at the tympanic membrane.

Compliance

Compliance is one component of acoustic admittance and is a measure of the mobility of the tympanic membrane and ossicular chain. It is the reciprocal of the stiffness of the middle-ear system.

Component tympanometry

Tympanometry involving the measurement of two components – for example, susceptance and conductance.

Measurement plane tympanometry

When the acoustic immittance is measured in the 'measurement plane', at the tip of the probe.

Middle-ear pressure

The pressure of the air enclosed within the middle-ear space, measured in decaPascals (daPa).

Multifrequency tympanometry

When two or more probe tone frequencies, or a swept-frequency probe tone, are used to measure the tympanogram.

Peak compensated static acoustic immittance

The compensated static acoustic immittance measured when the external auditory meatal pressure is at that which corresponds to the peak of the tympanogram.

Static acoustic immittance

The acoustic immittance of the middle ear at a steady and specified pressure.

Tympanogram

A graphical display of acoustic immittance with respect to the ear canal pressure.

Tympanometric gradient

A mathematical description of the slope of a tympanogram. Various methods of calculating the gradient have been suggested in the literature.

Tympanometry

The measurement of acoustic immittance at varying positive and negative pressures within the external auditory meatus.

References

Babonis T, Weir MR, Kelly PC, Krober MS (1994) Progression of tympanometry and acoustic reflectometry. Findings in children with acute otitis media. Clinical Pediatrics 33: 593-600.

Barnett ED, Klein JO, Hawkins KA, Cabral HJ, Kenna M, Healy G (1998) Comparison of spectral gradient acoustic reflectometry and other diagnostic techniques for detection of middle ear effusion in children with middle ear disease. The Pediatric Infectious Disease Journal 17: 556-9.

Block SL, Pichichero ME, McLinn S, Aronovitz G, Kimball S (1999) Spectral gradient acoustic reflectometry: detection of middle ear effusion in suppurative acute otitis media. The Pediatric Infectious Disease Journal 18: 741-4.

Bluestone CD, Cantekin EI (1981) Current clinical methods, indications and interpretations of Eustachian tube function tests. Annals of Otology 90: 552-62.

Bluestone CD, Klein JO (1995) Otitis Media in Infants and Children. 2 edn. Philadelphia: Saunders.

British Society of Audiology (1992) Recommended procedure for tympanometry. British Journal of Audiology 26: 225-57.

Brooks DN (1969) The use of the electroacoustic impedance bridge in the assessment of middle ear function. International Audiology 8: 563-9.

BS EN 60645-1 (1995) Audiometers - Part 1: Pure-tone Audiometers. London: British Standards Institution.

BS EN 61027 (1993) Specification for instruments for the Measurement of Aural Acoustic Impedance/Admittance. London: British Standards Institution.

Douniadakis DE, Nikolopoulos TP, Tsakanikos MD, Vassiliadis SV, Apostolopoulos NJ (1993) Evaluation of acoustic reflectometry in detecting otitis media in children. British Journal of Audiology 27: 409-14.

Harsten G, Nettlebladt U, Schalen L, Kalm O, Prellner K (1993) Language development in children with acute otitis media during first three years of life. Follow up study from birth to seven years of age. Journal of Laryngology and Otology 107: 407-12.

Hirsch JE, Margolis RH, Rykken JR (1992) A comparison of acoustic reflex and auditory brainstem response screening of high risk infants. Ear and Hearing 13: 181-6.

Holte L, Margolis RH, Cavanaugh (Jr.) RM (1991) Developmental changes in multifrequency tympanograms. Audiology 30: 1-24.

Hunter LL, Margolis RH (1992) Multifrequency tympanometry: current clinical application. American Journal of Audiology 1: 33-43.

Jerger J (1970) Clinical experience with impedance audiometry. Archives of Otolaryngology 92: 311-24.

Keefe DH, Levi E (1996) Maturation of the middle and external ears: acoustic power-based responses and reflectance tympanometry. Ear and Hearing 17: 361-73.

Kemaloglu YK, Sener T, Beder L, Bayazit Y, Goksu N (1999) Predictive value of acoustic reflectometry (angle and reflectivity) and tympanometry. International Journal of Pediatric Otorhinolarngology 48: 137-42.

Lucae A (1867) Ueber eine neue method zur unterzuchung des gehoerorgans zu physiologischen und diagnostichen zwecken mit hulfe des interferenzotoscopes. Archiv fur Ohren, Nasen und Kehlkopfheilkunde 3: 186-200.

McKinley AM, Grose JH, Roush J (1997) Multifrequency tympanometry and evoked otoacoustic emissions in neonates during the first 24 hours of life. Journal of the American Academy of Audiology 8: 218-23.

Marchant CD, McMillan PM, Shurin PA, Johnson CE, Turczyk VA, Feinstein JC, Panek SM (1986) Objective diagnosis of otitis media in early infancy by tympanometry and ipsilateral acoustic reflex thresholds. Journal of Pediatrics 109: 590-5.

Marchbanks RJ, Martin AM (1984) Theoretical and experimental evaluation of the diagnostic potential of the tympanic membrane displacement measuring system. Memorandum of the Institute of Sound and Vibration Research No 652.

Margolis RH (1993) Detection of hearing impairment with the acoustic stapedius reflex. Ear and Hearing 14: 3-10.

Margolis RH, Heller JW (1987) Screening tympanometry: criteria for medical referral. Audiology 26: 197-208.

Metz O (1946) The acoustic impedance measured on normal and pathological ears. Acta Otolaryngologica 63: 1.

Metz O (1952) Threshold of reflex contractions of muscles of the middle ear and recruitment of loudness. Archives of Otolaryngology 55: 536-43.

Meyer SE, Jardine CA, Deverson W (1997) Developmental changes in tympanometry: a case study. British Journal of Audiology 31: 189-95.

Paradise JL, Smith CG, Bluestone CD (1976) Tympanometric detection of middle ear effusion in infants and young children. Pediatrics 58: 198-210.

Samuel M, Burge DM, Marchbanks RJ (1998) Quantitative assessment of intracranial pressure by the tympanic membrane displacement audiometric technique in children with shunted hydrocephalus. European Journal of Pediatric Surgery 8: 200-7.

Shurin PA, Pelton SI, Finkelstein J (1977) Tympanometry in the diagnosis of middle ear effusion. New England Journal of Medicine 24: 412-17.

Sprague BH, Wiley TL, Goldstein R (1985) Tympanometric and acoustic reflex studies in neonates. Journal of Speech and Hearing Research 28: 265-72.

Sutherland JE, Campbell K (1990) Immitance audiometry. Primary Care 17 (2): 233-47.

Sutton GJ, Gleadle P, Rowe SJ (1996) Tympanometry and otoacoustic emissions in a cohort of special care neonates. British Journal of Audiology 30: 9-17.

Teele DW, Teele J (1984) Detection of middle ear effusion by acoustic reflectometry. In Lim DJ, Bluestone CD, Klein JO, Nelson JD (eds) Recent Advances in Otitis Media with Effusion. Philadelphia: Becker BC, pp. 237-8.

Terkildsen K, Scott-Nielsen S (1960) An electroacoustic impedance measuring bridge for clinical use. Archives of Otolaryngology 72: 339-46.

Terkildsen K, Thomsen KA (1959) The influence of pressure variations on the impedance of the human ear drum. A method for objective determination of middle ear pressure. The Journal of Laryngology and Otology 73: 409.

Vanhuyse V, Creten W, Van Camp K (1975) On the W-notching of tympanograms. Scandinavian Audiology 4: 45-50.

Vincent VL, Gerber SE (1987) Early development of the acoustic reflex. Audiology 26: 356-62.

Weatherby LA, Bennett MJ (1980) The neonatal acoustic reflex. Scandinavian Audiology 9: 103-10.

West W (1928) Measurement of the acoustical impedance of human ears. Post Office Electrical Engineers Journal 21: 293.

Chapter 9
Hearing aid systems

PHILIP EVANS

Introduction

A hearing aid is a device that processes sound in such a way as to make the information it conveys more accessible to the user. It is an integral part of the receptive communication chain, which includes the signal source and the listener. It should be seen as only one important part of a programme to minimize disability and handicap arising from hearing impairment by optimizing the partially hearing or deaf user's access to acoustical information.

A hearing aid will not restore normal hearing because it cannot fully overcome the complex fundamental impairments of auditory function (especially in sensorineural hearing impairment), including raised hearing thresholds, poor frequency and temporal resolution and reduced dynamic range. However, optimum communication will be achieved only by the provision of the most appropriate aid. The nature of the acoustic environment and the features that are likely to be most important to the user need to be considered when choosing the aid. The type and extent of auditory impairment of the user and the integrity of his or her other sensory modalities will also influence the choice. When the hearing impaired person is a young child, cognitive, linguistic and physical development and the family environment are important additional factors.

In the form with which most people are familiar, the hearing aid makes ambient sound louder across a limited frequency range. However, signal processing beyond uniform linear amplification is necessary for most hearing impaired children because of the characteristics of their hearing losses and the conditions under which they will be likely to use their aids. Amplification may vary with frequency, to suit the audiometric configuration of the child, or to limit the masking of informative sounds by ambient noise. Various forms of automatic gain control may be used to ensure that amplified sound is received by the child with optimum audibility and comfort and generally does not exceed his or her loudness discomfort level. It may be considered appropriate to amplify sounds preferentially from a particular direction or source (for example, a single speaker), to improve the detection and recognition of important sounds in background noise.

However, signal processing may not be limited to providing the hearing impaired child with an altered acoustical stimulus. Salient features of the acoustical environment, such as frequency and temporal information can be presented to the child through vibrotactile stimulation. Direct electrical stimulation of the acoustic nerve through an implanted device can be used to produce auditory perception of important acoustic features. Environmental aids can be chosen to signal specific environmental sounds (for example, doorbell or telephone) to the child visually. Each of these can be used to fulfil the aim of providing acoustic information to the hearing impaired child in an optimum way. It is important that the audiologist should be sufficiently aware of the requirements, capabilities and limitations of the child in selecting or recommending the most appropriate device. Vibrotactile aids and electrical stimulation systems will be discussed briefly at the end of this chapter and elsewhere in the book. Most of the subsequent discussion will concentrate on the electroacoustical hearing aid, which is by far the most common device fitted.

Hearing aids have generally been designed as either auditory prostheses or communication aids. An auditory prosthesis is intended to provide reasonable hearing in a range of acoustical environments, with minimum adjustment by the user. Until recently, the limited capabilities of such devices made them most suitable for people who are frequently in relatively benign auditory environments (with low noise and reverberation), or who have physical or cognitive difficulties that might make manipulation of controls difficult. Elderly hearing impaired people have been the main users.

A communication aid is envisaged as a device that allows the user to manipulate the processing of ambient sound to achieve an optimum input to the disordered auditory system, in varying acoustical environments. It may include some user-accessible controls for altering the performance of the aid and may be used with additional pieces of equipment to extract the maximum acoustic information from the environment. This concept was seen to be most appropriate for hearing impaired people with a need for optimum speech recognition in various listening conditions, including difficult environments with high noise or reverberation levels or multiple speakers. School-age children are generally included in this group. Certainly, no observer of a school unit for hearing impaired children can fail to be impressed by the competence and confidence with which the children manipulate their aids, including complicated radio aid systems, for maximum benefit.

For pre-school children, both types of aids are needed at different times. In infancy, auditory learning encompasses all types of acoustic stimuli in situations that allow the child to develop an understanding of the relationship between sound and everyday events or activities. Speech is only one aspect of the acoustic environment, albeit an important one. Much of the time, the very young infant is exposed to speech in relatively quiet conditions. The child needs to be provided with as 'natural' an auditory input as possible, without the necessity for (or the possibility of) frequent manipulation of controls. The older pre-school child is more likely to be involved in speech-centred activities in poor acoustical conditions (for example, in a playgroup or nursery) but must still have the opportunity of exposure to the general auditory environment.

With the development of increasingly sophisticated forms of control and acoustical processing, and the recent advent of digital signal processing in hearing aids, the distinction between the two types of devices is becoming blurred. Increasingly, aids can be programmed with two or more amplification configurations for optional selection by the user in differing conditions. Digital amplification allows comprehensive signal processing that, in some hearing aids, includes the facility to distinguish sounds with speech-like acoustical characteristics from other sounds, with the potential for noise suppression. With precise setting of amplification characteristics to the user's audiometric configuration according to a programmed fitting protocol, and automatic adjustment in response to environmental conditions, digital aids generally have few user-operated controls. It is inevitable that nearly all hearing aids will use digital signal processing within the next few years, with the benefits of improved reliability and reduced manufacturing and servicing costs.

The hearing aid as a system

The instrumental provision that is made for the hearing impaired child should be regarded as a system comprising several components. The system as a whole must be effective and efficient but each of the components should be chosen to be optimal for the child, as well as being well matched with the other components. In some cases, components of a system have to be obtained from a single supplier. This has the advantage of ensuring compatibility and so may be preferable even when not essential. However, the selection of components from different suppliers allows updating of the system as technical advances in individual components occur.

The system may be relatively simple or quite complex. Figure 9.1 shows a simplified schematic representation of a basic hearing aid, wholly worn by the user. It consists of:

- a microphone to detect the ambient sound;
- a variable amplifier;
- a receiver, or miniature loudspeaker, to convert the amplified electrical signal back to sound;
- a battery to provide power to the amplifier and, perhaps, the microphone.

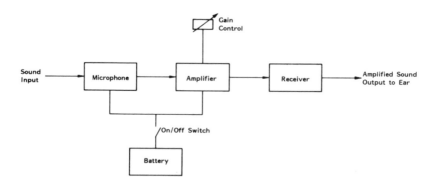

Figure 9.1. Schematic representation of a simple hearing aid.

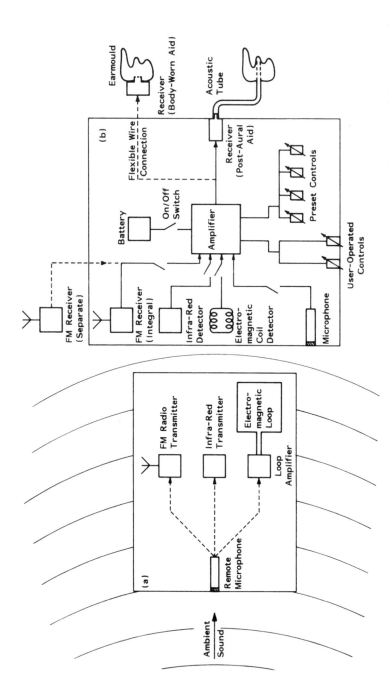

Figure 9.2. Possible components of a hearing aid system. Area (a) shows various forms of a remote microphone-transmission system. Area (b) encloses components which may be included in a single unit worn by the hearing aid user. See text for further explanation.

Most hearing aid systems worn by children are considerably more complex, particularly in the educational environment. Figure 9.2 depicts various possible elements of a hearing aid system that may be provided for a child.

The enclosed area (b), and the components connected to it, include elements that will normally be worn by the child. In a post-aural or intra-aural aid the audio-frequency receiver (a miniature loudspeaker) is usually contained in the same case as the rest of the aid. In a post-aural aid it is connected to an earmould by a plastic tube. The functions of the earmould are to retain the tip of the tube (and hence the sound output of the hearing aid) at the optimum position in the external meatus, to provide a secure fitting of the aid on the ear and to maintain an effective acoustical seal with the meatal wall. In an intra-aural aid, all or most of the items in the area (b) are fitted within the earmould itself. The receiver for a body-worn aid is external to the main body of the aid, being connected directly to an earmould by means of a spring-clip and to the main unit by a flexible lead.

The 'amplifier' will almost certainly consist of more than one stage of amplification and is likely to include several separate processing elements. In a digital signal processing aid there will be an analogue-to-digital converter (ADC) in which the fluctuating output voltage from the microphone, due to the varying acoustical input, will be continuously sampled or digitized before amplification and other processing. A digital-to-analogue converter (DAC) will change the digitized (and processed) signal back into analogue form before a final amplification stage and output to the receiver.

The hearing aid controls shown in Figure 9.2 may include some that are accessible to the user (usually an ON/OFF switch, a gain or volume control and, perhaps, a tone control). Others are intended to be pre-set by the clinician and usually take the form of screwdriver-operated switches or potentiometers (sometimes referred to as trimpots or trimmers) to alter the frequency-gain characteristic and the maximum output of the aid. Increasingly, however, hearing aids are adjusted by connection to a computer, allowing more accurate settings and reducing the number of relatively expensive, bulky and fault-prone control devices.

The area delineated (a) in Figure 9.2 encompasses components that may be present in a system using a remote microphone to provide an optimal signal (usually speech) to the hearing aid user in adverse listening conditions. The output of the microphone may be relayed to the child's aid by infra-red radiation, or by radio-frequency or audio-frequency electromagnetic transmission. In the case of a radio system the child's FM radio-frequency receiver may be integral with the rest of the aid or separate from it. Infra-red light detectors and audio-frequency electromagnetic coil detectors are virtually always fitted into the same case as the rest of the aid.

The concept of the hearing aid system includes all components involved in the fitting of the aid to the child, as well as the elements involved in the processing and transmission of acoustic information. A fault in a single component will reduce the effectiveness efficiency of the system and may cause the communication chain to the child to be impaired or broken altogether. It is therefore imperative that the system is checked frequently and that any faulty component is replaced immediately.

Types of hearing aid systems

Until recently, hearing aids were generally not designed with young children in mind, largely because they represent a very small proportion of hearing aid users. The situation has improved over the last decade and there are now several miniature aids with a range of output characteristics, often with optional facilities and accessories to meet the special needs of hearing impaired children. However, many remain ergonomically unsuitable for young children. When selecting a hearing aid system for a child the audiologist, working in partnership with the parents and the specialist educational support staff, must consider the child's needs in terms of:

- style;
- size;
- features;
- amplification characteristics;
- access to controls.

These aspects are not mutually independent. A specific style of hearing aid may be chosen because of the features required, but it may have implications in other areas (such as size). Selection of hearing aids will be discussed in the next chapter. The following sections will consider the options available to the audiologist.

Style

Post-aural

The post-aural or behind-the-ear aid is currently the most common style provided for hearing impaired children in Britain. Miniaturization of components has allowed a range of aids that are sufficiently small and lightweight to be fitted to pre-school children. Nevertheless, many post-aural aids are too big and heavy to fit securely on the pinnae of infants, particularly very young babies, whose pinnae may be quite floppy, due to lack of development of the cartilaginous tissue. A satisfactory fitting can be achieved in most cases by selecting an aid from the range of very small, light models that are available. Where necessary, proprietary retention loops can be used to hold the aid in position. If the pinnae are too floppy to support such a device, it may be necessary to secure the aid to the side of the child's head by the use of double-sided tape designed for use on skin, which is available from most large pharmacies and many hearing aid suppliers.

The incorporation of all of the electronic components in a single unit makes the post-aural aid reasonably resistant to damage. Nevertheless, its performance is likely to be impaired if it is dropped onto a hard surface. As an additional precaution, there are proprietary devices available to attach the aid to the child's clothing to prevent it from being damaged or lost if it does fall off the child's ear.

The circumaural placement the post-aural aid puts the microphone close to the 'natural' position for auditory input. Binaural fitting provides a close approximation to normal stereophonic stimulation, with its attendant theoretical advantages for directionalization of sound and signal detection in noise. However the close proximity of the microphone to the receiver requires great care to be taken to ensure sufficient acoustic isolation to prevent feedback, particularly in aids with high levels of amplification. Well-fitting earmoulds are, therefore, essential.

Development of components, in particular the electret microphone, has given the post-aural aid the potential for high gain over a wide frequency range. The performance of the aid can be manipulated by the incorporation of user-operated or pre-set controls and, in some cases, by substitution of different earhook tubes. Increasing miniaturization makes controls less accessible and more difficult for parents to read and manipulate, particularly while the aid is on the child. Hearing aids are increasingly designed to be set by connection to a computer, with few controls accessible to the child, but parents still need to be able to check that the aid is switched on and that the volume control (if it exists) is adjusted correctly.

Although the post-aural aid system is reasonably robust it is prone to failure in various ways.

A frequent problem is likely to be blockage of the acoustic tube connecting the aid to the child's earmould, by condensation arising from the high humidity of the external meatus. This may be sufficiently controlled by drying the earmould overnight in a warm dry place, such as an airing cupboard (not a hot oven!). When the condensation is excessive, causing blockage of the acoustic tube, the earmould should be detached from the aid and blown through by miniature bellows (available from most hearing aid suppliers) to clear the drops of moisture. The most common internal faults are likely to be corrosion of the battery terminals or control switches (hastened by the high humidity engendered by perspiration, particularly when the aid is covered by hair) and failure of the microphone suspension, usually caused by impact of the aid on a hard surface. Corrosion will cause increased electrical noise interference or intermittent function. Damage to the microphone suspension will give rise to increased distortion of the amplified sound or internal acoustic feedback.

Intra-aural aids

Intra-aural or in-the-ear aids fit wholly within the concha and the external meatus. All of the components of the aid are contained within an earmould that fills all or part of the concha and extends some way into the ear canal. The microphone, volume control and battery compartment door are fitted in the flat outer face of the device. There is some evidence that the placement of the microphone within the pinna gives significant advantages for sensitivity to high-frequency sounds and the localization of sound sources. However, the close proximity of the microphone and receiver limits the available gain of intra-aural aids because of the increased risk of acoustic feedback, so that they are generally suitable only for mild-moderate hearing losses. Although increasingly popular with hearing impaired teenagers, they are generally regarded as unsuitable for young children. The frequent need to replace the earmould for a growing child (and, hence, to re-case the aid itself) makes the intra-aural aid rather impractical, even though some manufacturers offer to undertake the re-casing free of charge within a specified period following initial purchase of the aid.

The controls of the aid are difficult to see and inaccessible to parents and teachers when the child is wearing the aid. Furthermore, the position and small physical size of the intra-aural aid means that it is not usually possible to include some facilities that may be useful for young children in a nursery class environment or the home. Neither a coil detector for electromagnetic loop systems, nor a radio frequency receiver, can be fitted into very small intra-aural aids. Even a socket for direct input from an externally worn FM radio receiver is not practicable in most cases because of the awkward placement and limited space on the face-plate of the aid. Nevertheless, for a child with a deformed or floppy pinna, which is unable to support a post-aural aid, an intra-aural fitting may exceptionally be considered if the hearing impairment is only mild.

The aesthetic advantages are rarely an issue with pre-school children themselves, but a reluctant parent may be more willing to encourage their child to use the aid if an intra-aural fitting is offered. However, the clinician should resist parental pressure to provide a young child with the most extreme version of an intra-aural aid, in which the device sits wholly within the ear canal. Such a device, generally referred to as an intra-meatal or completely-in-the-canal (CIC) aid, is likely to give minimal benefit to the child and cause significant practical difficulties for the parents and teachers.

Body-worn aids

Body-worn aids do not have any significant acoustic advantages over modern post-aural aids and are now fitted to young children only in exceptional circumstances, usually when the pinna is absent, deformed or excessively floppy, so that the child cannot wear a post-aural or intra-aural aid. A body-worn aid is heavy and cumbersome, and must be fitted in a harness, which the child wears on his or her chest. This placement makes the body-worn aid susceptible to 'body-baffle', causing a relative low-frequency emphasis due to the absorption of high-frequency energy by the child's clothing and body tissues and the reflection of low-frequency energy back to the microphone. The microphone is usually fitted into the top of the aid, rather than the front, in order to pick up the child's own voice most effectively. This makes it vulnerable to damage from spilt food, dribble and vomit. Most manufacturers of body-worn aids provide plastic covers to protect both the microphone aperture and the control switches, which are usually also placed on the top of the aid. This has the additional benefit of preventing the child from playing with, or accidentally knocking, the control switches.

The most common cause of failure of this type of aid is loss of electrical continuity of the flexible lead, which connects the receiver to the main unit, most often at the junction with one of the plugs at either end. The lead is highly vulnerable to damage, especially by being pulled by an inquisitive young child. The most effective way of checking the integrity of the lead is to replace it with a new one. Parents of a child who uses a body-worn aid should be supplied with several leads as they will undoubtedly have to replace them frequently. To minimize problems it is important to use the correct lead as specified by the manufacturer and to ensure that it is properly fitted.

Another problem with the body-worn aid is the size of the receiver. When fitted to a young infant it may be larger in diameter than the back-plate of the child's earmould and thereby cause irritation by abrasion of the pinna. Many receivers are also too heavy to be supported adequately by the earmould in the flaccid pinna of a baby, with the result that the earmould tends to be pulled partly or wholly out of the meatus. Both these problems may be solved in most cases by fitting a miniature receiver, but even that may be too large for a very young baby. Some hearing aid manufacturers will supply a circumaural clip to help to hold the receiver and earmould in place.

Bone-conduction aids

In a child with abnormalities of the external ear it may be difficult or impossible to fit a post-aural, intra-aural or body-worn aid. An absent or rudimentary pinna will preclude a post-aural fitting. The insertion of an earmould may be difficult in an unusually narrow or malformed external meatus and will obviously be impossible in a child with meatal atresia (absence of an external ear canal). In such cases, a bone-conduction aid may be fitted to transmit sound energy to the cochlea by vibration of the skull and, hence, the otic capsule. Such an aid may also be useful in a child with a large conductive component in his or her hearing loss, or with a chronically discharging ear, which prevents consistent use of aids with a conventional earmould.

A bone-conduction aid fitting may be in the form of a body-worn aid with the normal receiver being replaced by a vibrator, which is usually fitted to a sprung steel headband. The limitations outlined for a conventional body-worn aid apply in this case. Alternatively, the device may be entirely head worn. Proprietary systems are available but they tend to be too large for a young child. A better arrangement is to have a post-aural aid adapted by the supplier, who will remove the aid's receiver and fit a lead and a bone-conduction vibrator instead, with all components mounted on a lightweight headband.

The interface of the vibrating receiver with the skin causes considerable distortion in the signal and the relatively large mass of the moving-coil transducer in the bone vibrator limits the output of the system because of the large amount of energy required to drive it. The latter limitation is rarely a problem as the system is most frequently used in children with congenital conductive hearing loss and normal cochlear function. In such cases minimal amplification of ambient sound is required, but the aid will still need to have moderately high output in order to overcome the inertia of the transducer. More serious drawbacks are the lack of aesthetic appeal of the bone-vibrator fitting, physical discomfort, lack of firm connection, and the difficulty in keeping the headband in place. In very young infants, in whom the sections of the skull have not yet fused, the pressure exerted by a headband is undesirable. An acceptable temporary alternative arrangement is to fit an adapted post-aural aid system onto a sweatband or cap, with the aid and the vibrator mounted with Velcro[tm] patches.

Bone-anchored hearing aids

A conventional bone-conduction aid is now rarely considered for long-term use by children. Surgical treatment may allow the use of a normal post-aural or intra-aural aid with an

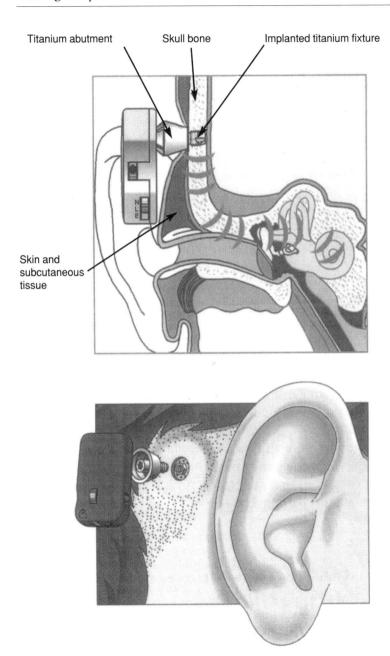

Titanium abutment   Skull bone   Implanted titanium fixture

Skin and
subcutaneous
tissue

Figure 9.3. Bone-anchored hearing aid (BAHA). The output of the sound processor is transmitted to the skull bone, and hence to the cochleae, through a percutaneous screw and abutment. In the upper diagram, for clarity, the sound processor is shown in front of the pinna. In reality, the BAHA is fitted behind the pinna, as in the lower diagram. (Courtesy Entific Medical Systems. Amended by permission.)

electroacoustic receiver. Where permanent bone-conduction amplification is necessary, a bone-anchored hearing aid (Figure 9.3) should be considered. In this, the transducer is fixed to the skull by a titanium screw and activated by direct connection to the body-worn amplifier. The device provides more reliable sound transmission, higher sound intensities and markedly better sound quality than a conventional bone-conduction aid. As the system includes a percutaneous fixture on which the device is fitted, there is a need for regular, meticulous cleaning to prevent the risk of infection. Due to limited skull-bone thickness and changing skull size, bone-anchored aids are not often fitted to children under five years of age, although younger children are increasingly being considered as candidates.

Spectacle aids

In this style, the hearing aid is incorporated into a spectacles frame and is designed for convenience for people with both visual and auditory impairments. Binaural amplification may be provided. Usually, the output of the aid is delivered to the ear in the same way as with a post-aural aid, i.e., through an acoustic tube fitted into an earmould. Alternatively, a bone vibrator may be fitted into the tip of the spectacles frame, where it lies against the mastoid process, providing a neat solution when a bone-conduction aid is required. However, neither version is commonly used with young children, because of the permanent linking of the aid to the spectacles, both of which are likely to require frequent repair or replacement.

CROS systems

In CROS (contralateral routing of signals) systems (Harford and Barry, 1965), the microphone and receiver of the system are separated and placed on opposite sides of the head. The basic system consists of two units, similar in appearance to a pair of post-aural aids, usually linked by a flexible lead. One of the units contains a microphone and amplifying elements and the other contains only a receiver. In a more advanced system, the output from the amplifier may be transmitted to the receiver unit by electromagnetic induction or FM radio. Such a system is used primarily in cases of unilateral or markedly asymmetrical hearing loss, to overcome the lack of sensitivity to sounds on the side of poorer hearing by amplifying and transmitting them to the better-hearing ear. Many variations of the basic system exist and the reader is referred to Dillon (2001a) for a description of them.

CROS systems are not often fitted to young children. Common experience is that children with unilateral hearing impairment generally manage satisfactorily without hearing aids. Children with markedly asymmetrical binaural losses are usually fitted unilaterally with an aid on the better-hearing ear, but may benefit from a BICROS system in which microphones on both sides are connected to a single aid on the better-hearing ear. It could be argued that young children are more suitable candidates for CROS aids than adults with acquired unilateral or asymmetrical losses as they learn faster and are more adaptable to new stimulus configurations. However, the more complicated systems may be ergonomically unsuitable for children and confusing for parents. The number of appropriate CROS fittings may also be limited by a fear that an 'incorrect' auditory representation of the world will be developed irreversibly by the child.

Optimization of signal-to-noise ratio

It is common experience that, in general, we hear better in quiet conditions than in noisy environments. Noise interferes with the detection and recognition of sounds that are important or useful to us. In order to hear best what we want to hear, the *signal-to-noise ratio* needs to be optimal. That is, the intensity of the sound of interest (commonly speech) should be well above that of the background noise. Which sounds are important ('signals') and which are not ('noise') will depend partly upon the circumstances in which we are listening and our priorities. 'Background' environmental sounds may be important for a child's development of auditory awareness of the world, particularly if he or she is in a position to see or touch the sources of the sounds. The same environmental sounds may disrupt the child's perception of a particular sound source (for example, a single speaker).

Noise may arise indirectly from the signal itself as well as from other sources. In many everyday environments, echoes that are caused by reflection of the signal off hard surfaces reach the child's ear with an appreciable time delay after the arrival of the sound along the shortest (direct) path and constitute noise with respect to subsequent elements of the signal. In addition to causing temporal confusion, the echoes have a masking effect upon signal components arriving at the same time by the direct path. The longer travel paths of the echoes and the higher absorptive capacity of air for high-frequency sounds mean that the echoes consist primarily of low-frequency energy, which may mask simultaneous softer sounds, with a tendency to a greater masking effect on high-frequency sounds. Where speech perception is concerned, this may cause weaker high-frequency components to be masked by low-frequency voiced sounds.

Reduced frequency and temporal resolution, which are characteristic of sensorineural hearing impairment, considerably exacerbate the deleterious effects of background noise on speech (Glasberg and Moore, 1989). Speech recognition of all children is reduced in background noise, but markedly more so for those who are hearing impaired (Finitzo-Hieber and Tillman, 1978). Hearing impaired listeners need a much higher signal-to-noise ratio than normal hearing listeners to achieve a similar level of speech recognition, especially if the background noise is fluctuating in frequency or amplitude (Peters et al., 1998), as is the case when there are other speakers in the vicinity.

In order to achieve maximum benefit from a hearing aid, it is important that the signal-to-noise ratio should be maintained at the highest possible level. There are several technical approaches to improving the signal-to-noise ratio in hearing aid systems but they all involve reducing the sensitivity of the system to sounds which are likely to constitute noise or selectively increasing the input level of sounds which are regarded as 'signals' (for example, the voice of a relevant speaker).

Some improvement may be achieved through the design and function of the amplification and signal-processing components of the aid, and this will be discussed later. However, best results are achieved by ensuring that there is a high signal-to-noise ratio at the input to the system.

A conventional hearing aid with a standard integral microphone will amplify all environmental sounds indiscriminately and more-or-less equally, within the limits of its frequency response. In a *remote microphone system*, the microphone is placed close to the preferred speaker to pick up speech without significant contamination by noise or reverberation effects. Figure 9.4 illustrates the signal-to-noise advantage offered by a remote microphone system. The signal is

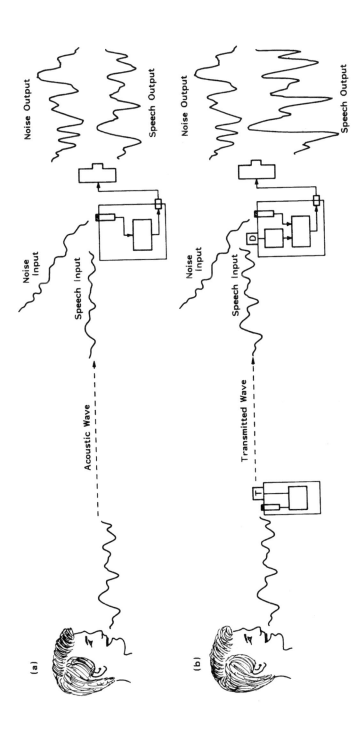

Figure 9.4. The signal-to-noise advantage offered by a remote microphone system. In (a), the speech acoustic wave reduces in intensity as it travels through the air to the hearing aid microphone. The amplified speech output is of a similar intensity to the amplified background noise. In (b), the low-gain remote microphone detects the speech with little noise contamination and the signal is passed to the transmitter (T). The transmitted signal-to-noise ratio is substantially increased and may be further enhanced by switching off the environmental microphone(s) on the child's aid.

amplified and transmitted to the child through one of several means. The hard-wired speech-training unit is still favoured by some teachers and speech therapists when working with individual children because of its excellent high-fidelity performance (Markides et al.,1980), but it has largely been superseded by more convenient systems as hearing impaired children are increasingly being taught in mainstream educational environments.

Electromagnetic induction

In this system the amplified output from the remote microphone activates a wire loop to create a fluctuating audio-frequency electromagnetic signal within a defined area. Most conventional hearing aids are provided with a switchable integral 'telecoil' (usually labelled 'T' on the function switch) to detect such a signal, sometimes with the optional simultaneous function of the environmental microphone (usually denoted 'MT'). The remote microphone may be connected directly to the loop amplifier, or a body-worn radio microphone may be used to allow the speaker freedom of movement. British Standard BS EN 60118-4 (1998), which is technically equivalent to IEC (1981a), specifies the magnetic-field strength required in loops for hearing aids and the National Deaf Children's Society has published a fact sheet giving guidelines for the installation and use of induction loops (NDCS, 1998a). Although the loop system is cheap and can be highly effective in reducing the adverse effects of environmental noise, it has several disadvantages:

• the electromagnetic field tends to be uneven and can 'spill over' into adjacent areas, with the possibility of detection by children outside the loop;
• the efficiency of the system depends partly on the orientation of the telecoil with respect to the loop, so that the strength of the induced signal may vary as the child's head moves;
• the telecoil may pick up noise from other sources of electromagnetic radiation, such as control equipment for fluorescent lighting;
• the electromagnetic transduction process is sometimes found to cause a relative reduction in low-frequency signal strength, compared to the performance of the aid with the environmental microphone.

For these reasons, the loop system is now rarely used in school and nursery classrooms, although it is widely fitted in public halls, churches and theatres for the benefit of hearing aid users. It offers little advantage for the hearing impaired child at home, except for connection to the audio output of a television set to provide a low-noise condition for viewing.

Infra-red transmission

Infra-red transmission can be used in remote microphone systems. The output of the microphone is fed into an infra-red transmitter, which may be worn by the speaker. The child wears a unit that detects the infra-red transmission and provides an audio-frequency signal, usually for direct input to the child's own hearing aid. The system avoids the spill-over disadvantage of the electromagnetic loop system as the infra-red signal is contained within the walls of the room. It is, however, susceptible to interference from strong sunlight and is therefore not suitable for use outside or in rooms with large windows that allow in a lot of direct sunlight. The body-worn transmitter also requires the speaker and the child to be facing each other for successful reception. A variation of the system uses a set of transmitters, usually placed at the corners of the room to ensure complete and even coverage. Infra-red systems have not gained as much popularity in educational settings in the UK as in continental Europe but are increasingly being used in other applications, such as television listening aids and concert halls. NDCS (1998b) gives further information about their installation and use.

FM radio transmission

In the most popular type of remote microphone hearing aid system used with children in the UK, the output of the remote microphone is conveyed to the child by frequency-modulated (FM) radio transmission. Three forms of FM hearing aid systems are available:

- The radio receiver worn by the child may be integral with a hearing aid in a body-worn unit (Figure 9.5). The hearing aid frequently has two independent channels, each with its own environmental microphone, in addition to the input from the FM receiver. Usually the environmental microphones and the radio receiver can be selected independently or can be

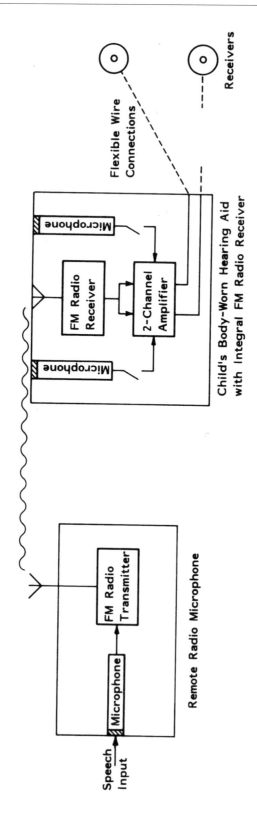

Figure 9.5. A radio/hearing aid system in which the radio receiver and the hearing aid are in the same unit.

operated together. The aid outputs are connected by wire leads to button receivers as in a conventional body-worn aid fitting.

- The radio receiver may be worn separately, to allow the child to use conventional hearing aids (usually post-aural) independently of the FM system (Figure 9.6). The connection between the radio receiver and the hearing aid(s) should preferably be by *direct audio input*, using a wire lead. BS (1999) and IEC (1999) specify electrical characteristics for the electrical input circuits in hearing aids. Manufacturers use connection devices (often referred to as 'shoes'), which are unique to their own systems, but BS (1997) and IEC (1996) specify dimensions for a standard plug and socket for coupling of the lead to the connection device. The lead itself (which may include an aerial for the radio receiver) is generally specific to each aid, so it is advisable to obtain connection equipment from the hearing aid manufacturer or supplier. The electrical input circuit of the hearing aid can also be used for direct connection of other audio devices such as radios, tape recorders or microphones. Some circuits provide a convenient means of incorporating the aid into a CROS system. For aids that do not have a facility for direct connection to a FM radio receiver, indirect input is possible. Usually this takes the form of electromagnetic induction, with the aid's telecoil being activated by an electromagnetic field generated by a neck-worn loop connected by wire to the radio receiver. However, the technical problems discussed earlier for electromagnetic loop induction apply to this approach and the system is cumbersome.

- A miniature FM receiver has recently been developed for direct connection to a post-aural hearing aid, by plugging into the standard electrical socket of the direct input shoe. The aerial is internal to the device, which is light, convenient and less vulnerable than systems using connection leads. However, it is currently provided predominantly for young people of school age.

FM radio transmission offers many advantages for use with young children, particularly in schools and nursery environments. It can operate over considerable distances (several hundred yards) with little or no hindrance from solid objects, so that the child is not constrained in a limited area. It is

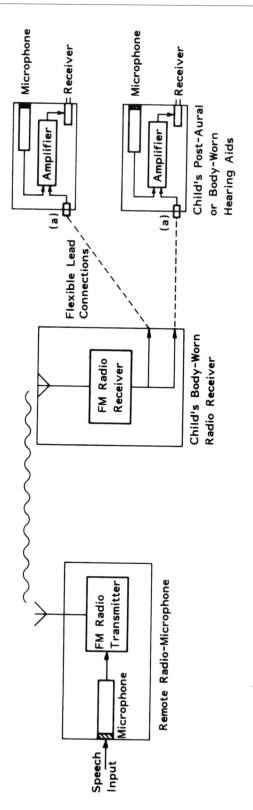

Figure 9.6. A radio/hearing aid system in which the radio receiver and the hearing aid(s) are worn separately by the child. The electrical input socket (a) will usually accept inputs from other electroacoustic devices.

rarely subject to interference. Spillover or cross-talk between channels used by children engaged in different activities is avoided by the use of different transmission frequencies. Currently, up to eight frequencies are designated for the sole use of FM radio hearing aid systems in the UK (depending upon the technical specification of the equipment) and many more are available, though with a slight risk of interference from other types of radio transmission systems (RA, 2001). In most systems, different frequencies can be selected by a simple change of an oscillator module and some allow the child to switch between the selected module frequency and another fixed frequency. This is useful in an educational environment, where one channel (the fixed frequency) can be common to all children in a group and each child can have his or her own channel for private communication with the teacher.

The radio aid is an effective and convenient device for providing the child in school or nursery with high-quality speech input with minimum noise interference. In Britain, it is seen largely as an educational aid and is usually provided by the local education authority. Its advantage for the child at home is less clear, as signal-to-noise ratios are generally good and there are few competing speakers. It is important that the limitations and disadvantages of the system are understood, to avoid its abuse by parents and teachers. If the young infant is too often distant from the speaker or the source of an environmental sound that is clearly audible to him through a radio aid system, his audio-spatial awareness could be impaired. Parents need to be aware that a child using a radio aid cannot be relied upon to recognize warnings and instructions at a distance. The convenience of the system may also encourage some parents or teachers to disturb the hearing impaired child at play in an intrusive way that would not be possible otherwise, or with a normal hearing child. The system needs to be used thoughtfully and carefully.

Components of hearing aid systems

Microphone

Most hearing aids are fitted with integral microphones. Other forms of input were discussed in the previous section. The progressive miniaturization of hearing aids, together with the demand for high power output, has led to a requirement for a microphone that:

- is highly sensitive;
- is small and light;
- has a flat frequency response;
- is stable and robust;
- has a low power requirement.

Such qualities are found in the electret microphone, which is now almost universally fitted to hearing aids. The microphone has a metallized, thin plastic diaphragm, supported on strips of permanently charged dielectric material (electrets), which forms a capacitor in conjunction with a metal backplate in which the electrets are fixed. Incoming sound waves cause the diaphragm to move relative to the backplate, thus changing the capacitance of the device and generating a small fluctuating current. A field-effect transistor (FET) amplifies the current for input to the main amplifier. The response of the electret microphone is relatively flat over a wide frequency range (typically 200 Hz to 7,000 Hz) and the small mass of the diaphragm gives it high sensitivity to acoustic stimuli. At the same time, the device has a low sensitivity to mechanical vibration (for example, due to movement of the wearer of the aid), is robust against physical damage and is largely unaffected by magnetic fields. The last property makes it particularly suitable for incorporation into miniature hearing aids, in close proximity to receivers.

Most hearing aid microphones are omnidirectional – that is, they are more-or-less equally sensitive to sound from any direction. In order to improve the signal-to-noise ratio, *directional microphones* have been developed for post-aural aids to provide relatively greater sensitivity to sounds arriving from in front of the hearing aid wearer than from other directions (Figure 9.7). The directionality is achieved by providing a second port for entry of sound energy into the microphone behind the diaphragm. Lower sensitivity to sound arriving at the rear port, together with the incorporation of an acoustic delay in the travel time of sounds from the rear port to the diaphragm provides selective reduction in sensitivity to sounds from behind the user through cancellation of the acoustic energy at the diaphragm. It should be noted that the extent of directionality specified by manufacturers, under laboratory conditions is not always achieved in everyday use.

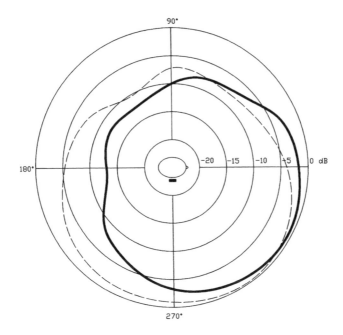

Figure 9.7. Typical relative sensitivity of a hearing aid with a directional microphone (———) compared with the same aid with an omnidirectional microphone (- - - -). Position of hearing is indicated by ▬ .

Placement of the microphone inlet is of some importance. In post-aural aids the inlet may be at the bottom of the aid but is most often at the top (facing forwards) because of the slight directional advantage and small improvement in high-frequency amplification afforded by forward-facing microphones. They are all prone to wind noise, but manufacturers usually fit windshields to reduce the problem. The position of microphones in body-worn and intra-aural aids has been discussed previously.

Receivers

Electromagnetic receivers (earphones) are almost universally fitted in hearing aids, because of their efficiency and high power-handling capabilities. They are generally designed to have a fairly flat response but it is over a narrower frequency range than electret microphones, particularly at high frequencies. For this reason, the receiver tends to be the limiting factor in the overall response of the aid. Generally, the higher the output capability of the receiver, the narrower the frequency range and the less smooth the frequency-gain characteristic of the aid. Receivers introduce 'peaks' into the frequency response.

The insert receiver of a body-worn aid is external to the main unit. Both standard and miniature receivers are available for most models, with varying power outputs and frequency ranges. Although standard receivers tend to have slightly higher power output, the practical fitting problems mean that they are generally unsuitable for young children. Receivers fitted to aids with push-pull amplifiers have three-hole sockets for the lead plug, whereas others may have only two holes. In some cases, the polarities of the plug and socket are important and the correct alignment is usually ensured by unequal pin size.

The internal receivers of post-aural aids are, of course, not able to be changed by the user. Different power or frequency-range requirements are met through a much wider range of models than is available with body-worn aids. The construction of the internal receiver differs somewhat from that of the insert receiver (apart from being smaller) but the performance characteristics of the two types are not substantially different.

Bone conduction receivers work on a similar principle but the vibrations of the receiver diaphragm are transmitted by direct coupling to the case of the receiver. The flat surface of the case, placed in contact with the head, causes the skull to vibrate so that the cochlea is stimulated directly through the vibration of the bony otic capsule.

Amplification and processing components

Hearing aids are amplifying devices, intended to make a wider range of sounds accessible to the hearing impaired user. However, because of the complex nature of sensorineural hearing impairment, more complicated processing than simple linear amplification is usually needed if the amplified sound is to be presented to the hearing impaired child at a comfortable level and with maximum effect. The increasingly common use of prescriptive hearing aid selection procedures requires accurate adjustment of the amplification characteristics and processing strategies of hearing aids to meet the specific needs of the individual child. Although conventional *analogue* hearing aids can achieve satisfactory outcomes in most cases, the recent introduction of *digital signal processing* into hearing aids allows wider application and greater precision in hearing aid performance.

Analogue hearing aids

In an analogue hearing aid the electrical signal from the microphone FET is fed into the main amplifier to produce an output of greater power, but which follows the fluctuations of the input signal. After any required modification, the amplifier output is fed into the receiver to be converted back to sound. The design aim for the main amplifier of a hearing aid is usually to achieve an acceptable balance between the output power required and the efficiency of the device in terms of battery power requirement. The amplification (or *gain*) is achieved in different ways, depending on the type or *Class* of amplifier.

Many high-powered analogue hearing aids incorporate a so-called Class B amplifier (also known as a *push-pull amplifier*). This directly amplifies the output signal from the microphone and has two separate amplifying elements in the output stage, operating in such a way as to maximize the current through the receiver. Both post-aural and body-worn aids are available with the capability for maximum output levels in excess of 140 dB SPL, suitable for the most profound hearing losses.

As Class B amplifiers are bulky and not very efficient, high-powered analogue hearing aids are generally relatively large and consume battery power at a high rate. To achieve greater efficiency, most other current analogue hearing aids have a Class D amplifier. This achieves amplification by using the output signal from the microphone to modulate the pulse duration of an electrical pulse train of constant voltage. The intensity of the acoustical output of the aid varies according to the duration of the pulses.

One significant drawback with any analogue amplifier is that its maximum output is limited to a specific level. With high input or gain levels the output becomes constant. The effect is to flatten the peaks and troughs of the amplified waveform (Figure 9.8). This so-called *peak-clipping* is used as a form of output-limiting in some hearing aids, but it has the disadvantage of introducing marked distortion into the output signal, giving rise to a noticeable 'roughness' in the sound quality. Note that the hearing aid receiver may also introduce peak-clipping into intense output signals, due to mechanical limitations of the receiver.

(a)   (b)

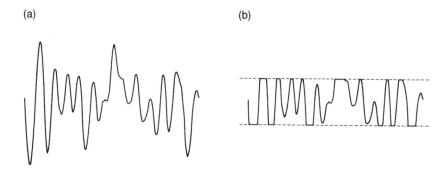

Figure 9.8. Peak-clipping of a waveform. When the amplifier signal (a) exceeds the maximum amplitude output limits of the amplifier, shown by the dashed line in (b), the peaks and troughs of the waveform are 'clipped'.

Digital signal processing aids

Digital signal processing (DSP), which is used extensively in a wide range of electronic and audiovisual applications, was introduced into commercial wearable hearing aids in the mid-1990s. In a digital aid, the amplification and processing of the acoustical signal is undertaken by a computer. As the computer cannot act directly on the acoustical signal (or the analogue electrical waveform arising from the microphone), an *analogue-to-digital converter* samples the microphone output to produce a series of discrete measurements of the size (power) of the signal (Figure 9.9). In order to obtain an accurate representation of the incoming signal, the sampling frequency must be at least twice the maximum frequency in the signal. Hearing aids are expected to cover a frequency range up to about 10 kHz, so the sampling frequency needs to be at least 20 kHz (that is, at least one sample every 1/20,000 second), to avoid any information in the signal being lost. The samples are then assigned numbers in a pre-determined scale, which covers the full range of possible power values. As the numbers need to be integers (whole numbers), each sample is assigned the number (the *digital code*), which is closest to its actual value. Finally, the digital codes are changed into binary digit (*bit*) numbers comprised of sequences of 0 and 1 values that are recognizable by the computer and can be subjected to arithmetical operations to achieve the amplification and processing required.

After processing, the digital signal needs to be reconverted to an acoustic signal. The *digital-to-analogue conversion* in a

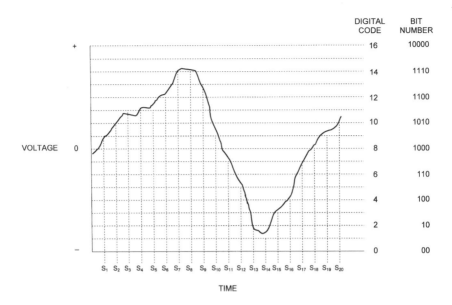

Figure 9.9. Digital sampling of an electrical analogue output from a microphone to produce a series of *binary digit* ('bit') numbers which is a numerical representation of the acoustic waveform. Each sample (s_1, s_2, s_3, ...) is assigned the *digital code* integer value closest to its actual value. The digital code values are represented as bit numbers in the signal processor in the hearing aid.

hearing aid is usually achieved by changing the digital signal to a sequence of discrete power values, which are used to activate the receiver. The mechanical inertia of the receiver smoothes out the stepwise changes in power, to produce an acceptable acoustical output.

Digital signal processing in hearing aids offers many potential advantages over analogue amplification, although not all may be realizable or useful in practice, at least where young children are users.

- Digital signal processing allows more precise control over the performance of the aid, to meet the needs of the individual user. The value of this depends partly on the validity of prescriptive fitting procedures, and the accuracy with which hearing thresholds can be measured in young infants.
- Digital signal processing uses battery power more efficiently than analogue amplification, at least when providing high power output. However, as processing becomes more complex, power use will increase. Nevertheless, the lower

power requirement of DSP aids enables them generally to be made smaller than analogue aids of similar performance (though size will continue to be limited by the microphone and receiver, and the need for the aid to be practical to be worn by the young child).

- Unlike an analogue amplifier, DSP does not produce internal noise, and therefore presents a 'cleaner' acoustical signal to the hearing aid user.

- Digital signal processing is more reliable than analogue amplification. This, together with the fact that the processor is more readily incorporated entirely on an *integrated circuit,* means that DSP aids are inherently cheaper to produce and maintain than analogue aids of broadly similar performance. Digital hearing aids are currently more expensive than analogue aids because manufacturers have only recently started to produce DSP aids in large quantities and need to recover their considerable development costs.

- Digital aids are capable of more complex processing than analogue aids. However, it is not yet entirely clear what types of processing (and, even less, exactly what processing algorithms) are likely to be beneficial, especially for young hearing impaired children.

- Digital signal processing allows storage of more than one programme of settings, for different performance of the aid in different conditions. Where the user selects these, the facility is likely to be of greater benefit to adults than to young children. However, it is possible to incorporate automatic selection of the processing strategy, dependent upon the acoustical characteristics of the sound input to the aid.

- In some types of DSP aids, it will be possible to import new forms of signal processing which may be developed in future (the user will retain the hardware, but will change the software). This should significantly reduce the costs of upgrading the user's aid provision.

Compression amplification

The narrowing of the dynamic range of hearing in sensorineural hearing impairment and its implications for hearing aid provision have been recognized for many years (Steinberg and Gardner, 1937; Pascoe, 1978). Ideally, amplification characteristics need to be chosen to ensure that the hearing aid output always falls within the reduced dynamic range of the user. The aim is to ensure that:

- most sounds should be presented to the user at a comfortable listening level;
- low-intensity sounds should be presented at a just audible level, which may require higher gain;
- amplified high-intensity sounds should be presented at a level below the user's loudness discomfort level, which may require lower gain.

This implies that the hearing aid may need to process input sound in different ways, depending upon its input intensity. Different fitting procedures approach the issue in various ways and the exact amplification characteristics required may be expected to vary with the characteristics of individual users' auditory functions.

Most hearing aid fitting procedures aim to ensure that the maximum output of the aid does not exceed the user's loudness discomfort level. For any young child, the aid should have an efficient output-limiting device to prevent excessive amplification when the child is in noisy environments. In many analogue aids, output-limiting is achieved by adjusting the peak-clipping level of the main amplifier but this causes distortion that can be quite unpleasant, at least for patients with mild-moderate hearing impairment, and can affect speech recognition adversely.

Compression amplification, more properly termed automatic gain control (AGC), is generally a preferred approach to output-limiting and is necessary to ensure appropriate levels of gain for input sounds of low and medium intensities. In a hearing aid AGC amplifier, the gain of the amplifier is varied automatically by a feedback loop, which senses the magnitude of the signal at a particular point in the circuit. A generalized input-output curve of an AGC amplifier is shown in Figure 9.10. Above a certain input level, the lower AGC limit, the gain of the amplifier is reduced for increasing input level. The output level rises more slowly, eventually becoming almost constant at high input levels. The lower AGC limit is sometimes adjustable through an internal pre-set control. In hearing aids with *wide dynamic range compression* the lower AGC limit is close to normal threshold intensity so that the compression occurs across most

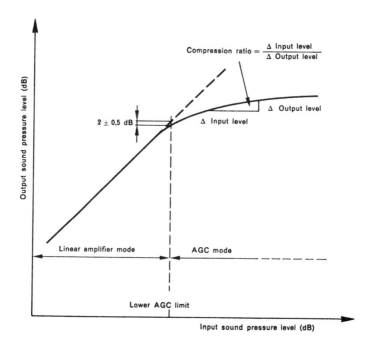

Figure 9.10. A generalised input-output curve of an amplifier with automatic gain control (AGC). The *lower AGC limit* is defined as the input sound pressure level at which there is a reduction in the gain of 2 ± 0.5dB with respect to the gain in the linear mode. Source: BS (1996).

or all of the input level range. In some hearing aids the gain for near-threshold sounds is increased to make them audible to the hearing impaired listener.

Single-channel compression aids measure the input sound level as a whole, across all frequencies, but this may not provide satisfactory performance for a child whose hearing impairment is markedly different in different frequency regions. Multi-channel compression aids are now widely available (particularly with digital signal processing), allowing different amplification characteristics for different frequency bands.

The effect of AGC on the performance of the hearing aid depends partly upon the point in the circuit at which the signal level is monitored (Figure 9.11). In input-controlled compression, the amplifier gain is dependent upon the signal level just before the user's gain (volume) control. Thus the maximum output of the aid depends upon the setting of the volume control (Figure 9.12). In output-controlled compression, the signal level is monitored after the volume control. The

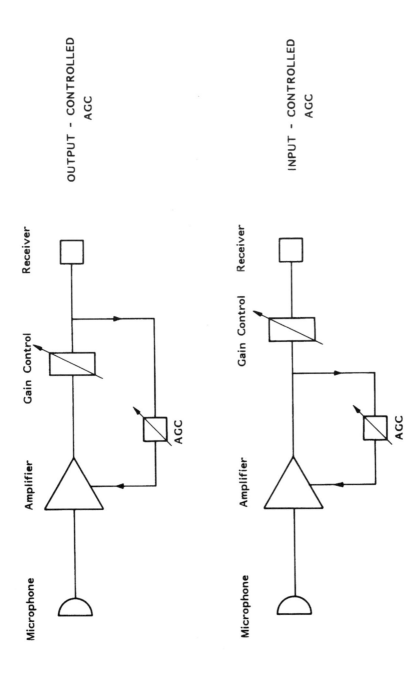

Figure 9.11. Schematic representation of output-controlled and input-controlled AGC circuits.

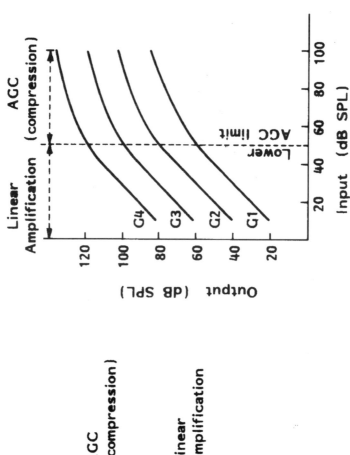

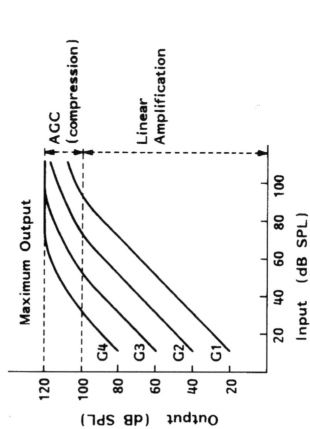

Figure 9.12. Effect of the gain control setting (G1–G4) on the maximum output of a hearing aid with output-controlled or input-controlled compression amplification (AGC).

setting of the volume control may influence the output indirectly (by modifying the amplifier gain through the feedback network), as well as directly through its attenuating function, but does not alter the pre-set maximum output of the aid. Each of the two types of AGC circuit has advantages and disadvantages and is best suited for a particular requirement. One aim may be to maintain the output of the aid within a narrow range around the user's most comfortable listening level, in spite of widely varying input levels. This is most likely to be required for patients whose dynamic range of hearing is markedly restricted, because of the effect of excessive loudness recruitment. In this case, input-controlled compression is preferable as the input signal to the user's gain control can be made to vary within a pre-determined narrow amplitude range, allowing the user to set the output to a preferred level, which may change with the type of listening task and the ambient conditions. A second application of AGC can be predominantly to restrict the maximum output of the aid to a level that is below the loudness discomfort level of the user. In this case, output-controlled AGC is preferable. Input-controlled compression is probably more appropriate for the responsible older child, who will be able to adjust his aid to suit himself in various circumstances. Generally, the pre-school hearing aid user cannot do this and there is a risk that the volume control may inadvertently be knocked by the child, causing the output of the aid to exceed the child's loudness discomfort threshold when high input sound levels occur. Output-controlled compression is useful in preventing this, but a better alternative might be to fit an aid with both input-controlled compression and a maximum output control (usually a peak-clipping device).

Although compression amplification distorts the signal less than peak-clipping, it has limitations. The attack time and recovery time of the AGC circuit, at the onset and cessation respectively of a sound exceeding the lower AGC limit, must be carefully set. It is important to minimize the risk that the early part of a loud sound will be amplified excessively, while ensuring that transient stimuli do not trigger the AGC unnecessarily. Similarly, abrupt release of the compression can be disconcerting for the hearing aid user, but the reduced gain should not be prolonged to the extent that subsequent quiet sounds are not heard. This is particularly important when listening to speech, to avoid the suppression of soft unvoiced phonemes by the action of the compression circuit in response to louder voiced sounds. (If this is a frequent problem, it suggests that the lower AGC limit is set too low.) For most single-channel compression aids, attack times are usually in the range 0.5–20 ms and recovery times in the range 60–150 ms.

In multi-channel aids, attack and recovery times may vary across channels. Some recent aids include a feature in which the attack and recovery times depend upon the ambient sound levels.

Compression amplification is a complex area, with many aspects that are beyond the scope of this chapter. For comprehensive coverage of the topic the reader is referred to Dillon (2001b).

Controls

Most analogue hearing aids include components to enable the performance of the amplifier to be altered. A volume control is nearly always provided to alter the amount of gain provided by the amplifier. A tone control may be included to change the slope of the frequency response (the relative amount of amplification in various frequency regions). As well as the external controls provided to allow the user to alter both of these functions, many aids also have internal pre-set controls, which are usually altered by screwdriver, to allow the clinician or teacher to set limits within which the user may vary the performance of the aid. Peak-clipping or compression facilities are nearly always adjusted by internal controls.

Any user-adjustable controls must not be easily accessible and vulnerable to exploratory manipulation by infants. Where necessary, control covers are usually available. Older pre-school children may be encouraged to adjust some controls (at least the volume control) themselves. The settings of user-adjustable controls should be clearly and unambiguously marked in accordance with international standards (for example, IEC, 1983f) so that the parent or teacher of a hearing impaired child can ensure that the controls are set correctly.

Increasingly, however, hearing aids are fitted with few or no controls accessible to the user. In the late 1980s, most major manufacturers started to produce *digitally programmable analogue aids*. These use analogue amplification technology but are controlled by digital circuitry. The absence of bulky trimmers allows the aids to be made smaller, while the digital controls offer greater precision and flexibility in the adjustment of the function of the devices. The clinician makes the initial settings, using a simple computer connected to the aid, but most aids of this type allow users to adjust their aids by remote control using various forms of transmission. This facility is useful for elderly users, who may find it difficult to manipulate switches and other physical controls fitted in hearing aids, but it is clearly not suitable for young children because of the potential difficulty of ensuring consistent settings. For this reason, and because of their relatively high cost, digitally programmable analogue aids have not been fitted widely to children in the UK.

Digital signal processing has virtually eliminated the need for user-accessible controls in hearing aids. These aids are adjusted by connection to a computer, according to fitting formulae that are usually determined by the manufacturers and based upon published fitting procedures. They require the input of the hearing threshold values (and, sometimes, the loudness discomfort levels or most comfortable listening levels) of the user. The intention is to set the aid's performance optimally for the user, according to the fitting formula adopted, though it is usually possible for the clinician to change some of the performance parameters. As DSP aids usually include single-channel or multi-channel compression, and use processing strategies that are intended to ensure that the aid output always falls within the dynamic range of the user, there is little need for them to have user accessible controls and most do not. For young children, this is beneficial, as it helps to ensure consistent performance of the aid, prevents accidental alteration of the functional parameter values and reduces the risk of damage. However, as no prescriptive fitting formulae are validated on very young children, it is important not to assume that the settings of the aid are optimum for the individual child. The clinician, taking advice from the parents and specialist educational staff, must monitor the child's aided performance and behaviour carefully.

Batteries

Most aids are powered by disposable batteries (more accurately termed primary cells) of various types. Currently, the Department of Health authorizes National Health Service hearing aid departments to supply most types of disposable batteries free of charge to patients using hearing aids provided by the NHS. These will include nearly all children, whether fitted with standard NHS aids or 'commercial' aids. All the batteries are also easily obtainable through retail outlets.

The significant features of a battery are:

- dimensions (shape and size)
- nominal voltage
- voltage stability over time
- energy density or capacity, measured in milliampere-hours (mAh)

The nominal voltage depends on the electrochemical system used. The service life of a battery depends greatly upon the power demand of the individual hearing aid and the use made of it by the child. However, the battery life can be estimated by dividing its capacity (in mAh) by the nominal current taken by the hearing aid (in mA). The current drawn from a battery affects its voltage. In use, the voltage of the battery is slightly lower than its nominal voltage, but this is allowed for in the design of hearing aids. However, excessive current demands, which may occur in very loud ambient noise, may cause the battery voltage to drop sharply, adversely affecting the performance of the aid.

Body-worn aids generally use the familiar AA cylindical battery with a nominal voltage of 1.5 volts. Two types are available: manganese- alkali and the cheaper carbon-zinc type. The manganese-alkali cell is preferable, because of its better voltage stability over time and its higher capacity. It will last up to twice as long as a carbon-zinc cell in service in the same aid. The rechargeable nickel-cadmium cell of the same size is not recommended, because of its lower nominal voltage and much smaller capacity.

Post-aural and intra-aural aids use the smaller 'button'-type cells, which are used to power many small electronic devices, such as cameras, calculators and watches. They use various electrochemical systems and are available in several sizes. For hearing aids the cells are usually of zinc-air type, which have a nominal voltage of 1.4 volts. The electrochemical function of the zinc-air cell depends upon the ingress of air through a number of small holes in the case. The size of the holes limits the current that the cell is capable of providing, but there are so-called *high performance* versions, for use with high-powered hearing aids, which have high current demand.

Table 9.1 lists the properties of the various types of cells, with their International Electrotechnical Commission

Table 9.1. Properties of common hearing aid batteries.

Type	IEC designation	Department of Health code	Electrochemical system	Nominal voltage (v)	Approximate capacity (mAh)	Diameter (mm)	Length/height (mm)
Cylindrical	R6	–	Carbon-zinc	1.5	1000	14.5	50.5
	LR6	CP6	Manganese-alkali	1.45	2200		
	PR41	CP41	Zinc-air	1.4	90	7.9	3.6
'Button'	PR44	CP44			400	11.6	5.4
	PR48	CP48			170	7.9	5.4
	PR70	CP79				5.8	3.5

designations and Department of Health codes. Figure 9.13 shows their typical discharge curves in use. Zinc-air cells have much flatter discharge curves in use than either of the cylindrical cells. The zinc-air cell maintains a nearly constant voltage until the end of its life, when the voltage falls rapidly. Both types of cylindrical cell lose voltage steadily in use. As the gain and maximum output of an aid depend partly upon the voltage available from the battery, a body-worn aid can be expected to show deterioration in performance over the lifetime of its battery. As the battery nears the end of its life the sound output of the aid will become increasingly distorted.

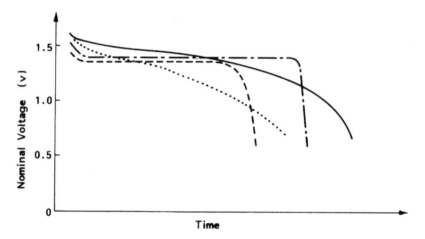

Figure 9.13. Typical discharge curves of various types of primary cells: carbon-zinc ············ ; manganese-alkali ———— ; mercuric oxide - - - - -; zinc-air —·—·— .

For maximum shelf life, batteries should be stored in cool, dry conditions. They should be kept in their packs until use to avoid the possibility of short-circuiting which will not only rapidly deplete the battery, but in some types will cause dangerous overheating, with a risk of fire. All batteries should be stored out of the reach of young children. The air-seal of a zinc-air cell should not be removed until the battery is about to be fitted into a hearing aid.

The battery compartments of hearing aids tend to be sources of problems, particularly with young children. They are often too easily opened by children, with the risk of loss of the battery or its ingestion by the child. Litovitz and Schmitz (1992) found that hearing aids are the most common intended use of batteries swallowed by children. In a third of such cases, the children removed the batteries from their own aids. Reilly (1979) and

Nolan and Tucker (1981) warned of the risk of young children swallowing mercuric oxide cells, the cases of which are particularly prone to fragment in such circumstances (Litovitz and Schmitz, 1992). Mercuric oxide cells should never be provided for hearing aids fitted to young children. The NHS no longer provides mercuric oxide cells and many battery manufacturers have stopped making them because of their environmental impact and high toxicity. However, if a child is known or suspected to have swallowed a battery of any type, medical advice should be sought urgently.

Young children should always be fitted with hearing aids with locking mechanisms on their battery compartments. Most major hearing aid manufacturers provide them routinely, or as optional facilities. Unfortunately locking mechanisms are often abused and easily damaged, more often by careless adults or older siblings than by the young hearing aid users themselves! If a locking mechanism is malfunctioning, it must be repaired as soon as possible. Carers should be advised that, when a locking mechanism is damaged, the battery compartment should be taped shut.

The potential malfunction of the aid due to corrosion of the battery terminals, mentioned earlier in respect of post-aural aids, applies also to all other types of aid. If the problem is minor, the terminals can be cleaned by rubbing gently with a rubber eraser.

Some types of hearing aid systems, particularly those employing remote microphones, are fitted with rechargeable batteries and often require special battery chargers provided by the manufacturers. Generally, the batteries require recharging after 6–12 hours of continuous aid use, though this depends greatly upon the gain setting. Removable rechargeable battery packs are preferable to permanently wired-in batteries as they offer the convenience of being able to continue using the aid (with a freshly-charged pack) while the exhausted battery is being recharged, which may take up to 12 hours.

Checking and measurement of the performance of the system

Aims

When hearing aids are fitted to a child, three forms of assessment are needed to ensure that the provision is appropriate and beneficial:

- the aids must be shown to be functioning correctly, according to the manufacturer's specifications;
- the fitting should be shown to have achieved the intended change in the child's auditory perception;
- it should be demonstrated that the provision, as part of a programme of support for the child and his or her family, has effected a significant reduction in the child's disability.

All three elements must be ongoing and involve interaction between the clinician, other professionals and the child's parents. The third element is beyond the scope of this chapter. So, too, is much of what is involved in the second element, which is a validation of the hearing aid selection procedure or fitting formula used in choosing and adjusting the aid for the child.

Every hearing aid should be checked electroacoustically to ensure that it meets the performance specifications given by the manufacturer, including the effects of adjustment of the controls. This should be done before the aid is fitted to the child and subsequently at regular intervals, not exceeding one year. The aid should also be checked whenever a fault is suspected and again when it has been repaired. Listening to the aid is a valuable test, and parents and special education support teachers should be encouraged to do this every day, along with a visual check of the condition of the aid. The most effective way of doing this is with a listening tube or *stethoclip,* which can be used with any type of hearing aid except a bone conduction fitting. For use with a high-output aid the stethoclip should be fitted with a damper, to allow the listener to check the aid at middle- and high-volume settings, without being exposed to excessively high noise levels. For bone conduction aids two checks are necessary. The aid should be listened to, with the sound quality and output with the existing bone vibrator transducer (placed on the listener's mastoid) compared with those obtained with a new transducer. The microphone and amplifying components of the aid should also be checked, using a stethoclip, with the bone vibrator replaced by an appropriate conventional receiver. The parent and teacher should be warned about the high acoustic output that is likely when this is done. Any suspected fault in the bone vibrator or the lead is best dealt with by its immediate replacement by a new component.

Electroacoustical measurements

Subjective checks will identify only the more obvious faults and, in particular, will not detect the inevitable deterioration in performance of the hearing aid as a result of wear in the controls and transducers. The clinician must also carry out electro acoustic measurements, using equipment similar to that shown schematically in Figure 9.14. The hearing aid is placed into a sound-attenuating test box, in which a sweep-frequency pure-tone or other signal is generated, with its microphone inlet sited within a target area. The sound pressure level of the test signal in the target area is maintained at a specified level by a control microphone and feedback loop, or by data derived from previous calibration. The receiver outlet of the hearing aid is connected to a coupler, which is a cavity of standard design, in which a microphone is fitted to detect the output of the aid. The output is analysed and the results are displayed, usually on a chart recorder. In most modern test systems all the components shown in Figure 9.14 are contained in a single unit, which may be portable. The equipment manufacturer's instructions for the placement of the hearing aid and the procedures for measurement of its performance must be followed precisely, to ensure accurate results. Specifications for the measuring equipment, test conditions and the procedures to be used are given in IEC (1983a) and IEC (1983d).

The purpose of the coupler is to provide a standard air volume in which to measure the output of the aid for comparison with other data. Two forms of coupler are generally in use, a 2 cm^3 coupler conforming to IEC (1973) and an occluded ear simulator conforming to IEC (1981b). The ear simulator is a device that is designed to have the same acoustic impedance as the average normal adult ear. Various designs are available but they all differ from the 2 cm^3 coupler in having side-branch cavities connecting with the main cavity. The sound pressure at the measurement microphone is intended to be similar to that which would be generated by the hearing aid at the eardrum of the average adult ear. IEC (1981b) describes arrangements for coupling various types of hearing aids, receivers and ear inserts to the ear simulator. Hearing aid manufacturers may publish performance specifications measured in either (or both) a 2 cm^3 coupler or an ear simulator and it is important to use the appropriate device when checking a hearing aid.

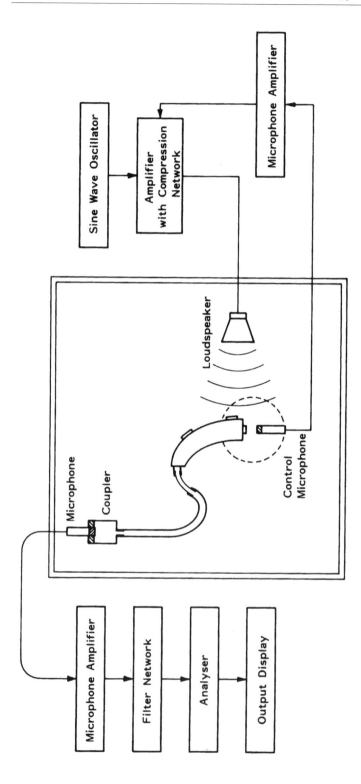

Figure 9.14. Schematic diagram of equipment for electroacoustic measurements of hearing aid function. The control microphone and feedback loop may be omitted and the stimulation level maintained accurately by digitally-stored calibration data. The test signal may be a pure-tone, a frequency-modulated tone, narrow-band noise, random broad-band noise, or weighted broad-band noise.

The test signal used in the measuring equipment needs to be appropriate for the functional characteristics of the aid being tested. Swept pure-tones are suitable for aids with linear amplification, or with single-channel compression and a relatively flat broad-frequency response. However, pure-tones will give misleading results when used with aids with multi-channel compression, or with single-channel compression and a filtered frequency response. Modern hearing aid measurement devices increasingly include broad-band (often speech-shaped) noise signals, which are more appropriate for these types of aids. The devices are able to calculate the gain in each frequency region for different intensities.

Measurement parameters

The standards IEC (1983d) and IEC (1983a) recommend and define performance measurements which should be made for comparison with manufacturers' specifications, or between different hearing aids or different control settings, respectively. Some hearing aid manufacturers give specifications in accordance with the American National Standard (ANSI, 1996), which differs in some respects from the IEC specifications. When checking an aid against the manufacturer's specifications, it is obviously important to ensure that the test conditions (for example, control settings, input levels and receiver type) are as shown on the specifications. The main measurements of interest are likely to be:

- basic frequency response;
- full-on acoustic gain frequency response;
- frequency response for an input SPL of 90 dB;
- effect of control settings on the performance of the aid;
- compression amplification characteristics;
- measurement of amplitude non-linearities (distortion);
- measurement of internal noise of the aid.

Basic frequency response

The frequency response of an aid is the sound pressure level developed in a standard coupler or ear simulator by the hearing aid, expressed as a function of frequency. It gives an indication of the way in which the output sound pressure level (SPL) of the aid (in dB) varies with frequency, for a specified gain control setting and input sound pressure level. IEC (1983a) defines a basic frequency response measured with an input sound pressure level of 60 dB and with the gain control set to produce a specified output at a reference frequency. If the input level is then varied, a family of curves is produced, called the comprehensive frequency response, showing the input-output characteristics of the hearing aid over its full range of operation (dynamic range). Figure 9.15 shows a typical comprehensive frequency response for an aid.

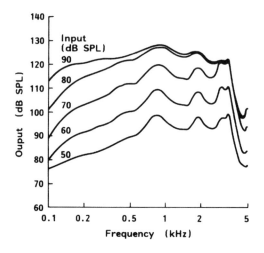

Figure 9.15. A comprehensive frequency response of a hearing aid. The basic frequency response is the 60dB input curve. When the gain control is set to maximum, the 60dB input curve is the *full-on acoustic gain frequency response* and the 90dB input curve is the *OSPL90 frequency response*.

Full-on acoustic gain frequency response

This is a frequency response measured with the gain control set to maximum, other controls set as required and with an input sound pressure level of 60 dB. The gain at any frequency is the difference between the input SPL and the measured output SPL. The maximum gain will be measured when all other controls are set to give the highest output. In some cases 60 dB input SPL will cause the aid to go into saturation, so that the gain measurements will be incorrect. If this happens the input should be set to 50 dB. If the aid is operating in a linear input-output condition, the output for 60 dB SPL input will be (10±1) dB above the output for 50 dB SPL input at any frequency.

Frequency response for an input sound pressure level of 90 dB

This is the frequency response obtained with the gain control in the maximum setting and with a 90 dB SPL input. It is abbreviated to OSPL90. Usually, any other controls are set for maximum gain and maximum output. In ANSI (1987) this measure is termed 'saturation sound pressure level for 90 dB input sound pressure level' (SSPL90) and is usually taken to be an indication of the maximum output of the aid. However, IEC (1983a) notes that the maximum output may occur at a single frequency with a higher input SPL and is best determined by measurement at discrete frequencies rather than with sweep-frequency measurement.

Effect of control settings on the performance of the aid

The effect of changing a control setting may be measured either to determine whether it is appropriate for the user or to check for a suspected fault in the control. The effect of each control should be measured in the mode which best reflects its function. Each control should be assessed separately except when it is specifically desired to measure the change in frequency response with a combination of control settings (perhaps as part of a hearing aid selection procedure). The effect of the tone control should be measured with respect to the basic frequency response. The function of the user gain control or the pre-set gain control should be assessed relative to the full-on acoustic gain frequency response, by adjusting the control to give progressively lower gain, while keeping the input SPL constant. The effect of altering a pre-set maximum output (peak-clipping) control should be measured with respect to the OSPL90 frequency response. Figures 9.16 to 9.18 illustrate the typical effect of these controls.

The effects of acoustic modifications to the performance of a hearing aid (such as venting of the earmould, insertion of acoustic dampers into the tubing, or the creation of a horn-effect tube in the earmould) can be measured similarly. The measurements must be made with an ear simulator and the tip of the earmould must be fixed into the inlet of the simulator as specified in IEC (1981b). Figure 9.19 illustrates the effect of insertion of a damper into the tubing of an aid.

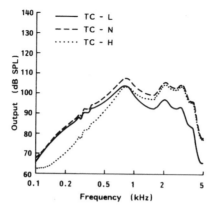

Figure 9.16. Effect of the tone control setting (TC) on the basic frequency response of a hearing aid.

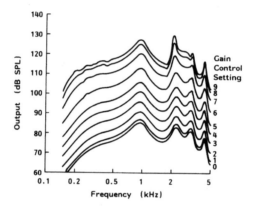

Figure 9.17. Effect of the gain control setting on the output of a hearing aid. The curve with gain control setting 9 is the full-on acoustic gain frequency response of the hearing aid. Note that the function of the gain control is not necessarily linear with respect to its nominal setting.

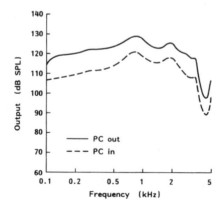

Figure 9.18. Effect of the maximum output control setting (PC) on the OSPL90 frequency response.

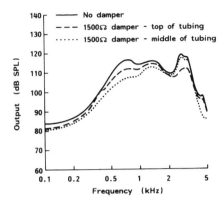

Figure 9.19. Effect of insertion of a 1500Ω damper into the tubing of a hearing aid, measured in an ear simulator conforming to IEC (1981b). Input 60dBSPL.

Compression amplification characteristics

The measurement of the characteristics of a pre-set automatic gain control (AGC) is described in IEC (1983b) and BS (1996). Most modern hearing aid measurement systems include this facility. The measurements that are most likely to be of relevance are onset (attack) and offset (recovery) times and the input/output functions. It may be difficult, or misleading to try to measure these in hearing aids in which the parameter values vary with ambient noise characteristics. The advice of the manufacturers of the hearing aid and the test equipment should be sought in such cases.

Measurement of amplitude non-linearities (distortion)

Distortion arises from limitations in the functions of components of the aid and is present in all systems. Its effect can be seen as the failure of the aid to reproduce faithfully the waveform of the input signal. It will be present to some extent in any new aid, but is likely to increase over the lifetime of the aid, or as a result of damage to individual components. It causes the sound input to have a rough quality and can give rise to loss of clarity. Frequency distortion occurs largely as a narrowing of the bandwidth of the output. Few hearing aids provide effective amplification outside a frequency range of 200–5,000 Hz (though some digital aids are specified as having an extended high-frequency response). Amplitude distortion results from the generation of energy at frequencies that were not present in the input signal. It takes two main forms:

- *Harmonic distortion* is the generation of frequencies which are integer multiples of frequencies which are present in the input signal. For a frequency $f_1 = xHz$ in the input signal, the hearing aid will generate energy at frequencies $2f_1$, $3f_1$, $4f_1$, . . . ($2xHz$, $3xHz$, $4xHz$ . . .) etc. Generally, the amplitude of the harmonics decreases towards the higher harmonics. Many commercial instruments are capable of separately measuring second-order ($2f_1$) and third-order ($3f_1$) harmonics, which are likely to be most troublesome. Some instruments provide a measure of total harmonic distortion (THD), which is largely the combined effect of the second-order and third-order harmonics. There are no standards specifying the allowable harmonic distortion in hearing aids, but high-quality aids will usually not exceed a THD value of 5 per cent.
- *Intermodulation distortion* occurs when two frequencies of similar amplitude are simultaneously present in the input to the aid. Intermodulation distortion products may be of higher or lower frequency than either of the two input frequencies, but only those of lower frequency are likely to be noticeable. Few hearing aid test systems provide facilities for measuring intermodulation distortion and there are no standards specifying allowable limits in aids.

It is important to remember that distortion is markedly increased when a hearing aid amplifier is operating at saturation output, due to the effect of peak-clipping. Distortion measurements must be made under conditions outlined in IEC (1983a) to ensure that the hearing aid is not at saturation output. As an aid will be more likely to reach saturation output if the gain control is set near maximum, it is important to choose an aid that will provide sufficient gain for the child with the gain control set about halfway.

Measurement of internal noise of the aid

If the internal noise level of the hearing aid is suspected to be unduly high, measurements should be made in accordance with IEC (1983a). It is important to ensure that ambient noise is not sufficiently high to influence the result.

In situ measurements

Hearing aid gain measured in an ear simulator or a 2 cm^3 coupler in a test box is called *transmission gain* and is a measure of the input/output function of the aid. Such measurements do not describe the performance of a hearing aid fitted to a hearing impaired person, as they do not take account of the effect of the aid and earmould on the acoustical characteristics of the outer ear, the variations in the dimensions of individual ears, or the diffraction and reflection effects of the head and body of the user on the sound field. The real gain of a hearing aid in use can be defined and measured in different ways.

Insertion gain is defined as the difference between the sound pressure in the external meatus with the hearing aid present and the sound pressure when the hearing aid is absent. To calculate the average insertion gain, it is necessary to make measurements of hearing aid performance in an occluded ear simulator fitted into a manikin, which is placed in a known sound field. An international standard (IEC, 1990) specifies the construction and required properties of a manikin, which should represent the head and upper torso of the adult human, with dimensions corresponding to the anthropometric medians derived from combined male and female populations. Another standard (IEC, 1983d) describes the conditions and methods of measurement of simulated *in situ* hearing aid performance.

Although hearing aid manufacturers sometimes publish insertion gain specifications for their aids, it is important to realize that the performance of an aid may be significantly different in use. For a start, people generally use their aids when wearing clothing and before they lose all their hair, neither of which the manikin has! More importantly, most individual hearing aid users do not conform to the average dimensions represented by the manikin. The differences are likely to be particularly significant for pre-school children. Similarly, the acoustic impedance of the occluded ear simulator is intended to represent that of the average adult ear and will be different from that of the smaller ear of a pre-school child. The actual output sound pressure of a hearing aid in a young child's ear is likely to be substantially greater than that measured in an ear simulator (Moodie et al., 1994). As there is a risk that the difference may cause the output to exceed the child's loudness discomfort level, measurement in a ear simulator (or a 2 cm^3 coupler) should not be relied upon when setting the maximum output of the aid. Unfortunately, neither a 'baby manikin' nor a child-sized ear simulator is available.

The only satisfactory way to determine the amplification of an aid when fitted to a child is to measure it in use. This can be done either by means of a probe microphone measurement system or by measuring the child's aided and unaided performance, on various behavioural or electrophysiological tests.

Probe microphone measurement systems are now available with many hearing aid test devices. These involve placing a probe-tube microphone into the child's external canal, with or without the hearing aid in place, to measure the sound pressure level at a particular point in the ear canal. With a probe microphone system, two types of measurement are possible. The first is an individual measure of insertion gain, which is the difference between the SPL values measured in the child's ear canal, with and without the aid system in place, for various frequencies. The second is the *real ear aided gain,* which is the difference between the SPL values, measured inside and outside the child's ear canal, while the aid is being worn by the child. Various hearing aid fitting procedures require one or other type of probe microphone measurement.

Although probe microphone measurements undoubtedly represent a major step forward in the measurement of hearing aid performance, the practical difficulties for their use with young children, particularly in a busy clinic, should not be underestimated. Manufacturer's instructions should be followed carefully in order to avoid discomfort to the child and to obtain reliable results.

Aided and unaided threshold measurements, using sound field stimuli with visual reinforcement audiometry or so-called 'play audiometry', can be used to obtain insertion gain values. The approach may be more acceptable than probe-tube microphone measurements in some (perhaps many) cases, but gives limited information and is less accurate.

Recent developments in digital hearing aids allow *in situ* threshold measurements to be made through the hearing aid itself, thus combining the benefits of probe-tube measurements and aided threshold measurements. The programmed AGC characteristics of the aid, adjusted automatically according the thresholds measured, ensure that appropriate gain is applied for all input levels and frequency regions. Such an approach probably offers the most satisfactory solution to *in situ* gain measurement in children.

Alternative forms of personal aids to hearing

Vibrotactile aids

These take the form of wearable (usually wrist-worn) devices that present acoustic information to the wearer through vibrotactile stimulation. They are likely to be of particular benefit to profoundly deaf children who may derive little advantage from conventional hearing aids. Vibrotactile aids generally provide information relating to acoustic energy in one or more limited frequency bands of importance in speech perception. The fundamental frequency of laryngeal vibration is usually cued to give voicing information. Higher frequency bands may be monitored to give cues to sibilant production and first or second formant frequencies. The reader is referred to Summers (1992) for a full description of tactile aids. Few published data are available for the use of vibrotactile aids by pre-school children where neural plasticity and learning capacity may be expected to make them particularly successful users. However, there are significant practical problems in the fitting of vibrotactile aids, whose are cumbersome and prone to frequent damage when fitted to young infants.

Artifical auditory stimulation

The implantation of devices in profoundly and severely deaf people, to stimulate the acoustic nerve directly, is now available in many centres worldwide. Various systems are available, using one or more stimulating electrodes and one or more channels of acoustic information. The electrodes are activated by a signal processor that either filters the sound input into one or more frequency bands, or extracts and codes specific acoustic features in the sound input. The electrode may be implanted in the cochlea or may be extra-cochlear, usually placed on the promontory of the middle-ear cavity. Tens of thousands of patients, a majority of whom are children, have now been implanted worldwide with excellent outcomes. Processing strategies, electrode technology and criteria for candidature are all undergoing rapid change as a result of research developments and clinical experience. Previous reluctance to fit children, for practical and ethical reasons, has generally been replaced by a view that severely hearing impaired children are likely to be the most successful users, if they are fitted in their early pre-school years. Cochlear implantation is covered in detail in Chapter 11 of this book.

References

ANSI (1996) Specification of Hearing Aid Characteristics. ANSI S3.22-1996. American National Standards Institute.

BS (1996) Hearing Aids. Methods for Measurement of Electroacoustical Characteristics of Hearing Aids with Automatic Gain Control Circuits. BS EN 60118-2. British Standards Institution.

BS (1997) Hearing Aids. Dimensions of Electrical Connector Systems. BS EN 60118-12. British Standards Institution.

BS (1998) Hearing Aids. Magnetic Field Strength in Audio-frequency Induction Loops for Hearing Aid Purposes. BS EN 60118-4. British Standards Institution.

BS (1999) Hearing Aids. Characteristics of Electrical Input Circuits for Hearing Aids. BS EN 60118-6, Edition 2, British Standards Institution.

Dillon H (2001a) CROS, bone-conduction and implanted hearing aids. In Hearing Aids. Sydney: Boomerang Press (Thieme).

Dillon H (2001b) Compression systems in hearing aids. In Hearing Aids. Sydney: Boomerang Press (Thieme).

Finitzo-Hieber T, Tillman T (1978) Room acoustic effects on monosyllabic word discrimination ability for normal and hearing-impaired children. Journal of Speech and Hearing Research 21: 440–58.

Glasberg B, Moore B (1989) Psychoacoustic abilities of subjects with unilateral and bilateral cochlear hearing impairments and their relationship to the ability to understand speech. Scandinavian Audiology Supplement 32: 1–25.

Harford E, Barry J (1965) A rehabilitative approach to the problem of unilateral hearing impairment. Contralateral routing of signals (CROS). Journal of Speech and Hearing Disorders 30: 121–38.

IEC (1973) Specification for a reference coupler for the measurement of hearing aids using earphones coupled to the ear by means of ear inserts. IEC 60126. Geneva: International Electrotechnical Commission.

IEC (1981a) Hearing aids. Part 4. Magnetic field strength in audio-frequency induction loops for hearing aid purposes. IEC 60118-4. Geneva: International Electrotechnical Commission.

IEC (1981b) Specification for an occluded-ear simulator for the measurement of earphones coupled to the ear by ear inserts. IEC 60711. Geneva: International Electrotechnical Commission.

IEC (1983a) Measurement of electroacoustic characteristics. IEC 60118-0. Geneva: International Electrotechnical Commission.

IEC (1983b) Hearing aids with automatic gain control circuits. IEC 60118-2. Geneva: International Electrotechnical Commission.

IEC (1983c) Hearing aids. Part 3: Hearing aid equipment not entirely worn on the listener. IEC 60118-3. Geneva: International Electrotechnical Commission.

IEC (1983d) Hearing aids. Part 7: Measurement of the performance characteristics of hearing aids for quality inspection for delivery purposes. IEC 60118-7. Geneva: International Electrotechnical Commission.

IEC (1983e) Hearing aids. Part 8: Methods of measurement of performance characteristics of hearing aids under simulated in situ working conditions. IEC 60118-8. Geneva: International Electrotechnical Commission.

IEC (1983f) Hearing aids. Part 11: Symbols and other markings on hearing aids and related equipment. IEC 60118-11. Geneva: International Electrotechnical Commission.

IEC (1990) Provisional head and torso simulator for acoustic measurements on air conduction hearing aids. IEC 60959. Geneva: International Electrotechnical Commission.

IEC (1996) Hearing aids. Part 12: Dimensions of electrical connector systems. IEC 60118-12. Geneva: International Electrotechnical Commission.

IEC (1999) Hearing aids. Part 6. Characteristics of electrical input circuits for hearing aids. IEC 60118-6. Edition 2. Geneva: International Electrotechnical Commission.

IEC (2000) Primary batteries – Part 1: General. IEC 60086-1. Geneva: International Electrotechnical Commission.

IEC (2001) Primary batteries – Part 2: Physical and electrical specifications. IEC 60086-2. Geneva: International Electrotechnical Commission.

Litovitz T, Schmitz BF (1992) Ingestion of cylindrical and button batteries: an analysis of 2382 cases. Pediatrics 89(4): 747-57.

Markides A, Huntington A, Kettlety A (1980) Comparative speech discrimination abilities of hearing-impaired children achieved through infra-red, radio and conventional hearing aids. Journal of the British Association of Teachers of the Deaf 4: 5-14.

Moodie KS, Seewald RC, Sinclair ST (1994) Procedure for predicting real-ear hearing aid performance in young children. American Journal of Audiology 3(1): 23-31.

NDCS (1998a) Loop Systems. Helpful hints on installation and troubleshooting. London: National Deaf Children's Society.

NDCS (1998b) Personal/Infra-red Systems. Guide to what features to look for. London: National Deaf Children's Society.

Nolan M, Tucker IG (1981) Health risks following ingestion of mercury and zinc air batteries. Scandinavian Audiology 10: 189.

Pascoe D (1978) An approach to hearing aid selection. Hearing Instruments 29(6): 12-16.

Peters RW, Moore BCJ, Baer T (1998) Speech reception thresholds in noise with and without spectral and temporal dips for hearing-impaired and normally hearing people. Journal of the Acoustical Society of America 103(1): 577-87.

RA (2001) UK Radio Interface Requirement 2030. Short Range Devices (Version 1.1). Radiocommunications Agency.

Reilly DT (1979) Mercury battery ingestion. British Medical Journal 1: 859.

Steinberg JC, Gardner MB (1937) The dependence of hearing impairment on sound intensity. Journal of the Acoustical Society of America 9: 11-23.

Summers I (1992) (ed.) Tactile Aids for the Hearing Impaired. London: Whurr.

Chapter 10
Hearing aid selection and evaluation for pre-school children

Roger Green

Introduction

The task of fitting a hearing aid to a hearing impaired child demands a great deal of skill and sensitivity on the part of the clinician. Audiology is a discipline that draws on many areas of knowledge, from physics to psychology, from medicine to management. The clinician needs to combine all of these, along with his clinical experience of what works, if a successful fitting is to be achieved. The subject is complex and there is not space in one chapter to cover all aspects in detail. The aim is rather to highlight some of the important central issues in order to generate a better understanding of the ideas that underpin the practice of hearing aid selection and evaluation with pre-school children.

To that end this chapter will discuss first the selection of hearing aids, in terms of both psychoacoustics and ergonomics, and then proceed to discuss the evaluation of the fitted hearing aid, both in the clinic and in the field.

The habilitation process

A fundamental point is that hearing aid fitting in pre-school children should not proceed in isolation, but rather as part of a structured habilitation programme. The organization of this programme will vary from centre to centre, but will almost always involve trans-professional working between clinical and educational audiologists, paediatricians, ENT, speech and language therapists and others.

Hearing aid issue usually happens in the early days after diagnosis, when families are still battling to come to terms with the diagnosis.

The shock and the grief that they feel may come out in a range of emotions including sadness, anxiety, confusion and depression. They may find it impossible to accept that their child can be less than perfect and even deny that there is a problem.

Eventually there will be recognition that the problem is real, but this may come very gradually. Emotions may turn to guilt, or anger. They may find themselves looking for someone to blame, themselves, the doctors, the nurses, the audiology team, even the phases of the moon. They may have a sense of helplessness and isolation. They will look for any sign from the professionals that things are not as bad as first thought. A tiny improvement in one test result may send them away from a test session elated with relief and hope, hope that can easily turn to despair when the improvement is not maintained.

Even when acceptance gradually emerges, parents will find themselves cycling back through the whole range of emotions, taking two steps forward and one step back.

Against this stormy background, the clinician is trying to fit hearing aids, explain their use and care, and expecting the parents to quickly become experts in hearing aid management. The clinician understands the need for the aid, and the benefits it will bring. The parents may hate it. It is the first visible proof that their child has a real problem, that the experts have not got it wrong, that this is something permanent. It is an unsightly chunk of plastic, hung from their child's ear and advertising to the whole world that their child is disabled. They don't like to look at it, to touch it, even to have it in the house. Little surprise then that the early months of hearing aid use may not be a smooth passage. (Green, 1999)

It therefore takes time and sensitive support to help families to adjust to their children's hearing impairment. Furthermore, the benefits provided by modern assistive devices, and the opportunities provided by early identification of hearing loss mean that we are now in an excellent position to get children on the road to communication early and effectively. Evidence and clinical experience both demonstrate how well children's speech, language and communication can progress with good early support.

This chapter specifically covers the fitting of hearing aids, but it is important to remember that parents need to come to an informed decision about which mode of communication they wish to pursue with their child – for example a signing, total communication or aural approach. Part of the habilitation process is to help them to reach that decision. Again, early identification gives us the ability to inform this decision at an early stage.

The habilitation process exists to support parents through the stages to acceptance and a positive attitude, to work with them to develop the child's communication skills, with the hearing aid assisting in that process where it can, to monitor the child's overall development, and to investigate the possible causes of the hearing loss. The National Deaf Children's Society in the UK has published several quality standards dealing with the habilitation process and related issues (National Deaf Children's Society, 1994, 1996, 1999, 2000). The most recent, National Deaf Children's Society (2000) is an excellent, succinct but comprehensive and detailed coverage of this area and is highly recommended reading.

Hearing loss is a long-term problem. The child will come into the clinic from time to time, even quite frequently in the early months following diagnosis. The family, though, will be with the child 24 hours a day, seven days a week. The role of the habilitation team is to support the family and to enable them to become increasingly well informed about their child's hearing loss and the options open to them as more information unfolds. It is the family that must decide when they wish to start with hearing aids, when cochlear implantation may be worthwhile, when to introduce sign as the preferred mode of communication. However they must be able to make properly informed choices. It is the clinician's role to work with them and support them, and to let the information unfold over time in a manner that suits the family. It is important to keep the family informed as to what is happening, in clear language free of unnecessary jargon, to be sensitive to the social and cultural differences in different families, and to the influence and perceptions of the wider family network.

This approach to habilitation has been encapsulated in the term 'family-friendly service'. In the UK, this is not simply a platitude but a written set of guidelines about what a service should have in place before it can truly call itself family friendly (see Baguley et al., 2000).

Who should be fitted?

There are varying views among clinicians about what constitutes a 'significant' loss, or a loss that would benefit from aiding. A consensus statement developed by the Pediatric Working Group of the Conference on Amplification for Children with Auditory Deficits (1996) in the US serves as a useful description of the principles and procedures that should be applied when fitting hearing aids to children. It deals with who should be identified, how they should be assessed, what hearing aids should be fitted and how. It states for example that hearing aids should be fitted to children with thresholds equal to or poorer than 25 dB HL. For children with milder loss, unilateral loss, rising loss or high-frequency loss above 2,000 Hz, it states that aiding should be considered on a case by case basis.

Selection and evaluation

It is necessary to clarify the difference between the processes of selecting and evaluating a hearing aid. When a child presents with a hearing loss that requires amplification, the clinician is faced first with the problem of selection,[1] that is of choosing from a large number of possible hearing aids (and hearing aid settings) the aid that is most likely to provide optimum benefit for that child. This requires an understanding of exactly what amplification is to achieve. Do we want to return auditory thresholds to 'normal' across the frequency range, or is it sufficient simply to make speech audible? How much emphasis do we give to the range of frequencies that make up the speech spectrum? Some sort of more-or-less explicit and more-or-less precise target for amplification is at the heart of most hearing aid selection strategies, and we will look at these in more detail shortly. We also need a means of selecting from the range of aids at the clinician's disposal one that is likely to provide the specified electro acoustic characteristics.

Once the first-choice aid is selected and fitted, it then requires evaluation. Evaluation is the process of assessing the performance of the aid when worn by the child, both in the clinic and out in the real world. The child may be tested wearing the aid, using a number of possible test procedures. Where there are shortcomings in performance, the aid will need modification or replacement until a satisfactory match is achieved.

In essence, then, the hearing aid fitting procedure includes the following stages:

---

[1] Strictly, there are three aspects of selection, namely prescription, selection and verification. Prescription means setting target hearing aid outputs, usually based on some prescription philosophy – this will be covered later in the text. Selection means choosing and setting up an aid to match those targets. Verification means confirming that the selected aid does deliver the target outputs.

- measurement of hearing impairment;
- specification of the ergonomic and electroacoustic characteristics of the hearing aid;
- selection and setting up of a hearing aid to give the required characteristics;
- fitting the aid;
- evaluation of the performance of the aid when worn by the child;
- modification of the selected aid as necessary.

Although these stages are usually sequential and rather separate with adults, with children there is often a considerable amount of back-and-forth movement between the stages. For example, with infants the initial prescription may be based on very limited information, perhaps one or two approximate threshold measures. The selected aid is very likely to need modification as more information about the degree of impairment is obtained in the weeks and months following the initial fitting.

Procedures used in the selection and evaluation of hearing aids for young children have historically been based on work done with adults or older children. Adults can provide two kinds of information that pre-school children usually cannot. First they provide a (relatively) accurate set of psychoacoustic measurements that can be used to both select and evaluate the hearing aid. Second, they provide verbal feedback as to their satisfaction with the hearing aid and their perception of its benefits. Pre-school children provide audiometric information, which is often a lot less precise. This is particularly true of infants in whom the early audiometric profile may be very approximate – perhaps no more than a click auditory brainstem response (ABR) threshold and some behavioural observation. Pre-school children are not usually sufficiently articulate to tell us what they think of the aids we have given them. We may have to rely on other behavioural indications, such as the child refusing to wear the aid, and even then the reasons for rejection may not be clear. For example, an aid may be rejected because it is too loud, or too quiet, or the mould uncomfortable.

Hearing aid selection – acoustic factors

A great deal of work has been done in recent years to try to establish the optimum amplification characteristics for any particular hearing loss. This work has generated a plethora of hearing aid prescription procedures. In essence, a prescription procedure uses measurements of the audiometric profile to prescribe hearing aid gain and maximum output characteristics. Gain prescription is usually based on amplifying the speech spectrum so that it falls in the patient's 'comfort zone'. Differences in prescription arise from different approaches to the frequency weightings used (for example, more-or-less low frequency to combat upward spread of masking, background noise; the use of different speech spectrums, and so forth). Maximum output prescription is based both on the need to prevent intense sounds becoming uncomfortably loud for the patient, and also to protect the ear from further damage.

Two prescription procedures in particular are comprehensively researched and have become popular in clinical practice. These are the National Acoustics Laboratory of Australia (Byrne and Dillon, 1986; Byrne et al., 1990) NAL prescription and the desired sensation level (DSL) prescription of Seewald and colleagues (Seewald, 1995). Essentially, these prescription philosophies have taken what is known about hearing impaired psychoacoustics to derive hearing aid gain and maximum output prescriptions for any particular set of audiometric thresholds. There is not sufficient space here to look at the different philosophies in detail, and the reader is referred to the literature for further information. It is useful to know the practical implications of using these procedures and there are some important points of principle that need to be understood.

The NAL, DSL and others generate target figures for the gain required at each frequency to make the speech spectrum audible at that frequency, given a particular degree of hearing loss. They also give target maximum output figures for the hearing aid.

It is possible to use, say, DSL with either a table of corrections, or a computer-generated set of targets. The latter is most common and certainly the easiest and least error prone. The clinician inputs a set of audiometric thresholds and the software calculates the required hearing aid gains and maximum outputs at the threshold frequencies.

These figures are entered into the software, and the target gain and maximum output figures obtained. Figure 10.1(a) shows these target gains and maximum output figures for a moderate hearing loss displayed in graphical form.

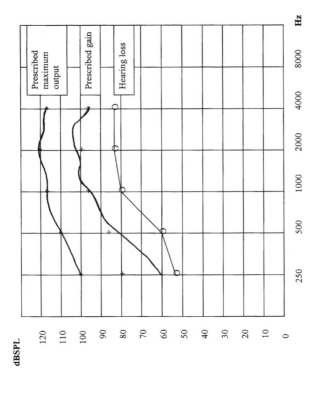

Figure 10.1(b). As 10.1(a) but now including the measured gain and maximum output from a hearing aid.

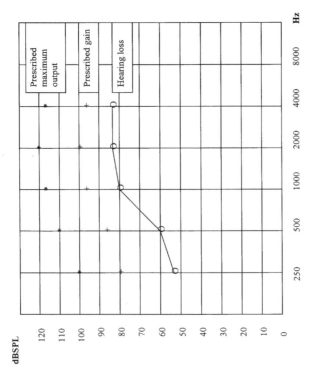

Figure 10.1(a). Gain and maximum output for a moderate hearing loss as prescribed by DSL.

A hearing aid is then selected and adjusted to best match these targets. Figure 10.1(b) shows the gain and maximum output measured on the selected aid. (In this example, the clinician will see that a reasonable match has been achieved but some fine-tuning will be necessary.)

In practice, the process is not so simple, and it is important to be aware of what else needs to be taken into account.

Threshold measurements

In young children, audiometric thresholds may be obtained in many ways (behavioural observation, VRA, distraction, play audiometry) and using a variety of input transducers (hand-held sound field, loudspeaker sound field, insert earphone, headphone). These methods are not necessarily equivalent and the thresholds generated by them may not be closely related to audiometric zero in dB HL, which is our 'standard' audiometric unit. For example, an eight-month-old child with the same hearing as a three-year-old may not give the same measured response levels if the former is tested with sound field VRA and the latter under headphones.

Whatever transducers are used, they must be calibrated and the units clearly stated. Insert earphones and headphones can be calibrated in dB HL. Sound field systems are often calibrated in dB A or dB SPL, though Benyon and Munro (1993) make a convincing case for calibrating sound field in dB HL where possible, and provide correction factors for doing so.

Desired Sensation Level requires the nature of the transducer and test arrangement to be specified. It then adjusts the prescription, taking these factors into account.

Age and ear canal acoustics

The prescription targets are based on averages. However there are two important ways in which the output of a hearing aid into individual ear canals will depart from that average.

First there are general, age-related effects. Younger children have smaller ear canals than older children and adults, so the hearing aid will behave differently when fitted to them. Typically the smaller the canal, the greater the sound intensity, and the greater the high frequency emphasis. Figure 10.2, taken from a study by the author, demonstrates this effect. It compares the output of a hearing aid measured in the ear canals of adults and children. The measurements are averaged for seven adults and four children (all under two years of age). The output in the child ear canals is shifted in frequency and reaches a maximum level of some 7 dB higher than in the adult ear canals. DSL supplies age-related correction factors which will take these differences into account.

Second, each individual ear canal is different, causing further individual variation in the amplification characteristics of the hearing aid. Figure 10.2 also shows one individual trace from a child. This trace demonstrates the considerable individual differences that can arise.

There are two ways to take account of the age and individual difference effects of the ear canal discussed above. The initial hearing aid selection is usually carried out without the child

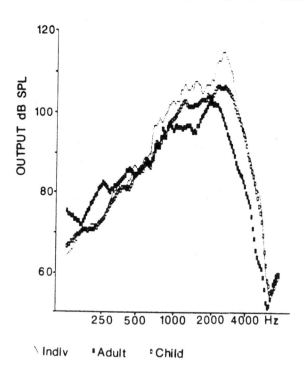

AID OUTPUT INTO EAR CANAL – CHILDREN V ADULTS

\ Indiv   ▪ Adult   ▫ Child

Figure 10.2. Plot of the output of a hearing aid into the ear canal, averaged for a group of adults (n = 7) and a group of young children (n = 4). Also shown is the output for one individual child.

being present (i.e. the aid is being selected ready for the first fitting.) The aid outputs are therefore measured in a test box, using a coupler. When the child's age is entered, the prescription will correct the targets by the average real ear effects for that age.

Individual differences can be accommodated if we know how the aid's performance in a coupler compares with its performance in the individual ear. If we can measure the difference between the sound level generated in a coupler and in the individual ear, then we can correct the coupler measured output by this 'correction factor'.

The correction factor is called the real-ear/coupler difference (RECD). The patient does need to be present for this measurement, but it can be made on a session prior to the fitting session. A fixed input sweep frequency signal is played into the ear, usually through a special foam insert (though the patient's earmould can be used if they have one). The ear canal level of the signal is measured using a calibrated probe tube microphone also placed in the ear canal. The same input signal is then played through the same transducer into the coupler, and the signal level measured by the coupler microphone. The differences between the real ear and coupler measures represent the RECD correction factor. All subsequent hearing aid measures in the coupler can then be corrected by this amount.

Non-linearity

Prescription procedures have been modified to incorporate non-linear hearing aids. For example, wide dynamic range compression (WDRC) hearing aids are based on the principle that cochlear damage usually causes abnormal growth of loudness. While sounds of low intensity may not be heard, sounds of high intensity can be very loud to the damaged ear. In order to make all sounds audible, the hearing aid will have to amplify different input levels by different amounts.

In a linear hearing aid the gain is the same regardless of the input (until high input levels trigger the output control circuitry). In a non-linear hearing aid, the gain varies with the input. Figure 10.3 illustrates this.

Figure 10.3 shows scales representing the dynamic range of hearing for a normal hearing person on the left and a hearing-impaired person on the right. The impaired dynamic range is smaller then the normal range. In Figure 10.3(a), a hearing aid

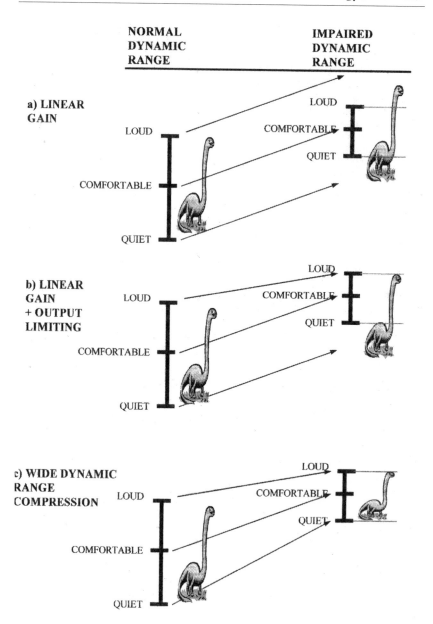

Figure 10.3. Wide dynamic range compression.

with linear gain is used to restore the comfortable levels for the impaired listener to normal. The gain of the aid is represented by the slope of the arrow. As the gain is linear, all input levels of sound are amplified by the same amount. As a result, loud sounds will exceed the patient's discomfort level, and quiet sounds will remain inaudible. In Figure 10.3(b), a hearing aid with linear gain and compression output limiting is used to keep high input level sounds from becoming uncomfortable by reducing the gain (shallower slope of arrow) for high inputs. Note, however, that quiet sounds are still inaudible. In Figure 10.3(c), a WDRC hearing aid is used to compress all input levels into the impaired listener's dynamic range. Low level inputs are given more gain (steeper arrow slope) and higher level inputs less gain. The whole input signal now becomes audible.

The term *compression ratio* is used to describe the extent to which the input range must be 'shrunk' to match the impaired listener's dynamic range. A compression ratio of, say, 2:1 means that a 20 dB input range is compressed into a 10 dB output range. The dynamic range, and so compression ratio, will often vary across different frequency ranges. Consider, for example, a patient who has a hearing loss, which is greater at high frequency. Typically the dynamic range for the low-frequency region will be greater than for the high-frequency region. The compression ratio will therefore need to be higher for the high frequencies. Wide dynamic range compression hearing aids usually have several frequency channels, each of which can have separately adjusted compression ratios.

The purpose, then, of WDRC hearing aids is to attempt to restore the normal sensation of loudness. An extension of the DSL fitting procedure (DSL I/O) works by calculating the compression ratio at each frequency based on the audiometric information. From this, it can then generate target gain or output curves for different inputs, as shown in Figure 10.4.

Eliminating background noise

Current generation hearing aids, including digital aids, are becoming increasingly sophisticated in their signal processing potential. One of the best ways to improve hearing is to reduce background noise, and it is probably just as important to find ways of doing this as it is to get a good prescription match – indeed some audiologists would say this is the most important thing. There are a number of ways of doing this:

- Signal processing – digital signal processing is beginning to enable the hearing aid to separate speech from background noise so that the speech can then be given differential amplification.

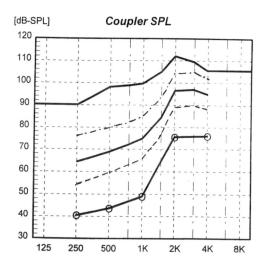

Figure 10.4. Output curves for a moderate hearing loss as prescribed by DSL I/O. The curves are for inputs of 50, 65 and 80 dB SPL. Prescription for maximum output is also shown. Note that the compression ratio increases (curves become closer together) with increasing hearing loss.
o/p for 80 dB i/p —·—·— ; o/p for 65 dB i/p ——— ; o/p for 50 dB i/p - - - - -

- Multiple microphones – directional microphones have been a feature of hearing aids for some time. Again modern processing has enabled dual or even multiple microphone arrangements to enhance speech in background noise.
- FM systems – these are still probably the most effective at reducing background noise, as they effectively move the sound source up to the ear. It is worth noting that many children are likely to use FM systems at some stage and whatever hearing aid is fitted needs to have provision for linking with an FM system.
- FM sound field systems – for older children with milder losses, a classroom fitted with a speaker that brings the teacher's voice to an individual loudspeaker close to the child can be useful. Sound delivered through an array of speakers in a classroom can in fact benefit all the children in the class.
- Understanding the problem – not high tech but if the family understands the added difficulties that background noise brings, they can take steps to avoid it, such as turning off the TV or radio when playing with the child, being close to the child when possible, so that their voice is louder than the surrounding noise.

Hearing aid selection – ergonomic factors

Hearing aids differ not only acoustically (in the sound they deliver) but also ergonomically (how easy they are to manage). Selection of ergonomic characteristics should proceed in parallel with selection of electroacoustic characteristics. The most carefully adjusted aid is of no use at all if it is too large or too cumbersome for the child to wear. Clinicians usually fit hearing aids in the uncluttered confines of their clinic. It is the parent who must manage the aid back in the real world, where hearing aids are worn on little ears, and little ears are fixed to little heads and bodies, and the owners of those little heads and bodies like to experiment with sand or water or jam, and to see how messy stewed prunes can really be, and to practise the art of hanging upside down from climbing frames, and to see if dogs like hearing aids...

The main ergonomic choices are listed below. They are not independent of each other or of electroacoustic considerations. Thus, for example, a body-worn hearing aid may be selected for its better low-frequency response as much as its easier management in a particular circumstance.

Hearing aid type (body-worn/behind-the-ear/in-the-ear)

Hearing aids worn behind the ear are the most commonly fitted to children in the UK. They can be made very powerful, and the increasing presence of active feedback control circuitry, particularly in digital hearing aids, along with improvements in earmould manufacture, mean that this power can be realized without prohibitive feedback. Such aids have greater cosmetic appeal than body-worn systems. However, body-worn hearing aids are still useful in some circumstances:

- for some profound losses, behind-the-ear aids may not be able to provide sufficient low frequency gain, and are more prone to feedback at high amplification levels;
- with infants, who spend much time lying down or with their head resting against pillows or parents, a behind-the-ear aid may be constantly dislodged. A body-worn system can be less of a problem in these early months of fitting, as the amplifier can be moved away from the child, for example hung on the side of the cot.

In-the-ear hearing aids are becoming increasingly popular. Generally they are less powerful than behind-the-ear aids and historically they have been less versatile, their small size limiting electroacoustic flexibility. Recent developments have seen considerable improvements in in-the-ear aids, but their use with pre-school children is still limited. They are not suitable for more severe losses, they do not work well with radio aids, and they cause problems with management (small, fiddly, no battery lock or volume control cover, frequent replacement). In-the-ear aids have obvious appeal to parents but they cannot always provide sufficient gain or frequency response. The clinician should strongly resist sacrificing electroacoustic performance for cosmetic appeal. If this is to be achieved against considerable parental pressure for something small and 'invisible', any explanations and demonstrations of the benefits of a correctly fitted aid will need to be clear and convincing.

Hearing aid size

As has been said, the great majority of hearing aids fitted to children are small behind-the-ear aids. These can now reach almost to the power of their larger predecessors, as well as providing the necessary range of facilities, such as direct input, directional microphones etc. Despite the small size of aids, difficulties are still experienced in keeping them in position on small ears. This can be helped with the use of paediatric earhooks, 'huggies' (small plastic loops that fit around the ear and to which the aid can be fastened), or 'toupee-tape' (sticky double sided tape which sticks the aid to the head).

All hearing aids fitted to children should have battery locks. Most hearing aid batteries today are zinc-air rather than mercury, but swallowing one can still give serious internal burns and the batteries may need to be surgically removed. It is therefore essential to keep prying fingers out of the aid by fitting battery locks. This will not completely solve the problem, as little teeth may do what little fingers did not. Therefore parents also need advice about safety with batteries.

Aids should also be fitted with volume control covers to prevent alteration of the volume control setting (accidentally or otherwise). It should be remembered that brothers and sisters are just as likely to play with a hearing aid as its wearer.

Bone conduction hearing aids

Occasionally a child needs to be fitted with a bone conduction hearing aid. These are fitted where there is a large conductive component to the loss. This may be caused by a canal atresia, where the ear canal is replaced by bone or cartilage. It may also be where there is a chronically discharging ear, a condition that can be aggravated by the presence of an occluding earmould. A bone conduction aid consists of a hearing aid (body-worn or behind-the-ear) connected to a special transducer which sits behind the ear on the mastoid bone. The transducer feeds sound directly to the inner ear by vibration through the skull, thus bypassing any middle-ear blockage. In some cases a bone-anchored hearing aid may be the method of choice. In this arrangement the transducer can be fitted to an abutment surgically implanted in the skull. This gives a better transmission of sound, and the smaller device has greater cosmetic appeal. It is not, however, usually suitable for very young children as the skull is still developing and the bone too thin to take an abutment.

Note also that where there is a conductive component to the hearing loss an appropriate adjustment needs to be made to the prescription.

Monaural/binaural fittings

There has, in the past, been some reluctance to fit binaural hearing aids (an aid in each ear). However there is now little doubt that it is best to adopt the approach that two hearing aids should be fitted unless there is a good reason for not doing so. The well-known comment that you do not go to the optician expecting to come out with a monocle still makes the point well. There are some specific advantages of binaural over monaural hearing that can be made accessible with binaural fittings. These include:

- localization – the direction of sound is more easily detected with two ears than with one;
- summation – sounds heard with two ears are a little (3 dB) louder, enabling the gain in both hearing aids to be slightly less than with one hearing aid;
- fusion – most real-life listening situations are at least partly reverberant and binaural hearing makes us less susceptible to the degrading effects of such reverberation on speech;

- unmasking - binaural hearing can make it easier to understand speech in noisy backgrounds, a particularly difficult task for the hearing impaired.

It is best to go for two aids at the outset where possible, as it is more difficult to introduce a second aid later on than it is to take one away.

Hearing aid selection – cosmetic factors

Children tend to be less conservative than their parents and when they are given the choice will often choose brightly coloured hearing aids with earmoulds to match. Younger children also like to add to the décor with coloured stickers. Some hearing aid companies supply sets of these (with illustrations of everything from sea horses to sunglasses) and they can be obtained easily in many shops. It is also possible to decorate the hearing aid casings individually, though care must be taken not to use paints that would damage the casing and invalidate the hearing aid warranty. Decoration includes everything from football team emblems to abstract art. It is also possible to embed, for example, miniature football team badges into the plastic of the earmould. There are also examples of hearing aids designed or decorated to act as fashion items, just as spectacles can be. This individualization is not a trivial activity. It can give children a greater sense of ownership, control and even pride in their hearing aids and can change them from being reluctant users to enthusiastic users.

Some parents are happy with bright colours. Others would rather use the colour to camouflage the aid as much as possible, at least in the early stages of fitting. It is worth noting, in this regard, that hearing aids are better camouflaged if their colour matches the hair colour rather than the skin colour. Hearing aids are available in black, grey, brown and beige to suit these ends.

Clinical evaluation

First fitting

The first fitting of a hearing aid is likely to be conducted against a background of mixed emotions from the family. Families take varying amounts of time to come to terms with the diagnosis of deafness, never less than months and often many years. At this early stage they may still be reluctant to accept the reality of the diagnosis, and that hearing aids really are a necessary step. Clinicians understand the need for the aid, and the benefits it will bring, but must be sensitive to the family's frame of reference. Families will have various expectations of the hearing aid, which may be anything on a continuum from assuming the hearing aid will do nothing for the child, to expecting the child to be transformed and speech to come pouring forth as soon as the aid is switched on.

It is probably ideal to proceed with hearing aids as soon as reasonably possible, but the decision must be that of the family and should not be forced on them. Indeed, if they are not yet ready to cope with hearing aids, it may be better to delay fitting them and concentrate on supporting the parents until they do feel ready to proceed.

It is probably best not to become too involved in evaluation at the first fitting. If the initial selection of the aid has been done carefully (and it is worth noting that this selection can be quite time consuming and should be done in advance of the fitting session) then much of the session itself can concentrate on the process of introducing the family to the aid. Evaluation usually begins in earnest at the first follow-up visit.

The first fitting visit should concentrate on checking the following:

- the moulds fit comfortably in the ear;
- the aids fit neatly behind the ears, not protruding, hanging loose or easily dislodged;
- the aid can be set to the correct volume without feedback;
- the family knows how to operate and insert the aids;
- the family knows about the use of batteries, battery locks and volume control covers;
- the family knows what volume setting to use;
- the family knows when the next appointment is;
- the family knows whom to contact with any questions;
- the family knows that there is no such thing as a 'silly' question.

Families need to be advised about how to introduce the child to the hearing aids. Generally the advice is for the child to begin wearing the aid gradually but consistently over the first few weeks to full time wear. Each family's experience will be different. Some children will quickly reach the point where they wear the aid all day; with others it will take much longer. It is probably best to advise against too rapid an increase to full-time wear in order to avoid physical discomfort of the ear (the 'new shoe' effect). One not uncommon pattern is that children go through a honeymoon period when they seem to accept the aid very well, followed by a period of defiant rejection. A firm policy, employing reward when the child complies, and gentle firmness and perseverance when they don't, usually pays off in the end.

Evaluation

Evaluation is necessary to check the child's aided performance. It can also be used to demonstrate to the parents that the aid improves the child's hearing and, where parental scepticism and resistance are met, to further convince them of the need for amplification.

Evaluation of the hearing aid fit includes both objective and behavioural measures.

Objective measures

The hearing aid outputs should be checked in a test box against the outputs obtained at the selection stage, to make sure that the aid is still functioning properly.

Real ear performance can be checked by measuring the aid's output while worn. This is done by inserting a probe tube microphone into the ear canal, and measuring the sound levels in the ear canal both with and without the hearing aid.

Behavioural

It is useful to the clinician, and reassuring to the parents, to measure how well the child hears when aided. Aided thresholds can be measured in exactly the same way as unaided thresholds (using behavioural observation audiometry (BOA), visual reinforcement audiometry (VRA), play audiometry, and so forth) and the results compared. It is useful to plot the results obtained in this way on an audiogram that also shows various real life sounds across frequency, including speech (see, for example, Figure 10.5, taken from Northern and Downs, 1991). The clinician can then talk through the audiogram with the family, highlighting the unaided/unaided differences and points

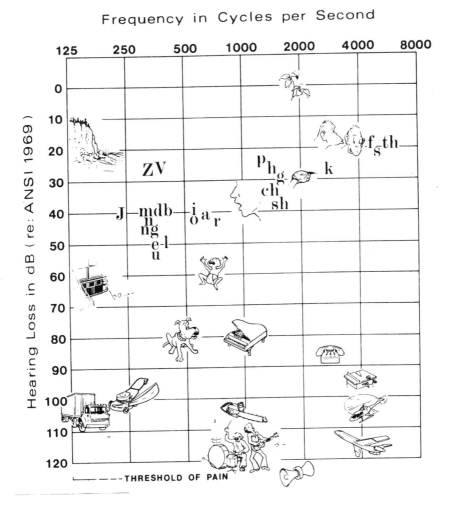

Figure 10.5. Pictorial audiogram.

where the aid may need further adjustment if some speech sounds are still not accessible. This audiogram should be given to the family as an important part of their record of the child's progress.

Tolerance can be measured by presenting sounds across frequency in ascending loudness until the child begins to show the early signs of distress – this must be done with caution as sudden presentation of a distressing sound may upset children to the point where they reject the hearing aids. Tolerance measures can also be recorded on the audiogram.

In addition to measurements using frequency-specific sounds (for example, warble tones and narrow-band noise) it is worth measuring responses to speech. For pre-school children who are not up to formal speech discrimination testing (such as the McCormick Toy Test) this will take the form of speech detection tasks, in which voice is presented at gradually increased levels until children respond in much the same way as they do to frequency-specific stimuli. Voice can be presented either live or through loud speakers. If the system is not calibrated, response levels can be measured using a sound-level meter. One major advantage of using speech signals to check the aided performance is that speech means far more to families than frequency specific sounds do, at least early in the habilitation process. They will often be more impressed by the results of tests using voice than by all of our whistles and beeps.

It is sometimes useful to carry out aided 'speech' detection using frequency specific phonemes, such as (from low to high frequency in order) 'ee', 'oo', 'aa', 'sh', 'ss', in order to demonstrate the audibility of such sounds when the child is wearing the aids.

Field evaluation

An important aspect of evaluation comes from observation of the child in the real world outside the clinic. The family will need to make frequent visits to the clinic in the early stages so that a picture of the child's aided performance can be built up gradually. At these sessions parents can be questioned in detail about the success of the fitting. In many services, there will also be support from the education service and their views become an important part of building up a picture of how the aid is helping.

Essentially we need to know two things. First, is the hearing aid doing any good? As Tucker and Nolan (1984) point out, this may not show up early in the fitting in terms of speech and language development. Rather it will be apparent from less specific behaviour, such as children being generally more responsive to sounds, more aware of noises they had previously ignored, being reluctant to take their hearing aids out and so on. Second, we need to know of any tendency the child may have to reject hearing aids and of what strategies we can best employ to get around this. Is the child upset by loud noises? Are the hearing aids rejected in certain situations (such as in a noisy playgroup)? This may imply that the aid is too powerful. Alternatively, is the child not showing signs of reacting to sound at home, or only to loud sounds? Does the child not react when called? Does he or she not appear to hear the television, the doorbell, a dog barking? This may be because the aid is not powerful enough, or not functioning correctly. The hearing may have changed (such as with a bout of glue ear) or the canals may be occluded with wax. Is the child reluctant to wear the hearing aids at all? This may be caused by poorly fitting earmoulds.

Information from observations in the field and in the clinic need to be pieced together to confirm the adequacy of the selected aids. Sometimes the two sets of information are complementary, for example not enough gain achieved according to clinical measurements and parents reporting little improvement in response to sound. In such situations steps must be taken to try to bring about a more satisfactory fitting. Sometimes the two sets of information may be contradictory, for example when the parents report no problems with tolerance but the child reacts vigorously to modestly raised speech and narrow-band noise in the clinic. In such situations it may be necessary to ensure, first, that the parents have understood exactly what is being asked and that they are not answering one question where the clinician is asking another. Audiologists are used to using a wide range of terms to talk about sound. Some of these terms have been taken from general parlance, but have come to mean quite specific things. Words such as 'frequency', 'intensity', 'tolerance' and so forth may mean something different to the non-clinician who usually has a much less sophisticated set of terms to deal with sound (at least in the early stages of habilitation). Misunderstandings can arise because of this. However, if contradictions remain then it is probably better to rely cautiously on the real-world performance of the child than on the less representative clinical results, until such a time as the contradiction can be resolved.

In practice, evaluation takes place in some form of hearing aid review clinic. In summary, these clinics are used to obtain the following information:

- Comments from the family, the visiting teacher, and, if he or she is old enough, the child, on the effects of the fitting. Comments are sought on wear time, apparent comfort, responses to sound when aided, changes in communication and tolerance problems.

- Ears are checked for wax occlusion, presence of effusion and so forth.
- Moulds are checked for damage, obstruction and fit.
- Aids are checked in the test box against targets, for gain/frequency response, maximum output and distortion.
- Real ear aided performance is measured with probe tube microphones
- Behavioural measures of aided performance, including tolerance, are carried out using frequency specific tones and speech.
- Behavioural measures of unaided hearing are repeated to confirm levels, check stability of hearing, and fill in information at missing frequencies.
- For older children, speech discrimination can be performed, although this is more useful as a demonstration to parents of aided benefit than as a means of confirming the adequacy of the aid or of choosing between different aids (Green, 1987).

The special challenges of early identification

Recent developments in hearing screening have made early identification of hearing loss much more common. Indeed, with good programmes of universal neonatal screening, some 90% of children with significant hearing loss are likely to be detected at birth (Davis et al., 1997). This has brought its own set of special problems.

How early should we be fitting hearing aids?

This is an important question. The practical problems of fitting hearing aids to infants are considerable. They spent much time lying down, giving great potential for feedback and dislodged hearing aids. Moulds will need constant replacement, requiring frequent trips into the department. Hearing aid selection and evaluation of the fitting are also difficult when the child is too young to give clear responses to sound.

Parents may be reluctant to have aids fitted before they have had a chance to enjoy their baby at home unencumbered by hearing aids. If the child has already been through a stormy neonatal period, the family may be even more reluctant to apply technology too soon.

Despite this, parents of hearing impaired children report a preference for diagnosis and hearing aid fitting as early as possible (Bamford et al., 1998). Furthermore, there is increasing evidence of the importance of auditory stimulation in the first six months of life (see, for example, Yoshinago-Itano et al., 1998). Each family will be different, and while, in principle, the earlier amplification is fitted the better, in practice it will be necessary to proceed at whatever rate the family wishes, as we have already stated.

Hearing aid selection in infants – some issues

The hearing aid fitting will only be as good as the information on which it is based. So how do we know what we are fitting to? How can we assess hearing in infants accurately?

There has been a recent development in establishing thresholds across frequency in the very young. Behavioural observation audiometry, carefully used, can give broad information about hearing loss with a degree of frequency specificity. Impedance audiometry and stapedius reflex testing can help reveal the presence of middle-ear effusion and conductive pathology, although impedance testing in the very young requires careful interpretation.

Some audiologists promote the use of frequency specific ABR testing, for both air and bone conduction ABR. For example Stapells and Oates (1997) suggest that, given appropriate recording techniques, ABR thresholds to low and high frequency tonal stimuli can give reasonable predictions of threshold, and bone conduction ABR can be used to establish the presence and extent of any air-bone gap (Stapells, 1998).

It is certainly the case that, until the child is old enough to give accurate behavioural responses (usually around six months), the 'prescription' is an approximation, because the estimates of threshold are an approximation. It is wise to err on the side of caution and not fit too powerful an aid at this stage. Too much volume can distress the child and cause the aid to be rejected as well as, in extreme cases, causing cochlear damage (see below). Powerful hearing aids also cause feedback in the ear more easily and so can be difficult to manage. However too little volume is also a problem. If the aid is not powerful enough, the child will not hear with it and is likely simply to reject the 'foreign object' in his ear. In order to ensure that the aid is at least broadly right, giving not too little and not too much amplification, it is necessary to check the fitting frequently in the early weeks, particularly with babies.

A separate class of problems relates to the fitting philosophy that we use with very young children who are pre-lingually hearing impaired. Many prescription methods are based on adult measurements. This means that the psychoacoustic information that is used to translate from the degree of hearing loss to the prescribed gain is based on measurements of loudness growth taken on adventitiously hearing impaired adults. It may be that pre-lingually deafened infants require different amplification strategies to adults. For example, there is some evidence that pre-lingual children need louder signals (Nozza et al., 1991) and more adventitious signal-to-noise ratios (Nozza et al., 1990) than adults do in order to learn to process speech. Prescriptions do not address this issue (Snik and Martin, 1998) and may underestimate the required gain. Dillon (1998), however, sounds a cautious note against using high-level inputs. He points out that protection of the cochlea from noise-induced damage is paramount and the intensity levels in small infant canals is already high. The issues are not resolved and the consensus is that more research is necessary.

Final comments

This chapter has concentrated on hearing aid fitting but it is important to realize that there is much more going on in hearing aid sessions than just matching an aid to a prescription target. As we have discussed, the whole process can be an anxious one for the members of the child's family. They may still be at the stage of coming to terms with the diagnosis of deafness, and have many unasked questions about its consequences. The hearing aid session should therefore be used to impart all the necessary information to them, and to allow them time to ask these questions. Indeed there is far more to cover than can be done in one or two sessions, and a co-ordinated long-term approach from the whole team of people involved in helping the family is the ideal.

It should be clear from this chapter that audiologists working with the hearing impaired child need to be versatile members of the rehabilitation team. They must understand in detail the hearing aids that are available and must know how to match the hearing aid to the child's needs, as well as being aware of the limitations of doing this. They must be sensitive to the feelings of the child and the family. The aid itself can provide an important link to communication, but every child and family needs to be helped to make that link work for them. For that to happen, the audiologist must work in close liaison with parents, teachers, speech and language therapists, doctors and all other caregivers involved with the child. Children can do amazing things, and with a little help from us, they can succeed in pulling the language rabbit from out of the hat.

References

Baguley D, Davis A, Bamford J (2000) Principles of family friendly hearing services for children. BSA News 29: 35-39

Bamford J, Davis A, Hind S, McCracken W, Reeve K (1998) Evidence on very early service delivery: what parents want and don't always get. In Seewald R (ed.) A Sound Foundation Through Early Amplification. Phonak AG.

Benyon G, Munro K (1993) A discussion of current sound field calibration procedures. British Journal of Audiology 27(6): 427-32.

Byrne D, Dillon H (1986) The National Acoustics Laboratories' (NAL) new procedure for selecting the gain and frequency response of a hearing aid. Ear and Hearing 7: 257-65.

Byrne D, Parkinson A, Newall P (1990) Hearing aid fitting and frequency response requirements for the severely/profoundly hearing impaired. Ear and Hearing 11: 40-9.

Davis A, Bamford J, Wilson I, Ramkalawan T, Forshaw M, Wright S (1997) A critical review of the role of neonatal hearing screening in the detection of congenital hearing impairment. Health Technology Assessment 1997: 1(10): 1-177.

Dillon H (1998) Fitting a wide dynamic range of speech into a narrow dynamic range of hearing. In Seewald R (ed.) (1998) A Sound Foundation Through Early Amplification. Phonak AG.

Green R (1987) The uses and misuses of speech audiometry in rehabilitation. In Martin M (ed.) (1987) Speech Audiometry. London: Taylor & Francis.

Green R (1999) Audiological management in the first eighteen months. In Stokes J (ed.) (1999) Hearing Impaired Infants: Support in the First Eighteen Months. London: Whurr, pp. 55-6.

National Deaf Children's Society (1994) Quality Standards in Paediatric Audiology. Vol. I: Guidelines for the Early Identification of Hearing Impairment. London: National Deaf Children's Society.

National Deaf Children's Society (1996) Quality Standards in Paediatric Audiology. Vol. II: The Audiological Management of the Child with Permanent Hearing Loss. London: National Deaf Children's Society.

National Deaf Children's Society and British Cochlear Implant Group (1999) Quality Standards in Paediatric Audiology. Vol. III: Cochlear Implants for Children. London: National Deaf Children's Society.

National Deaf Children's Society (2000) Quality Standards in Paediatric Audiology. Vol.IV: Guidelines for the Early Identification and the Audiological Management of Children with Hearing Loss. London: National Deaf Children's Society.

Northern J, Downs M (1991) Hearing in Infants. Baltimore: Williams & Wilkins.

Nozza R, Rossman R, Bond L, Miller S (1990) Infant speech sound discrimination in noise. Journal of the Acoustical Society of America 87: 339-50.

Nozza R, Rossman, R, Bond L (1991) Infant-adult differences to unmasked thresholds for the discrimination of consonant-vowel syllable pairs. Audiology 30: 102-12.

Pediatric Working Group of the Conference on Amplification for Children with Auditory Deficits (1996) Amplification for infants and children with hearing loss. American Journal of Audiology 5(1): 53–68.

Seewald R (1995) The Desired Sensation Level (DSL) method for hearing aid fitting in infants and children. Phonak Focus 20: 3–18.

Snik F, Martin H (1998) Fitting preschool and primary school children with hearing instruments: an evaluation of hearing aid prescription rules. In Seewald R (ed.) (1998) A Sound Foundation Through Early Amplification. Phonak AG.

Stapells D, Oates P (1997) Estimation of the pure-tone audiogram by the auditory brainstem response: a review. Audiology and Neuro-otology 2: 257–80.

Stapells D (1998) Frequency-specific evoked potential audiometry in infants. In Seewald R (1998) A Sound Foundation Through Early Amplification. Phonak AG.

Tucker I, Nolan M (1984) Educational Audiology. Beckenham: Croom Helm.

Yoshinago-Itano C, Sedley A, Coutter D, Mehl A (1998) Language of early and later deafened children with hearing loss. Paediatrics 102: 1161–71.

Chapter 11
Cochlear implants

SARAH FLYNN

Introduction

Cochlear implants are an alternative form of assistive device for those who receive little or no benefit from conventional acoustic hearing aids. They comprise a surgically implanted component and externally worn equipment. They operate by stimulating remaining auditory nerve fibres electrically thus bypassing absent or dysfunctioning hair cells in the cochlea or inner ear. The electrically induced nerve impulses are transmitted to the brain to produce a sensation of hearing (Figure 11.1). This chapter gives an overview of cochlear implant systems and describes the implantation process for deaf children.

Historical development of cochlear implants

The complexity and capability of cochlear implants has advanced considerably since the first clinically available device, the 3M/House implant, developed by House and Urban in the USA (House et al., 1976). This device, like the 3M/Vienna (Hochmair-Desoyer, 1986; Burian, Hochmair-Desoyer and Eisenwort, 1986) and UCH (Cooper et al., 1989) devices had one active electrode through which electrical stimulation was delivered. These single-channel devices were used in adults initially, and then children, giving auditory sensation which, for most patients, helped with lipreading (Simmons, 1966; Bilger, 1977).

Multichannel implants split the incoming signal into different speech features or frequency bands. This information is

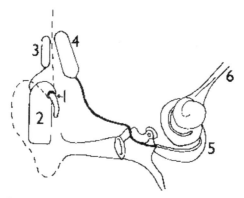

1. Microphone picks up environmental and speech sounds
2. Speech processor filters and compresses the input signal, and processes the intensity and frequency of sound into a suitable electrical code
3. Transmitter coil sends the signal to the internal implant via an FM carrier wave
4. Internal implant decodes the signal and sends it to the intracochlear electrodes
5. Current flows from the electrodes in the cochlea to stimulate the remaining auditory neurones electrically
6. The hearing nerve is activated and sends a signal to the brain which is interpreted as sound

Figure 11.1. Components of an implant system with a body-worn speech processor and their functions.

delivered to an array of electrodes located at different places along the cochlea. Multichannel implants thus aim to make some use of the tonotopic arrangement in the cochlea. The Ineraid (formerly Richards or Utah) multichannel implant uses continuous analogue (CA) processing, where the incoming sound is divided into frequency bands and these are delivered simultaneously to four active intra-cochlear electrodes according to their frequency (Eddington et al., 1978; Parkin and Stewart, 1988). The Nucleus 22 cochlear implant has 22 active intra-cochlear electrodes. Formant features of speech were extracted and delivered to different electrodes in a series of pulses, according to their frequency (Clark et al., 1987). Even though the speech was processed in different ways in both of these devices it was clear that, on average, patients derived more benefit from multichannel than single-channel implants (Gantz et al., 1988; Doyle, Pilj and Noel, 1991; Cohen, Waltzman and Fisher, 1993; Cohen and Waltzman, 1995; Eyles, Aleksy and Boyle, 1995). Speech processing for the Nucleus 22 implant changed to include high frequency information; the multi-peak (MPEAK) strategy (Von Wallenberg and Battmer, 1991) and later formant extraction was replaced with the spectral peak (SPEAK) strategy (Skinner et al., 1994).

Wilson et al. (1991) developed a new pulsatile strategy known as continuous interleaved sampling (CIS), which sampled and split the incoming sound into frequency bands that were allocated to different electrodes. This strategy allowed fast sampling of the incoming sound and rapid delivery of stimulus pulses. The improvements in speech perception with this fast-rate strategy were such that it is available as a processing strategy for most currently used implants (Wilson et al., 1995).

Cochlear implantation was initially restricted to adults with acquired hearing losses because it was thought that only those who had developed speech and language auditorily could make sense of the auditory signal provided by an implant. As the benefits of implantation in adults surpassed expectations, children with acquired hearing losses were implanted and later children with congenital hearing losses. The implantation of children has been a contentious issue because to obtain the most benefit with a cochlear implant the child must be implanted at a young age or after a short duration of deafness. Children, therefore, are often not mature enough to be involved in the decision to have an implant. There were also concerns as to whether pre-lingually deafened children would be able to make use of the sound signal conveyed by implants (Lane, 1995). Cochlear implants have, however, been successful with children with congenital and pre-lingually acquired hearing losses providing they are implanted early (Osberger et al., 1991a; Staller et al., 1991; Gantz et al., 1994; Miyamoto et al., 1995; Summerfield and Marshall, 1995; Osberger et al., 1996; Cohen and Waltzman, 1996; Miyamoto, Svirsky and Robbins, 1997; Tait and Lutman, 1994; Parkinson, El-Kholy and Tyler, 1998; Miyamoto et al., 1999a; O'Donoghue et al., 1998). Cochlear implants are now widely accepted as an appropriate form of help for profoundly deaf children and give them the option of participation in hearing and deaf society (Cohen, 1994; McCormick, 1991).

Cochlear implant systems

Components of cochlear implants

All cochlear implants comprise an internal implanted electrode array and an external microphone, speech processor and transmitter. The external components may be housed separately and connected with leads or cables such as the Sprint body-worn processor for the Nucleus CI24M, the CIS pro+ processor for the Medel Combi 40+, and the body-worn processor for the Clarion implant. The Tempo+ and Esprit behind-the-ear processors of the Medel Combi 40+ and the Nucleus CI24M implants, respectively, have the microphone set in the speech processor. The microphone of Clarion implant systems is housed in the transmitter coil. Table 11.1 shows the main features of the most widely used current cochlear implant systems.

Speech processors

Speech processors are individually set by the audiologist to suit each patient but also have user-operated switches on them. These switches turn the processor on and off and select the volume, sensitivity and program to be used. The volume switch changes the loudness but only within the range set by the audiologist with the implant software program. The sensitivity relates to the quietest sounds that are processed by the speech processor. If the sensitivity is set low only the louder sounds will be transmitted but if the sensitivity is set high a wide range of sounds from quiet right through to loud will be transmitted. A middle sensitivity setting is usually best for speech; if sensitivity is too low the quieter sounds of speech will be missed but if sensitivity is too high quiet background sound may appear disproportionately loud and make speech difficult to discern. The processor can store more than one program or map and the patient can switch between the programs. There are often warning lights, sounds or displays to alert users or their parents or teachers that there may be a fault with the processor, battery, leads or microphone.

Signal transfer

All current implant systems transfer the signal from the speech processor to the internal electrode array transcutaneously. The electrical signal is converted into a radio signal that travels across the intact skin and is decoded and delivered to the electrodes by the internal part of the implant system. The Ineraid implant uses percutaneous transmission via a plug or pedastal through the skin but infection around the plug and damage may limit the use of the implant and in the worse case result in reimplantation (Cohen and Hoffman, 1991; Eyles et al., 2000). The direct wire connection did, however, make the use

Table 11.1 Main features of cochlear implant systems currently in use.

Feature	Clarion	Nucleus 22	Nucleus CI24	Medel Combi 40+	Ineraid
electrode array	curved	straight	straight, contour or double array	straight either long, compressed or split	straight
number of intracochlear electrodes	16	22	22	12	6
number of channels	variable according to processor settings	up to 22	up to 22	up to 12	up to 6
stimulation mode	monopolar bipolar	(monopolar) bipolar common ground	monopolar bipolar common ground	monopolar	monopolar
speech processors and [strategies]	CII series processors* [CIS, SAS, PPS and new hybrid strategies]	Spectra [SPEAK] Esprit 22*	Sprint [SPEAK, ACE, CIS] Esprit* [SPEAK] 3G* [SPEAK, ACE, CIS	CISpro+ [CIS, n of m] Tempo+* [CIS]	Ineraid [CA] CISpro link [CIS]
Processor checking	Body-worn – indicator lights Post-aural – no	Spectra – indicator lights, signal check and monitor earphones Esprit 22 – signal check and monitor earphones	Sprint – indicator lights, monitor earphones and signal check Esprit and 3G – monitor earphones and signal check	Cis pro+ indicator lights, monitor earphones and signal check Tempo+* indicator lights and signal check	CISpro link indicator lights

The Nucleus 22 implant has been superseded by the Nucleus CI24 implant but there are many children still using the Nucleus 22 device. The Ineraid device is no longer made and most of the remaining users are adults. Monopolar stimulation is only available in newer versions of the Nucleus 22 implant. The * indicates a post-aural processor. The speech processing strategies shown in square brackets are as follows: SPEAK – spectral peak, ACE – advanced combination encoder, CIS – continuous interleaved sampling, SAS – simultaneous analogue stimulation, PPS – paired pulsatile stimulation, n of m – n spectral peaks of m channels, CA – compressed analogue.

of newer processing strategies easier to apply to the existing internal part of the implant. Transcutaneous systems usually use a magnet to hold the transmitter coil in place over the internal part of the implant.

Internal electrode array

The internal part of the implant system decodes the radio signal from the processor and delivers tiny electric currents to nerve endings in the cochlea via electrodes spaced along the electrode array inside the cochlea. The electrode contacts may be plates, discs or rings of metal that conduct the electricity. These are connected to wires running up to the main body of the internal implant. All of the internal implant except for the tiny contacts is hermetically sealed and covered in non-reactive material such as silastic to prevent body fluids from affecting the implant and to ensure that the electric current does not cause undesired stimulation. In order for an electric current to flow there must be an active electrode (positive pole) and an inactive, reference or ground electrode (negative pole). Charge flows from the active to the inactive electrode, thus inducing an electric current. Extra-cochlear electrodes are implanted under the muscle behind the ear or are positioned on the case of the implant body for use as reference or ground electrodes

The active electrodes of all current implant systems are intra-cochlear that is, they are inserted inside the cochlea, which does result in damage to the cochlea (Boggess, Baker and Balkany, 1989). Extra-cochlear systems are less invasive because all the electrodes are outside the cochlea but require more current to produce a sensation of sound. Performance with intra-cochlear devices has surpassed that with extra-cochlear stimulation (Hortman et al., 1989; Kasper, Pelizzone and Montandon, 1991). Different implant systems have different numbers of intra-cochlear electrodes; the Clarion has eight pairs of electrodes, the Nucleus CI24M has 22 electrodes and the Medel Combi 40+ has 12 electrodes. Electrode arrays are flexible and smooth to allow insertion into the cochlea without stress on the array. They vary in length and thus, in how far they can be inserted into the cochlea and in how far apart the electrode contacts are spaced. The Clarion implant had a coiled and now has a curved electrode array and special surgical tools are needed for insertion (Balkany, Cohen and Gantz, 1999; Filipo et al., 1999). The rationale for this design is to locate the active electrodes near to the modiolus or centre of the cochlea close to remaining neurones thus giving more specific stimulation of different regions of the cochlea at lower current levels. Techniques to locate active electrodes close to the modiolus are actively being researched and, if effective, are likely to produce further improvements in the speech perception of implanted patients. Split electrode arrays have been developed by MXM, Cochlear and Medel for use with ossified cochleae so that electrodes can be inserted at different locations in the cochlea (Bredberg et al., 1997; Richardson et al., 1999). The Combi 40+ implant, which has the longest electrode array, has the option of a compressed array, still with 12 electrodes but more closely spaced if insertion is likely to be difficult because of cochlear deformity.

Speech processing

In a normally hearing ear sound is coded by the firing of different numbers of neurones located in different places in the cochlea. Sound is differentiated by changes in loudness and pitch over time in a normally hearing human. The speech processor of the implant system codes loudness as current density that is related to the current level and duration of each individual pulse of electrical stimulation. Pitch is coded by separating the sound into different frequency bands that give rise to stimulation of different electrodes located along the cochlea. The apical region of the cochlea is more sensitive to low frequencies and the basal part of the cochlea is more sensitive to high frequencies. The range from just audible to the maximum comfortably loud level is the dynamic range and it extends from 0–120 dB in normally hearing people. For electrical stimulation in all implant systems this range is equivalent to about 10 dB to 25 dB of the acoustic range for normal hearing. The speech processor must, therefore, compress the incoming sound into the narrow range available for electrical stimulation. Compression and other aspects of processing the sound signal are implemented in different ways in different implant systems. The different methods of processing the sound and more particularly speech signal are known as sound or speech processing strategies and all aim to give the clearest possible speech signal.

Speech processing may be analogue where stimulation occurs on all channels simultaneously and continuously or it may be pulsatile where the sound signal is sampled, converted into pulses and delivered to different channels sequentially. The only current implant system that has the option of simultaneous analogue stimulation (SAS) is the Clarion implant (Battmer et al., 1999). The incoming signal is split into eight frequency bands that are delivered via eight electrode pairs in a bipolar stimulation mode to different regions of the cochlea. The Ineraid device, which is no longer made, used continuous analogue (CA) stimulation in a monopolar mode with four channels. The use of bipolar stimulation in the SAS strategy lessens current spread and thus reduces channel interactions which caused poor frequency discrimination in some Ineraid users (Dorman et al., 1990, Favre and Pelizzone, 1993). There is also the option of a hybrid strategy, the paired pulsatile strategy (PPS), with the Clarion implant. This strategy delivers paired pulses simultaneously to two out of eight channels at a time (Zimmerman-Phillips and Murad, 1999).

All other currently used speech processing strategies are pulsatile and fully sequential so that channel interaction is minimized. Pulsatile strategies fall into two broad categories: continuous interleaved sampling (CIS) and spectral maxima strategies. Continuous interleaved sampling comprises splitting the whole of the incoming signal into frequency bands and delivering the bands of stimulation to electrodes in different regions of the cochlea according to frequency (Wilson et al., 1991). The sound is sampled and pulses are presented at a fast rate in order to preserve as much as possible of the temporal features of sound. The CIS strategy is now widely used and is available as a programming option for most implant systems. Some Ineraid implant users now have access to the CIS strategy with adapted Medel processors (Wilson et al., 1995; Pelizzone, Cosendai and Tinembart, 1999; Kompis, Vischer and Hausler, 1999). There are, however, variations in the implementation of the CIS strategy in different devices. The number of channels, the spacing of electrodes, the rate of stimulation, the frequency range of the implant and the update or sampling rate can all influence individual patient's performance with the CIS strategy (Dorman and Loizou, 1998; Eddington et al., 1994; Nelson et al., 1995; Lawson et al., 1996; Wilson, 1997; Fishman, Shannon and Slattery, 1997; Brill et al., 1997; Kiefer et al., 2000).

Spectral maxima strategies are also known as 'n of m'; n number of maxima delivered to m number of electrodes. The speech processor analyses the incoming sound and picks out a pre-set number of maxima, that is, a certain number of the loudest frequency bands in the signal. Only these bands are delivered to electrodes along the array according to their frequency. Stimulation roves between the electrodes allocated frequency bands that coincide with the strongest frequencies in the signal at a given moment in time. The Nucleus advanced combination encoder (ACE) offers a spectral maxima strategy that typically uses eight or 12 maxima roving over 22 electrodes. The stimulation can be at fast pulse rates and programming options are very flexible. The ACE is available to Nucleus CI24M implant users with the Sprint (body-worn) and Esprit 3G (post-aural) speech processors. The spectral peak (SPEAK) strategy typically uses about six maxima roving over 20 electrodes and uses slower pulse rates. It is available for use with the Nucleus 22 and the Nucleus CI24M implants. An 'n of m' strategy is available with the Combi 40+ implant when used with the CIS pro+ (body-worn) processor. This fast rate strategy extracts up to eleven peaks from the incoming signal and these are used to stimulate up to twelve electrodes. Speech processing strategies for cochlear implants have been reviewed by Loizou (1998) and Wilson (1997).

Selection of a cochlear implant for use with children

Children are implanted early in their lives and will need to use their implant systems for many years. Some implant teams use more than one type of implant. There are three essential considerations for choice of device: safety, efficacy and long-term maintenance.

Safety

The implant should cause only the desired auditory stimulation and should not result in adverse effects to body tissue. The implant must also be impervious to body fluid and be biocompatible. In young children the implant must be able to accommodate skull growth. The insertion of the electrode array results in some trauma to the cochlea and fibrous tissue can develop around the drilled areas of the cochlea and the electrode array but no reduction in ganglion cell populations has been found (Terr, Sfogliano and Riley, 1989; Linthicum et al., 1991). Even the electrode array allowing the deepest insertion, up to 30 mm, has not resulted in further degeneration of neural elements (Gstoettner et al., 1997). Patients who have used implants long term have not shown any signs of deterioration in their responses as a result of chronic electrical stimulation. Investigations into the effects of long-term electrical stimulation indicate that there is beneficial effect on auditory neuronal survival (Miller, 1991; Leake et al., 2000). The safety and longevity of implants is related to the design, the quality of the components used and the quality and cleanliness of the manufacturing process. In the US the Food and Drug Administration (FDA) regulates trials of new cochlear implants whereas in Europe regulation is by the CE mark. Issues of safety and biocompatiblity are discussed in more depth by House and Berliner (1986) and Shepherd, Franz and Clark (1990). Brummer, Robblee and Hambrecht (1983) and McCreery et al. (1990) have studied safety aspects of electrical stimulation in the body.

Efficacy

Clinicians need to be confident that a particular implant will be more beneficial than non-invasive alternatives such as conventional hearing aids and vibrotactile aids. Auditory benefit occurs relatively quickly in adults with acquired hearing losses (Summerfield and Marshall, 1995; Tyler and Summerfield, 1996). For this reason most programmes wait until there is demonstrable benefit from new implants or processing strategies in adults with acquired hearing losses before using them with children. There is now a large body of evidence that shows that multichannel cochlear implants improve speech perception for suitable children but benefit accrues over significantly longer time periods than for implanted adults (Osberger et al., 1991a; Staller et al., 1991; Gantz et al., 1994; Miyamoto et al., 1995; Summerfield and Marshall, 1995; Osberger et al., 1996; Cohen and Waltzman, 1996; Miyamoto, Svirsky and Robbins, 1997; Tait and Lutman, 1994; Parkinson, El-Kholy and Tyler, 1998; Miyamoto et al., 1999a, O'Donoghue et al., 1998). For children and for adults there is wide variation in the level of individual benefit obtained. It is not possible to predict precisely, for any individual adult or child, the level of auditory skills that will be attained after implantation.

Long-term maintenance

Children will need to use their cochlear implants for many years. Successful outcomes from implantation are only possible if the implant can be used consistently. For the lifetime of the internal device the patient needs access to replacement external equipment and the means for the speech processor to be programmed. The external equipment of different implant systems is not interchangeable. Ideally new processors or strategies should be accessible to existing as well as newly implanted patients without the need for surgery to replace the internal part of the device. To provide this type of long-term support, cochlear implant manufacturers will, of course, need a high level of financial stability. Currently available implant systems do have some in-built flexibility, which could enable new developments in speech processing to be used by patients who are implanted now. Children using the Nucleus 22 device have been able to take advantage of better speech processing strategies with the MSP (mini speech processor) and later the Spectra speech processors, which are compatible with their internal electrode array (Von Wallenberg and Battmer, 1991; Cohen and Waltzman, 1995; Dillier et al., 1995; Shallop and McGinn-Brunelli, 1995; Cowan et al., 1995; Lenarz and Battmer, 1995; Sehgal et al., 1998). The Ineraid cochlear implant is no longer made but some Ineraid patients now use specially adapted CIS pro-speech processors which enable these patients to use the CIS strategy (Wilson et al., 1995; Pelizzone, Cosendai and Tinembart, 1999; Kompis, Vischer and Hausler, 1999).

Other beneficial features of implant systems for children

- Telemetry enables the clinician to detect electrode short circuits quickly from information sent back from the internal implant without the child needing to report any change in sound quality. With the Nucleus CI24M implant neural response telemetry (NRT) detects neural responses with electrically evoked compound action potentials (Abbas et al., 1999, Shallop, Facer and Peterson, 1999 and also see Chapter 7).
- Objective tests such as electrical auditory brainstem responses (EABR) (see Chapter 7) and electrical stapedial reflex measurements (ESRT) (Stephan, Welzl-Muller and Stiglbrumer, 1991; Battmer, Laszig and Lehnhardt, 1990; Hodges et al., 1999) are possible with most currently available implant systems. Tests can be carried out intra- and post-operatively and are particularly useful in the early stages of tuning the speech processor with young children.
- The external equipment should have tamper-proof battery compartments and switches, unplugable leads for ease of replacement, no sharp components and should be small enough for young children to use comfortably.

- Durability of the externally worn equipment is important in maintaining consistent device use. If there are frequent breakdowns the child will not be able to use the implant consistently. More staff time and larger stocks of spare equipment will be required if repairs and replacements are needed often.
- Batteries used by speech processors need to be available easily and locally to patients and should last at least all of the child's waking day because they may not always indicate when the processor is not working.
- Indicators of processor function in the form of lights or auditory signals allow parents and teachers to check the external equipment and alert them to faults, especially with young children who may not be able to report faults.
- Use of FM radio aids with implants is particularly important in educational settings where background noise can cause problems for implanted children (Wood, Flynn and Eyles, 2000). Other accessories may be available for use with loop systems, the television or for listening to music. Various pouches, harnesses, bumbags and belt clips are available from some manufacturers, which give the child different options for wearing the external equipment depending on their age and lifestyle.
- The presence of a magnet in the transmitter and internal implant is problematic for magnetic resonance imaging because of the torsion created by the strong magnetic fields used by MRI and shadow effects on the scans in the region of the implant (Portnoy and Mattucci, 1991). If the patient has a known medical condition that is likely to require the use of MRI there is a magnetless Clarion implant that is held in place by an earmould (Weber et al., 1999; Graham et al., 1999). The Nucleus implant has a magnet that can be removed with minor surgery if MRI is required (Heller et al., 1996). Trials with the Medel Combi 40+ implant have shown that MRI can be safely carried out under certain specific conditions (Teissl et al., 1998).

The cochlear implant team

In order to provide a good service to implanted children and to enable them to obtain the maximum benefit from their implants, many skilled professionals are involved from the stage of initial assessment through to long-term follow up. Various skills are brought together to provide a cohesive service. All team members should have input into the management of individual patients. Worldwide, team approaches to cochlear implantation have produced the best results for patients (Gersdorff, 1991). In the UK the development of specialist cochlear implant teams was stimulated by the department of health directly funding the first six teams to evaluate the benefits of implantation nationally (Summerfield and Marshall, 1995). There are now more teams, including several that implant children. To enable the development of a good level of expertise and experience, teams should be set up to implant a minimum of 10 patients per year and should comprise teams of personnel with a variety of skills (Quality Standards in Paediatric Audiology III, Cochlear implants for children, 1999.)

The requirements of a paediatric team differ from those of an adult programme (Fraser, 1991) and it should ideally comprise professionals experienced in working with young deaf children (Archbold, 1992). The paediatric only team may have a greater opportunity to develop specialist experience of working with young children. Working with implanted adults can, however, give valuable insights into hearing with an implant. Many teams run adult and children's programmes in tandem but for children's programmes, teachers of the deaf, access to an educational psychologist and staff experienced with young deaf children will be needed. With joint adult and children's teams transfer of school leavers to the adult programme is easy; the staff are familiar to the patients and teachers of the deaf are available should help be required in further education settings.

Although the composition of implant teams varies there should be a core of medical, audiological and rehabilitative personnel, usually otologists, audiological scientists, speech and language therapists and teachers of the deaf (Figure 11.2). The team is also likely to have input from, or access to, the specialities of radiology, medical physics and educational psychology. Technical/electronic support and the inclusion of a deaf person to act as advocate on the team is also beneficial. All team members will use their skills during the assessment, implantation and rehabilitation phases. For patients to benefit fully from the team approach the team needs to be interactive in deciding which patients are suitable for implantation and in maximizing progress and problem solving following implantation.

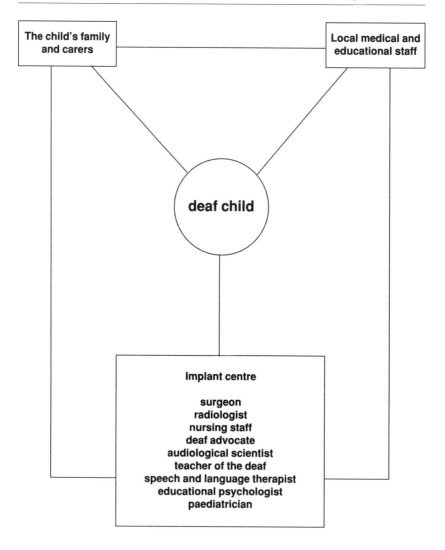

Figure 11.2. The composition of and interaction within a paediatric cochlear implant team.

Many teams use a key worker system where the child and their family are allocated one member of the team to act as their first point of contact and co-ordinate care for the child. This promotes a good relationship between the child's family and the team. The key worker has detailed knowledge of a particular child's progress and they can update other team members as necessary. In most teams one member of the team also takes on an overall co-ordinating role. Central to the team are, of course, the child and their family and carers who together with local education professionals play a major role in successful outcomes from implantation.

Assessment of candidates for implantation

A significant but small proportion of children with sensorineural hearing loss, estimated to be about 300 per year in the UK during the 1990s, are suitable for cochlear implantation (Davis, Fortnum and O'Donoghue, 1995). The process of selection for cochlear implantation should be regarded in the wider context of determining the best form of help for each hearing impaired child rather than a 'pass-or-fail' scenario. The implant team should be prepared to offer recommendations (and in some cases practical assistance) about the best form of help for each child. This could be an implant, a change of hearing aid, frequency transposition aids, tactile aids, or consideration of other management such as the introduction of manual communication. The assessment process may extend over several months. This gives opportunities for information giving and discussion with families and children, if they are old enough. Prior to deciding whether or not a child should be implanted it is important for families to be realistic about the benefit that an implant might give and appreciate the considerable commitment required from implanted children and their families to achieve the maximum benefit with the implant. Families need to be made aware of any restrictions such as avoiding contact sports and the difficulty of using MRI after implantation. They also need information about minimizing the possible effects of static electricity. Some implant teams operate a fast-track assessment for children who have acquired deafness after meningitis so that if the child is suitable for implantation the implant can be inserted before ossification occurs in the cochlea. The fast-track approach may also be considered for children with recently acquired hearing losses to retain auditory skills and prevent degeneration of auditory neurones. Considerable time must still be given for the provision of information and discussion but this can be concentrated into a shorter overall time period.

Audiological assessment

Performance with cochlear implants has improved with new devices and speech processing strategies to the extent that some children with severe hearing losses as well as those with profound hearing losses are now considered for implantation (Kiefer et al., 1998; Rubenstein et al., 1999). Cochlear implants can be effective for children with severe to profound hearing losses. The performance of implanted children, however, has not been shown to be better than that of hearing impaired children fitted with hearing aids who demonstrate good aided thresholds across the speech frequency range (Miyamoto et al., 1995; Osberger et al., 1991a; Osberger et al., 1996; Agelfors, 1998; Tait and Lutman, 1994; Snik et al., 1997; Spencer, Tye-Murray and Tomblin, 1998; Meyer et al., 1998). For this reason and because cochlear implants are invasive and expensive, careful audiological assessment of candidates is essential to determine accurately their best responses with bilateral hearing aids.

Children are tested behaviourally to determine their best response levels with and without hearing aids. Pure-tone audiometry, unaided sound field testing using conditioning techniques or using visual reinforcement audiometry (VRA) with very young children provide measures of the degree of hearing loss. Auditory brainstem electric response measurements and sometimes also electrocochleography are routinely used to confirm the degree of hearing loss. Prior to aided testing, the hearing aid settings and technical performance should be checked for satisfactory functioning. Well-fitting earmoulds are a necessity and new moulds should be obtained before the assessment if required. Adult candidates for implantation are assessed with tests of speech discrimination as well as aided sound field responses to determine the level of benefit they obtained from hearing aids (King, 1991). Many young severely and profoundly deaf children being considered for implantation have little or no memory of speech and are unable to carry out even the simplest speech discrimination tasks. It is, therefore, necessary to assess the potential benefit of hearing aids with sound field aided measurements using frequency-specific stimuli such as warble tones.

During the audiological assessment treatable components to the hearing loss such as middle ear fluid should be identified with otoadmittance measurements. After the resolution of any temporary conductive component the hearing levels, with and without hearing aids, need to be reassessed. The absence of stapedial reflexes confirms the presence of a sensorineural hearing loss providing there is no conductive element. The absence of otoacoustic emissions in an ear with normal middle-ear function is indicative of at least some cochlear dysfunction. The presence of an emission in an ear with a significant hearing loss could indicate auditory dysfunction at a higher level than the cochlea which may not be helped by a cochlear implant (Maxwell, Mason and O'Donoghue, 1999; Miyamoto et al., 1999b).

The tuning or programming of the speech processors of implant systems after implantation requires considerable threshold type testing using VRA or conditioned response test techniques. Although objective measurements help with initial settings there are not yet any objective or automated methods of precisely tuning the implant. Children, therefore, must demonstrate at pre-implant assessment the ability to change their behaviour in response to stimulation, to associate to visual rewards with auditory stimuli or carry out conditioned responses to stimulation through the implant. If children are not developmentally ready to complete the assessment, some practice with conditioning games can help before reassessment. Very young children have a limited attention spans and may not always respond at true threshold levels (the quietest sound level that they can hear at). The trend is for implantation to be carried out at younger ages to take advantage of the increased plasticity of the nervous system in young children. In order to achieve a full and accurate picture of a young child's potential with conventional hearing aids it is likely that more than one session may be required for audiological assessment.

If the child's hearing aids are inappropriate, alternative, suitable aids should be fitted. A trial period of several months will be required for the child to get used to the new hearing aids before reassessing the aided responses. In order to proceed with further cochlear implant assessment the benefit afforded by well-fitted hearing aids used consistently over a period of months should be less than that expected from implantation. Cochlear implants now have the potential to give aided responses at levels of 30–45 dB across the frequency range 250 Hz to 4 KHz. Conventional aids can often give some help at lower frequencies but aided responses are more likely to be poorer over the 2–4 KHz region with severely to profoundly deaf individuals. This frequency range is also particularly important for the perception and production of certain consonants (Boothroyd and Medwetsky, 1992). For this reason many paediatric programmes have now adopted guidelines of aided responses being worse than 55–60 dB across the frequency range 2 KHz to 4 KHz for continuing implant assessment (McCormick, 2001). In very young children, those with borderline hearing levels, or cases of possible progressive hearing loss monitoring over time and repeated assessments may be needed to obtain sufficient information about the benefit of hearing aids.

Radiological and medical evaluation

Radiological investigation is required to identify deformity or pathological changes within the cochlea. Two types of imaging are used; ultra high resolution computed tomography (CT) and magnetic resonance imaging (MRI). Computed tomography scanning shows the bony structures in the cochlea but does not always accurately predict the presence of ossification. Magnetic resonance imaging (MRI) can be used to show new bony growth and soft tissue (Harnsberger et al., 1987; Yune, Miyamoto and Yune, 1991; Gray et al., 1991; Bath et al., 1993; Woolley et al., 1997; Seidman, Chute and Parisier, 1994). If CT scanning indicates deformity to the cochlea, including narrowing of the internal auditory meatus, MRI may be helpful in determining the presence of the auditory nerve (Nadol et al., 1997; Maxwell, Mason and O'Donoghue, 1999).

Determining the presence of the auditory nerve is important because cochlear implants operate by stimulating auditory neurones to produce a sensation of hearing. The number of neurones required is still under investigation but research suggests that even those with few surviving neurones will gain some benefit from implantation (Terr, Sfogliano and Riley, 1989; Nadol, Young and Glynn, 1989; Fayad et al., 1991). Aetiology may effect the number of surviving auditory neurones or the auditory nerve, thus influencing outcomes from implantation. Poor outcomes are thought to be at least partially due to damaged or dysfunctioning auditory neurones. Promontory stimulation or round-window stimulation (Shipp and Nedzelski, 1991) is now rarely used as a measure of neuronal integrity because negative results did not necessarily relate to poor responses after implantation. A particular pathology or cochlear deformity may not necessarily be a contraindication to implantation, provided that the electrode array can be inserted into the cochlea. Information about aetiology may influence which device or surgical method is used. It may also be helpful in guiding expectations and enabling implant candidates and their families make more informed decisions about implantation.

Ossification of the cochlea can occur in post-meningitic patients who make up a significant proportion of children being considered for cochlear implants (Balkany, Gantz and Nadol, 1988; Harsnberger et al., 1987). If ossification or soft tissue (the precursor to ossification) is detected inside the cochlea it may be advisable to fast-track the implant assessment. Ossification does not necessarily preclude implantation but it may influence the choice of electrode array or ear for implantation. Implantees and their families need to be warned that the outcome of implanting an ear with ossification could be poorer than if the cochlea is patent. Thus, the outcome of radiological investigations will influence which ear is implanted, which device is used, whether fast-tracking is needed, expectations counselling and whether an implant is feasible at all.

Thorough medical evaluation is needed to assess the child's general health and fitness for general anaesthesia. Patients with medical conditions not necessarily related to their deafness have been successfully implanted but special arrangements may be needed for the anaesthesia and surgery (Gibbin, O'Donoghue and Murty, 1993; Axon et al., 1997; Szilvassy et al., 1998; Cinamon et al., 1997; Camilleri et al., 1999). Rehabilitation may have to be adapted to fit in with children's other needs if they have multiple disabilities. Detailed knowledge of other medical conditions allows for advanced planning to accommodate specific needs.

During the medical evaluation parents need time to discuss what implant surgery involves and the possible side effects. The risks of implant surgery are low and the same as for any other procedure that requires a general anaesthetic. Additional possible complications specific to implant operations are skin-flap infection or wound breakdown, compression or incorrect positioning of the electrodes, damage to the facial nerve, stimulation of the facial nerve (causing pain or twitching), altered taste, transient dizziness and rejection of the device by the body (Cohen and Hoffman, 1991; Niparko et al., 1991; Hoffman and Cohen, 1993; Luetje and Jackson, 1997; Miyamoto et al., 1996).

Educational and speech and language assessments

Professionals in the child's local educational setting will be very involved in rehabilitation after implantation and it is, therefore, valuable for staff from the implant team to make contact with and gain the co-operation of local professionals during the assessment. Local education staff may need information about cochlear implants and realistic expectations of performance following implantation. Local professionals may contribute information during assessment for implantation candidacy particularly if trials with new hearing aids are required. Information about children's responses to sound in every day life and use of hearing aids is a valuable addition to the formal testing carried out at the implant clinic. Baseline assessments of language status before implantation are important in determining future benefits from implantation and in guiding parental expectations (Archbold, 1992; Robbins and Kirk, 1996). Children from oral, signing and total communication backgrounds can be considered for implantation but after implantation a commitment to promoting the use of the auditory sensations provided by the implant facilitates progress with the implant (Meyer et al., 1998; Tait and Lutman, 1997; Tait, Lutman and Robinson, 2000).

Meeting with other implant users and deaf advocates

Members of the implant team are all well equipped to give implant candidates and their families information about cochlear implants, the results of assessments, the operation, tuning the device, rehabilitation and the level of commitment that the family must give for the implant to be successful. There is, however, great value in implant candidates and their families meeting other families of implanted children and implanted adults. Families of other implanted children can discuss their feelings about implantation and how they coped with the procedure. The implant candidate's family can also see a child making use of their implant in a real life environment. Implanted adults are better able to describe how they felt after the implant surgery, what sound is like through an implant, how it changes with time and processor tuning.

The author's team arranges for the families of implant candidates to meet with a deaf advocate who is a signing hearing aid user and also a social worker for the deaf. This gives families, particularly the majority where both parents are hearing and have had no prior experience deafness, the chance to explore wider issues of deafness in relation to implantation. Parents may also wish to meet families who have decided against implantation for their deaf children. Meeting with implant users and the deaf advocate can help other team members in promoting realistic expectations about cochlear implants. Information giving is an important and continuous part of the assessment procedure. Families of implant candidates need to appreciate that while the benefits of implantation may be considerable, rehabilitation is a slow process requiring a high level of commitment (Downs and Owen Black, 1985; Quittner, Thompson Steck and Rouiller, 1991).

The decision about whether to implant

A profile for the selection of children for implantation has been devised by Hellman et al. (1991) and brings together all the issues important for selection. This will include the results of tests and other information such as medical and radiological evaluations, local services and educational setting, the child's age and duration of deafness. If at all possible the child's feelings about implantation should be considered; this is not possible for young children but picture books and play activities can be used to inform young children about the implantation process. If implantation is recommended factors influencing the type of implant to be used and which ear to implant will be discussed and decided. Usually the cochlear implant team jointly decides whether a child is suitable for implantation but it is the child and family who ultimately decide whether or not to go ahead.

Cochlear implant surgery

The surgery required to insert the internal implant and electrode array varies slightly according to which device is used and the results of pre-operative scans. Accounts of the techniques used may be found in the manufacturers' surgical manuals. Detailed descriptions of surgical techniques are given by Webb et al. (1990), Clark et al. (1991), Balkany, Cohen and Gantz (1999), Filipo et al. (1999), Bredberg et al. (1997) and Colletti et al. (1999). Special tools may be used for the insertion of the electrode arrays and replica electrode arrays are available to allow the surgeon to test how far into the cochlea the electrode array can be inserted with each patient.

Surgical procedure

Children are usually admitted to hospital for three or four days. After general anaesthesia is administered the hair is shaved in the region of the incision.

* An incision in the shape of a C, a U or an inverted J is made in the shaved area to expose the section of the skull in which the body of the internal implant will be embedded. The skin flap is fairly large so sutures are remote from the implant body and this minimizes the risk of skin-flap complications.
* In order to gain access to the cochlea the mastoid bone, which lies behind the ear, is drilled to form a cavity.
* A bed is created in the skull in which to seat the implant body and a groove is made to house the electrode array lead wires.
* Holes are drilled for the ties that will be used to secure the implant body in position.
* The electrode array is inserted into the scala tympani via the round window niche, which may have been slightly enlarged by drilling, or via a hole drilled directly into the scala tympani. The electrode array is inserted gently into the cochlea. For split electrode arrays a further opening is drilled into the scala tympani so that the two parts of the electrode array can be inserted into different regions of the cochlea (Bredberg et al., 1997; Richardson et al., 1999). Ideally the whole electrode array is inserted but this may not be possible if ossification or soft tissue impede the electrode array as it curves round the cochlea. Although complete insertion is preferred not all electrodes have to be used and benefit may be gained from using a reduced number of active electrodes (Balkany, Gantz and Nadol, 1988; Balkany et al., 1996; Kirk, Sehgal and Miyamoto, 1997).
* The implant body is secured in position and the entrance/s to the cochlea are sealed around the electrode wires.
* The reference or ground electrode is positioned in the muscle under the skin behind the ear.
* The wound is sutured and a bulky pressure dressing is applied.
* The surgical procedure takes about two to four hours to complete.

The facial nerve passes close to the site of cochlear implant surgery but facial-nerve function can be monitored during surgery to minimize the risk of any damage. Patients with varying degrees of cochlear deformity have been successfully implanted except where there is complete aplasia or absence of the auditory nerve. The surgical technique may need to be modified because of unusual anatomy or it may not be possible to insert all active channels. There is a risk of cerebrospinal fluid leak but this can be controlled (Slattery and Luxford, 1995; Tucci et al., 1995; Luntz et al., 1997; Bent, Chute and Parisier, 1999).

During the hospital stay an X ray is taken to confirm the position of the electrode array in the cochlea. This is useful for the initial tuning so that electrodes outside the cochlea are not activated and can be used as a baseline for checking the implant position should there be any complications or trauma to the implant in later use.

Intra-operative measurements

Intra-operative measurements comprise checks of implant function and tests to demonstrate an auditory response to stimulation through the implant. All the latest generation of implants have telemetry, which enables signals to be transmitted back from the implant about electrode impedances and possible short circuits. The implant may be tested in sterile conditions prior to insertion to check for electrode shorts. Should any problem with the implant be discovered at this stage a backup device should be used. Telemetry carried out immediately after insertion may reveal high impedance temporarily for some electrodes but this may be due to air bubbles introduced during the insertion. These electrodes often come back into compliance with time (French, 1999). Towards the end of the operation objective measurements of auditory responses can be carried out to give an indication of which electrodes can give an auditory sensation. These measurements are electrical stapedial reflex measurements (ESRT), electrically evoked auditory brainstem responses (EABR) and, for the Nucleus CI24M implant, neural response telemetry (NRT).

Electrical stapedial reflex measurements are carried out after the implant has been positioned but before the middle ear is closed. The implant is stimulated on separate channels and the surgeon observes the contraction of the stapedius tendon via the operating microscope. The lowest level of stimulus at which the tendon is consistently observed contracting is the ESRT for that channel with the particular stimulus parameters used.

Using this technique, measurements can be made on several channels in five to 10 minutes. Electrical stapedial reflex measurements can be recorded using admittance meters to detect the response contralaterally (Battmer, Laszig and Lehnhardt, 1990; Stephan, Welzl-Muller and Stiglbrumer, 1991). For this method access to the contralateral ear is needed during the operation and an admittance meter. The presence of the ESRT is indicative of an auditory response to stimulation through the implant. The current level required to elicit the stapedial reflex is considerably higher than levels that will be used for initial stimulation.

Electrically evoked auditory brainstem response measurements can be recorded when the implant is in position (see also Chapter 6; Shallop et al., 1990). Auditory responses in the brainstem to electrical stimulation through the implant are recorded with scalp electrodes. Measurements can be carried out on several electrodes while the surgeon is suturing the wound and do not need to prolong the time period under anaesthesia. Electrically evoked auditory brainstem response measurements have been related to the upper level of the initial dynamic range of stimulation (Shallop et al., 1991) and also to the threshold for electrical stimulation (Mason et al., 1993) but these differences probably reflect different recording parameters and the small size of the dynamic range at the first stimulation. Both EABR and ESRT measurements are possible with the most widely used current generation implants.

Neural response telemetry is recorded by presenting stimulus pulses to an intra-cochlear electrode coupled to the ground electrode in the muscle and a nearby electrode coupled to the ground electrode on the implant case is used to record the response via the telemetry system. NRT measurements have the potential in helping with device tuning and selection of electrodes with the 'best' neural responses. The presence of an NRT response also indicates that the implant is causing stimulation of auditory neural elements (see also Chapter 6; Abbas et al., 1999; Shallop, Facer and Peterson, 1999).

All of the intra-operative measurements give some reassurance immediately after the operation that an auditory sensation can be elicited via the implant on the channels tested. Electrically evoked auditory brainstem response measurements can guide the first level of stimulation at the initial tuning session.

Surgical complications and reimplantation

Major surgical complications after implantation are rare and relate to rejection of the implant by the body, movement of the electrode array out of the cochlea, infection or major problems with the skin flap (Cohen and Hoffman, 1991; Daspit, 1991; Hoffman et al., 1991; Hoffman and Cohen, 1993; Luetje and Jackson, 1997; Miyamoto et al., 1996). In extreme cases the implant may have to be removed even though it may still be functioning (Hoffman et al., 1991, Balkany et al., 1999). Less severe complications such as dizziness (Dobie, Jenkins and Cohen, 1995), facial nerve damage and minor skin flap problems may be transient and, if not, can be treated conservatively. There may be damage to electrodes in difficult insertions or stimulation of active electrodes can result in pain, twitching or feeling down the face. Both of these problems can be resolved by deactivating damaged electrodes or those from which current spreads outside the cochlea (Niparko et al., 1991).

Should the implant fail, be rejected or be damaged due to trauma reimplantation is possible. The most common cause of reimplantation is device failure. Electrostatic discharge can occasionally cause device failure (Parisier, Chute and Popp, 1996). Balkany et al. (1999) report that device failure rates over five years are estimated at 1.5% for the Clarion and Nucleus devices. Parisier, Chute and Popp (1996) report a higher failure rate with the Nucleus 22 device used in children prior to modification of the implant. They report some of the key features indicative of possible device failure in children as fluctuations in threshold and comfort levels for more than six electrodes, need for frequent remapping, poor progress in auditory skills, extraneous noises reported by the child, sudden adverse stimulation, and more than three changes of external equipment in three weeks. Twomey and Archbold (1997) report that, of six implant failures in children, four were identified during tuning sessions at the clinic, one by the child and one by a speech and language therapist. The children continued to use their devices despite poorer performance and the experience of some discomfort when using the device. Failures can be sudden or gradual over long periods of time. The same study reported 21% children implanted with the Nucleus 22 device had at least one non-functioning channel. The stage at which intermittency or reduction in the number of electrodes compromises the auditory signal so that it is no longer possible to 'programme round' a problem and maintain an acceptable level of benefit is when the implant should be deemed to have failed. All the implant companies have their own data relating to implant failures but the figures are not expressed in the same way. Von Wallenburg and Brinch (1995) have expressed Nucleus 22 reliability on the basis of failures per cumulative years of use. Newer devices may appear to have lower failure rates because problems have not yet been identified and reported. Overall numbers of failures will be lower if fewer patients have been implanted with a particular device.

Reimplantation has been shown to be possible if a device failure occurs and in many, but not all, cases similar levels of performance are obtained from the second device (Gantz, Lowder and McCabe, 1989; Jackler, Leake and McKerrow, 1989; Cohen and Hoffman, 1991; Ray, Gray and Court, 1998, Balkany et al., 1999). Reduction in the length of insertion and thus in the number of active channels that can be used has, however, been reported for some patients undergoing reimplantation (Miyamoto et al., 1997). Histological evidence shows that the electrodes cause trauma but there is no evidence of any effect on remaining neural elements (Linthicum et al., 1991). This is reassuring since the dynamic range for electrical stimulation has been shown to be related to spiral ganglion cell survival (Kawano et al., 1998). The occasional development of a tissue sheath round electrode arrays must be taken into account in implant design so that explantation followed by insertion of a new electrode array is possible. Reimplantation after an implant failure is stressful for children and their families and they need rapid action in confirming device failure, information about the reason for the failure and advice on reimplantation (Twomey and Archbold, 1997). Children are now being implanted at a very young age and it is likely that they may need reimplantation at some point either because of device failure or to take advantage of new electrode designs and/or speech processing strategies.

Fitting and programming the speech processor

The externally worn components of the implant system (the transmitter coil, microphone, speech processor and connecting cables) are fitted three to four weeks after implantation when the wound has healed and the child has fully recovered from the surgery. The speech processor is tuned, programmed or mapped (Figure 11.3) to determine the characteristics of the electrical signal required to provide the best auditory percept for each individual. For speech understanding the implanted patient needs to be able to discriminate a range of different pitches and loudness levels from the electrical stimulation. The patient's performance will ultimately depend on many factors but appropriate tuning of the implant is the basis on which to build good auditory performance.

First the threshold (T or THR) of electrical stimulation must be measured for each active channel. This is the lowest current density that produces an auditory sensation. The maximum current level that the patient can tolerate without discomfort, referred to as the comfort (C) or most comfortable level (MCL), is then determined. The difference between the threshold and

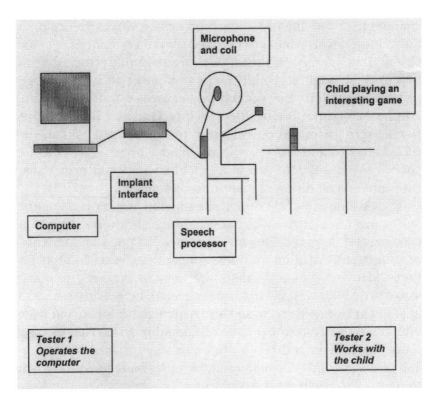

Figure 11.3. Clinic set up for tuning cochlear implants for young children. Tester 1 may operate the computer and implant interface in an observation room. Alternatively, depending on the child's age and the individual clinical situation, tester 1 may be in the same room as the child but out of their field of vision.

upper level of stimulation is the dynamic range. Threshold and comfort levels vary between patients and between different channels in the same patient. Lower thresholds and large dynamic ranges are associated with greater percentage of surviving neurones and better speech perception especially for vowel recognition (Pfingst, Spelman and Sutton, 1980; Kawano et al., 1998; Loizou, Dorman and Fitzke, 2000). It is, therefore, beneficial for patients to have their processor set to give them their largest comfortable dynamic range. Using the measurements of dynamic range the speech processor can be set so that speech and environmental sounds will be delivered through the implant within the audible range of electrical stimulation but avoiding levels that cause discomfort.

Different implant systems use a variety of units of current such as current amplitude, electrical decibels or arbitrary units relating to current density. The T and C levels for each individual will vary according to the speech processing strategy and configuration of active and ground electrodes used. Certain changes to the tuning of a speech processor, therefore, result in the T and C levels having to be remeasured. Equipment specific to each device is required for programming the speech processor in addition to a PC type computer with specialized software installed. The speech processor is connected to the computer via the device specific interface and the stimulus parameters (sometimes referred to as the map) can be transferred to and stored within a microchip memory in the speech processor. The latest generation of speech processors can store several different maps or programmes.

With young children, tuning the implant system is a lengthy and sometimes difficult process. Young children's attention span may be short and they may have had little or no experience of sound, thus making loudness judgements very difficult for them. Many test sessions, therefore, may be required to reach stable processor settings and testers need to be sensitive to small changes in behaviour as sound levels increase. Information from intra-operative testing can ensure that stimulation begins on a functioning channel that has produced some auditory sensation and give some indication of a suitable stimulation level at which to start. There are not yet any objective or automated techniques for fully programming the speech processor.

Pre-training

Some groups advocate pre-training of specific tasks such as on/off or big/small discrimination with vibrotactile or visual stimuli before initial stimulation through the implant (Mecklenburg et al., 1990; Huarte, Molina and Manrique, 1996). This may be advantageous but the tasks must not become tedious for the child prior to initial stimulation. The stimulus provided by the implant will be different from the pre-training stimuli and further conditioning to respond to the implant stimuli or associate it with a visual reward will still be required at the first tuning session. Test techniques appropriate for the developmental stage of the child can be identified prior to initial tuning.

Preparation for initial stimulation with the child's key worker and other staff who will be doing the tuning can be beneficial for children and their families alike. Prior to implantation the continued use of hearing aids, despite the little benefit they may afford ensures that the child remains accustomed to wearing an assistive device. The child should also be allowed to see, handle and wear a dummy speech processor and headset before initial stimulation so that the equipment is familiar and any fear of wearing it is overcome. Young children may be more relaxed if they are familiar with the clinic surroundings. Discussion with the key worker and videos of other children at initial stimulation can prepare parents for a wide variety of responses to initial stimulation; occasionally the child is pleasantly surprised but more common responses range from no outward response to great distress at even minimal stimulation. Most children, however, adapt quickly and begin to enjoy environmental sounds that they can associate with objects. For this reason pointing out objects that make sound and encouraging the child to experiment with sound and play with musical instruments during the initial tuning period can encourage the child to use their speech processor. Some children enjoy the sound of their own voices whereas others find this strange and initially, may be quieter when using their speech processor.

Choosing the parameters for stimulation

The choice of parameters used will depend on the speech processing strategies and stimulus modes offered by the particular implant and speech processor used. Surgery and the intra-operative test results can influence which electrodes are activated. Other parameters such as the number of channels, or spectral maxima, the stimulation mode and the rate of stimulation can be selected.

Speech processing strategy

Most of the latest cochlear implants and processors offer a choice of speech processing strategies. The CIS strategy is the first choice for most clinics using the Clarion and Medel implants. The Medel post-aural Tempo+ processor has CIS only. Other choices for the Clarion are the SAS strategy, which is often preferred by patients who have lower threshold and MCLs (Battmer et al., 1999) and the new paired pulsatile strategy. With the Medel CIS pro+ body-worn processor the n of m strategy may be used as an alternative to CIS. The Nucleus CI24M implant with the Esprit post-aural processor currently uses the SPEAK speech processing strategy only but the Sprint and Esprit 3G processors can support SPEAK, ACE and the CIS strategy. SPEAK and ACE are spectral maxima strategies but the ACE strategy is faster rate. Most clinicians choose either ACE or CIS if the Sprint or Esprit 3G processors are to be used because they offer faster stimulus rates that are likely to produce better results for most but not all patients (Lawson et al., 1996; Brill et al., 1997; Kiefer et al., 2000). Good results have been achieved with all the above strategies but it is not yet possible to predict the best strategy for each individual patient. It is, however, possible to change the speech processing strategy and parameters within a strategy if the patient is not making as much progress as expected. The T and C levels need to be remeasured if the strategy changes because the loudness percept will be different.

Stimulus mode

Electrical current flows from an active (intra-cochlear) electrode of the implant to a reference or ground electrode and any neurones within this electrical field will be stimulated to induce a sensation of hearing. Stimulus mode is the configuration of the active electrodes with the ground electrode/s. When the active and ground electrodes are located remotely, for example when active electrodes are inside the cochlea and ground electrodes are outside the cochlea, stimulation is monopolar. When active and ground electrodes are located in close proximity the stimulation mode is bipolar. All of the latest generation of cochlear implants can use monopolar stimulation and this is usually the first choice of stimulus mode for pulsatile sequential processing strategies because the current levels required are lower. Bipolar stimulation is used for the Clarion SAS strategy, which uses simultaneous stimulation; higher current levels may be required but there is less current spread with bipolar stimulation and, therefore, less chance of channel interaction resulting in confusing signals to implant users. The Nucleus device can use a variety of stimulation modes although the older Nucleus 22 device did not have a remote ground electrode for monopolar stimulation. A range of bipolar modes is possible depending on which electrode is designated the ground electrode. If it is the next-but-one electrode the stimulus mode is bipolar + 1, the next but two is bipolar + 2 and the next but three is bipolar + 3. The common ground mode was often used initially with children using the Nucleus 22 device because, prior to telemetry, electrode shorts were less likely to give an adverse stimulation in this stimulus mode. At any time with pulsatile strategies only one electrode is active and in common ground mode all the intra-cochlear electrodes not active at a given moment in time join to form the ground electrode; hence the common ground mode.

Choice of electrodes and channels

The audiologist can select which intra-cochlear electrodes will be used as active channels based on surgical outcomes and intra-operative tests. The term electrode refers to the physical contact through which the current flows whereas a channel is an electrode through which different information is sent; usually different frequency information. It would, thus, be possible, although not useful in practice, to send information from one frequency band to two electrodes that would then be acting as a single channel. Telemetry measurements show if there are any electrode short circuits and these electrodes can be deactivated before stimulation. Also any potentially active electrodes that could not be inserted into the cochlea are deactivated prior to initial stimulation. For initial stimulation an electrode that elicited a good neural (NRT) or auditory response (ESRT or EABR) is usually selected.

The audiologist may opt to use all the available active electrodes. Alternatively a number of channels may be selected for stimulation from a larger set of intra-cochlear electrodes. If eight channel CIS is to be used in the Nucleus device eight well spaced and well functioning electrodes are selected out of the 22 possible electrodes to be the eight channels. With ACE and 'n of m' spectral maxima strategies the number of maxima needs to be selected and the number of electrodes over which the stimulation will rove according to frequency will be selected omitting any problem electrodes. Intuitively it would seem better to have as many channels as possible to deliver different frequency information but with current implant designs and sequential stimulation there is a trade-off between the number of channels or maxima and the rate of stimulation such that more channels means that the stimulation rate has to be lower. Higher stimulation rates better represent the changes in the sound signal over time – the temporal features of sound – and have been associated with better speech perception performance. Dividing frequency information between more channels does, however, enhance the spectral information conveyed. There is evidence to suggest that a minimum of four channels should be used to give reasonable performance and between six to 10 channels is the optimum for speech discrimination, on average, with current implant designs (Eddington et al., 1994; Helms et al., 1997; Brill et al., 1997; Dorman, Loizou and Rainey, 1997; Fishman, Shannon and Slattery, 1997; Kiefer et al., 2000).

Threshold measurements

Threshold measurements are carried out using visual reinforcement audiometry (VRA) or conditioned response techniques that are described in detail elsewhere in this volume. These techniques are widely used in paediatric audiology and the technique used depends on the developmental stage of the child. During the early stages of stimulation in the very young child close observation of behavioural changes may be needed to determine when the child is perceiving stimulation. Behavioural responses to stimulation include stilling, touching the transmitter coil or side of the head, removing the coil, laughing, crying, or seeking parental reassurance. Thresholds must be obtained for all active channels and a wider variety of activities or visual rewards are likely to be required than with audiometric testing. Several sessions will probably be needed to complete all the threshold measurements with a young child. Not all channels have to be activated at the same time because the speech processor can allocate frequency bands to the available activated channels. The advent of telemetry allows any electrode shorts to be easily detected and deactivated. Also, the use of monopolar stimulation (ground electrode remote from the active electrodes) gives less variation in T and C levels on different channels. It is, therefore, possible to interpolate T levels for unmeasured thresholds in the early stages of stimulation providing that at least some T levels have been measured. It is, of course, advisable to measure the T level for each individual channel when possible to set the dynamic range more accurately.

Maximum comfortable level

Young children with implants will have had little or no experience of hearing prior to implantation and are unlikely to have developed a concept of loudness. To set the upper level of the dynamic range, the maximum comfortable level (C or MCL) the implanted child needs to indicate to the clinician the point just before the level of stimulation becomes uncomfortable. Young children are unlikely to be able to indicate when this level has been reached (MacPhearson et al., 1991). During the initial stimulation period it is advisable to set a very small dynamic range thus not allowing a discomfort level to be reached. Any sign of blinking, flinching, touching or attempting to remove the headset should be taken as a sign of discomfort and the level of stimulation reduced. Over subsequent sessions the child will become more used to stimulation through the implant and the dynamic range can be gradually increased to reach the maximum comfortable levels. The level of stimulation needs to be increased cautiously because there may be only a small difference in current level between the loud but comfortable level and painful stimulation.

Children who are more experienced at using their implants and older children can indicate when sound is okay or too loud, that is, they learn that they can indicate stop at any time and stimulation will be stopped. The next step is to carry out simple loudness scaling and indicate whether sound is okay, loud, or too loud, so that accurate C levels can be set and the whole dynamic range can be used. Games with loudness scales such as drawings of different facial expressions, different sized objects or coloured green amber and red lights to press on (red being for stop) can be used to illustrate the task and make it more interesting.

The C levels can also be estimated by using electrical stapedial reflexes recording the response in the contralateral ear (Hodges et al., 1999). The C level is usually set just below the reflex threshold. The child must be fairly still during the measurements but watching a video often helps. This procedure cannot be used in the early stages of stimulation because the C level may not yet be above the ESRT and thus stimulation at ESRT is likely to be uncomfortable. If there is any middle-ear dysfunction in the contralateral ear it will not be possible to record a response and in a minority of cases there will be no stapedial reflex. It is, therefore, essential to observe the child during this procedure to ensure that stimulation is not producing uncomfortably loud sound.

Speech processor activation

Once sufficient measurements are made a map or program is loaded into the speech processor. Most of the latest generation of implants have speech processors that can store more than one program. If the child does not like or does not do well with a particular program the parents have the option of using a previous or quieter program until further tuning can be carried out. The speech processor settings can be altered by user operated switches or buttons which work within the parameters set by the audiologist with the implant computer software. The warning lights or alarms should be set so that parents and teachers can be alerted to a flat battery or processor fault because young children will not always indicate if they hear a beep or see a light. An important part of the initial tuning period is explaining to parents and teachers, if present, how the external implant equipment functions, what the processor buttons do and basic troubleshooting such as changing leads and batteries in case of a fault.

Further measurements and tuning checks

Implanted children require regular tuning checks of their implant systems to carry out further measurements and refinements to the map and to check the functioning of the implant. As children become older and more used to the signal through the implant, they will be able to carry out T and C level measurements more accurately. They may also be able to carry out balancing of different channels to ensure equal loudness across different frequencies. It may be possible to identify channels that do not function optimally because of poor loudness growth or because the user experiences no difference in pitch perception between channels. Once identified, better results are usually obtained by deactivating less efficient channels so that a faster pulse rate can be used (Eddington et al., 1994; Lawson et al., 1996; Brill et al., 1997; Kiefer et al., 2000) thus selection of the 'best' channels may give improvements in performance. If progress is not as good as expected tuning changes can be made such as changing the strategy, filtering, pulse rate and overall frequency boundaries. Optimum representation of different loudness levels (influenced by the loudness growth functions of the implant system) can aid implanted patients' ability to discriminate phonemes (Zeng and Galvin, 1999). Lawson et al. (1996) found that eight out of 10 implanted subjects achieved better speech recognition results when the frequency range of the implant was extended up to 9,500 Hz. The allocation of frequency bands to different channels can also affect speech perception with cochlear implants (Fu and Shannon, 1999; Skinner, Holden and Holden, 1995). The flexibility of the latest generation of implants allows for customization of stimulus parameters but it is not yet clear which specific parameters will be best for each implanted individual.

Several tuning sessions will be required for the initial stimulation period with follow-up at least every few months during the first year after implantation. Gradually less changes to the map will be required. During the second and third years post-implantation, most centres see children at the clinic twice a year and thereafter on an annual basis. There may be additional appointments for fitting of FM radio aids and other accessories with the implant or if the stimulus mode or strategy needs to be changed. Regular monitoring of the implant system is required to monitor the functioning of the device in young children either using the telemetry systems of newer implants or by carrying out regular integrity checks with older devices (Parisier, Chute and Popp, 1996; Twomey and Archbold, 1997). The child will always need access to the implant centre for tuning and checking of the implant system and for medical check-ups. Figure 11.4 shows a procedure for fault finding and troubleshooting with implants for children. Good liaison between different professionals in the implant team and with

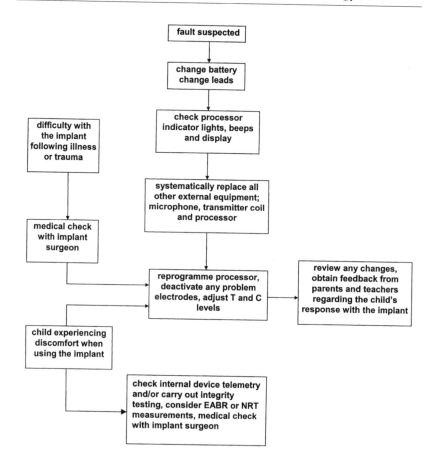

Figure 11.4. Flow diagram of a fault identification procedure for troubleshooting with cochlear implants used by children.

families and local professionals facilitates problem solving should a fault be detected.

Part of the tuning process is to assess how the child responds with the implant. This is done initially by measuring aided responses with the implant using age-appropriate test techniques such as VRA or conditioned responses. The aided levels should ideally demonstrate that the child is able to detect different frequency sounds including high frequencies within the speech frequency region. Speech discrimination by young children can be tested with speech sounds such as the Ling five sounds (Ling, 1988) and later the McCormick Toy Discrimination Test (McCormick, 1977; Ousey et al., 1989). Feedback from rehabilitation staff regarding changes in the child's auditory performance and their behaviour at home and school with the implant can also give valuable help assessing the child's auditory progress and determining whether the implant is well tuned. Improvements in performance show that the map is giving the child good access to sound but any drop in performance may suggest an equipment failure or inappropriate tuning. It should be noted, however, that children require a short time to get used to changes in the speech processor map. If the processing strategy or stimulus mode is changed the child will need time to adjust to the new sound signal and some retuning about a month later before the new settings yield improvements. Interchange of information about the children's progress with their implant and changes to the tuning of the implant between different staff on the implant team and local professionals can greatly facilitate the child in maximizing their benefit from the implant.

Rehabilitation

The tuning of the speech processor is just the first step in the rehabilitation process for the implanted child. Even with the latest implants and optimal tuning the implant cannot produce the same hearing sensation as normal hearing. Moreover, implanted children may have little or no memory of speech thus the process may be more one of habilitation than rehabilitation. Implanted children need help to learn to interpret and use the new sound sensation received via the implant so that it can be integrated into their everyday lives. Most of the time of implanted children is spent at home and at school with their families and local teachers. The rehabilitation efforts of the implant team need to be addressed not just to the children but to parents and all education professionals and carers associated with the children (Selmi, 1985; Geers and Moog, 1991; Archbold, 1992). Rehabilitation sessions may be divided between the implant centre, home and school. Important factors in effective rehabilitation include promoting appropriate expectations with the implant, ensuring consistent use of the device and enabling the child to learn to use the sound signal in a natural real life way. Rehabilitation should aim to immerse the child in auditory experience that is interesting and relevant to them.

Many rehabilitation methods appropriate for young hearing aid users are applicable to implanted children (Wood et al., 1986; Tait and Wood, 1987; Tait, 1987). Cochlear implants give a different sensation from conventional hearing aids in that implanted children experience a sudden, often overwhelming, onset of sound including good access to high-frequency sounds. More rehabilitation time is required around and immediately after the time of initial stimulation. Rehabilitation sessions may be combined with tuning sessions at the clinic initially but will also occur at the child's home and school. After the initial stimulation period an intensive period of weekly rehabilitation sessions involving parents and teachers may be offered at the child's home or school to launch the child in learning to use the new sound signal. The frequency of rehabilitation visits gradually decreases over time. Extra help may still be needed long after implantation if new programming strategies or new equipment (for example, FM radio aids, accessories or new speech processors) are introduced or if the child has a new class teacher or moves to a new school. This type of outreach rehabilitation is common and successful in the UK (Lutman et al., 1996). Some implant centres advocate intensive rehabilitation where the child and their family stay at the implant centre for an extended period of time (Bertram, 1996) or because of distance may offer home rehabilitation programmes (Tye-Murray et al., 1996).

The cochlear implant can only produce improvements in speech perception and production if the device is used consistently. Initially children may be reluctant to use the device and early rehabilitation may be directed at distracting children from the external equipment by interesting them with everyday sounds such as telephones ringing, doorbells, percussion instruments and the toilet flushing. The other factor aiding consistent use of the device is the early detection of faults in the external equipment and the speedy rectification of any faults. Local professionals and parents and carers need to be able to carry out basic troubleshooting and be able to change batteries and leads. Daily checks of implant function by checking processor indicator lights and a quick sound check of familiar words or the Ling sounds (Ling, 1988) is advisable when possible with young children. If a fault is suspected parents and teachers should be encouraged not to delay in contacting the implant centre so that replacement equipment can be issued quickly. Parents and the child's school should have spare batteries and leads so common faults can be remedied quickly. Many implant programmes run information days for parents and professionals to learn about troubleshooting and implantation generally. Young children are often not able to indicate that the device is not working, particularly if the fault is intermittent or there is a change in sound quality rather than no sound at all. Children may change in their auditory responsiveness or their behaviour may change. In these cases it is advisable to check the implant components.

Sound through the implant should be fun but is initially meaningless to the child. Play with noisemakers and musical instruments help children to enjoy using their device. Early responses to environmental sounds may be observed and children can be alerted to the source of the sound. Pre-verbal skills such as eye contact, turn taking and auditory processing are established first (Tait 1987; Tait and Wood, 1987; Tait and Lutman, 1994). Games can be used to reinforce and reward children in learning to distinguish on/off, loud and soft, single and repeated, short and long, high and low pitched sounds. Discrimination of environmental and speech sounds can then be developed in a more structured way. Considerable speech and language therapy is needed to develop the child's language skills further. Individual children have widely different language abilities at the time of implantation and it is important to use materials and methods that will produce communication but that will be appropriate to the child's language status and chronological age. This ensures that he or she has a realistic chance of success at each task but is also sufficiently interested in each activity to participate. Practical rehabilitation ideas for young, implanted children are discussed further by Somers (1991), Allum (1996) and Robbins and Kirk (1996).

Good communication style, particularly turn taking and autonomy, whether vocal or gestural prior to implantation, is likely to lead to better speech discrimination and intelligibility later (Tait and Lutman, 1997; Tait, Lutman and Robinson, 2000). Practical help in promoting positive communication skills between parents and their implanted children can be offered through Hanen courses (Manolson, 1992). These courses comprise individual family and group sessions with specially trained speech and language therapists. They also provide the opportunity for parents and children to meet with other families of implanted children who are learning to make the most of their implants.

Evaluation of progress in auditory perception and in speech and language development is an important part of rehabilitation and ensures that implanted children can reach their true potential with their implant. Specific strengths and weaknesses can be identified and the need for further tuning changes or particular aspects of auditory communication that need extra help can be highlighted. Methods of evaluation of implanted children's progress need to cover a wide age range and a wide auditory ability range. Video analysis techniques have been used to evaluate developing communication skills (Tait, 1987) and emerging spoken language (Osberger et al., 1991b). Rating scales such as the categories of auditory performance (CAP) (Archbold, Lutman and Marshall, 1995; Archbold, Lutman and Nikolopoulos, 1998) and the speech intelligibility rating (Allen, Nikolopoulos and O'Donoghue, 1998) can be used to demonstrate changes in responses to sound and speech intelligibility in everyday situations without the need to 'test' the child. Questionnaires for parents and teachers, such as the meaningful auditory integration scale (MAIS) (Robbins, Renshaw and Berry, 1991) give valuable information about the child's longitudinal functioning at home and school. Story telling is also being used to assess the language development of young implanted children (Starczewski and Lloyd, 1999). As the child gets older and more competent with the implant more formal speech perception and production tests can also be used (Tyler, 1993). It is important to test children with interesting test materials and to select tests that will not result in very poor scores or the child may become demoralized. More formal speech perception assessment quantifies improvements since implantation and can influence judgements about map settings and processing strategy.

Informing parents about the changes in the child's use of the implant and auditory communication ability will encourage parents to continue to support their children throughout the rehabilitation process. Progress may appear slow to parents despite pre-implantation expectations counselling but parents are very often pleased to see measured improvement in their children's functioning with the implant. The majority of implant centres view rehabilitation as an important aspect of implantation and paediatric programmes require considerably greater time and resources for rehabilitation than adult programmes (Tucci, Lambert and Ruth, 1990).

Outcomes of cochlear implants in children

Cochlear implants have now been used for considerable periods of time with adults and children. The lives of most implant users and their families have been transformed by access to some sound. Most enjoy improved speech perception with lipreading and a significant number are able to understand conversational speech without lipreading. Cochlear implants give access to environmental sounds and many implant users learn to discriminate between different environmental sounds. Some multichannel implant users are able to have limited conversations on the telephone (Cohen, Waltzman and Shapiro, 1989; Dorman et al., 1991; Giles, 1993) and enjoy music to some extent (McDermott and McKay, 1997; Fujita and Ito, 1999). There are, however, wide variations in the performance of individual implanted children, which is influenced by factors such as:

- age and duration of deafness;
- aetiology of deafness;
- type of device;
- mode of communication;
- participation in the rehabilitation programme.

Speech perception and production skills in implanted children

Much emphasis has been placed on the benefits of implantation in terms of speech perception and production in children because communication and language are so important for any child's education and quality of life. The rate of acquisition of speech and language skills and the level of benefit that accrues varies between individual children but some general trends have been identified. Adult implant users with acquired deafness can show up to 50% improvement in speech perception in the first month after implantation and the level of benefit is unlikely to continue increasing after 30 months of implant use (Tyler and Summerfield, 1996). Implanted children with post-lingually acquired deafness also show rapid improvement in speech perception during the first six to twelve months after implantation, after which benefit still increases but at a slower rate (Gantz et al., 1994; Robbins and Kirk, 1996). Children with congenital or pre-lingually acquired deafness show much slower improvement in speech recognition after implantation. Many do not show useful word understanding until they have used their implants for two to three years (Tyler and Summerfield, 1996; Gantz et al., 1994; Summerfied and Marshall, 1995; Allen and Dyar, 1997; Fryauf-Bertschy et al., 1997). Children have been shown to need two years of implant use before most were able to score in tests of vowel perception (Parkinson, El-Kholy and Tyler, 1998). Even longer time periods are needed before intelligible speech develops (Osberger et al., 1996; Allen, Nikolopoulos and O'Donoghue, 1998; Inscoe, 1999). Some young pre-lingually deaf implanted children eventually do as well as, or better than, post-lingually deafened implanted children (Gantz et al., 1994; Nikolopoulos et al., 1999; Miyamoto et al., 1995; Shepherd et al., 1997). Many studies of pre-lingually deaf children with implants show that speech perception and production skills gradually improve over several years and no plateau in benefit level is seen even five or six years after implantation (Waltzman et al., 1994; Allen, Nikolopoulos and O'Donoghue, 1998; O'Donoghue et al., 1998). The degree to which the significant improvements in auditory perception and spoken language lead to enhanced academic achievement in school and increased opportunity for personal fulfilment is not yet known.

The speech perception and production abilities of implanted children and those who use tactile aids or hearing aids have been compared. Implanted children have better speech recognition and intelligibility than children who use tactile aids (Osberger et al., 1996). Vowel production by implanted children is significantly better compared with children using tactile aids (Ertmer et al., 1997). Speech discrimination by implant users has been found to be better than speech discrimination by hearing aid users with an average hearing loss of 104 dB (Miyamoto et al., 1995). Meyer et al. (1998) found that speech perception scores of implanted children were similar to hearing aid users with average hearing losses of 101 dB after two years of implant use and equivalent to the scores of hearing aid users with average hearing losses of less than 90 dB after four years of implant use. Pre-lingual auditory behaviour of young cochlear implant users has been found to be akin to that of hearing aid users who went on to use audition successfully as their primary communication mode (Tait and Lutman, 1994). In a study of speech discrimination in noise hearing aid users achieved better scores than implant users despite having similar scores in quiet (Agelfors, 1998). This may have been because the hearing aid users had binaural hearing aids and had been using their hearing aids for longer. With long periods of cochlear implant use children use inflected endings more often than hearing aid users suggesting that implanted children will go on to develop better grammar than some hearing aided children (Spencer, Tye-Murray and Tomblin, 1998). The hearing level at which an implant is likely to give more auditory benefit than hearing aids may change as implant design improves further and results from young children implanted with newer devices become available.

Age and duration of deafness

Duration of deafness is one of the most important predictors of outcomes with cochlear implants (Tyler and Summerfield, 1996; Van Dijk et al., 1999). Post-lingually deafened children should be implanted as soon as possible once profound deafness has been confirmed to maximize the survival of auditory neurones (Miller, 1991). To minimize the duration of deafness congenitally or pre-lingually deafened children should be implanted at a young age. Children who have little or no experience of spoken language need to be able to make use of the sound signal from an implant to learn aural and spoken language rather than to reawaken a language that they already know. Children with congenitally or pre-lingually acquired deafness should be able to make better long term use of auditory input if it begins during the critical periods for language development (Ruben, 1997) and when there is still high plasticity of the central nervous system (Ryals, Rubel and Lippe, 1991; Shepherd et al., 1997).

Maturational delays in the P1 component of the late cortical potential in implanted patients have been shown to be equivalent to the duration of deafness. This suggests that profound deafness in young children prevents maturation of auditory pathways but that stimulation with cochlear implants permits maturation to resume (Eggermont et al., 1997). Many studies show that pre-lingually deaf children implanted before the age of three to five years old show better auditory skills than those implanted later in childhood (Waltzman et al., 1994; Miyamoto et al., 1999a; O'Donoghue et al., 1998; Summerfield and Marshall, 1995; Fryauf-Bertschy et al., 1997; Tyler et al., 1997). The rate of language acquisition in children implanted before the age of three can match that of their hearing peers. Profoundly deaf hearing aid users, in the same study, progressed at an average rate of five months per chronological year, thus falling further behind in their auditory language skills as they got older (Miyamoto, Svirsky and Robbins, 1997). Children implanted under the age of three years showed continuous steady improvement and scored higher on open set speech perception tests after two years of implant use than children implanted after the age of three (Waltzman et al., 1994; Miyamoto et al., 1999a). Children implanted between the ages of two and four years old have better word recognition than children implanted between the ages of four and nine years on average (Tyler et al., 1997).

Pre-lingually deafened adults and teenagers, show disappointing outcomes from cochlear implantation (Dawson et al., 1992). Children between the ages of five and 13 years old have been show to obtain benefit from implantation (Gantz et al., 1994) although outcomes may be poor if the duration of deafness is more than 10 years (Summerfield and Marshall, 1995). Implantation after the age of five years in pre-lingually deaf children has been found to give less functional benefit and these children may have more difficulty in adjusting to a cochlear implant (Fryauf-Bertschy et al., 1997). In a study of vowel perception by implanted children the lowest scores were obtained by children aged nine to fourteen years (Parkinson, El-Kholy and Tyler, 1998).

Children who have been deaf from early in life but who have used hearing aids and have developed oral communication skills may enjoy further gains in speech recognition with an implant even though they were implanted later (Kiefer et al., 1998; Rubenstein et al., 1999). Adults and children with some residual hearing tend to achieve better speech recognition than those with no residual hearing (Summerfield and Marshall, 1995; Van Dijk et al., 1999).

Aetiology

Children with congenital or acquired deafness can obtain similar levels of benefit from implantation provided that they are implanted at an early age or soon after the onset of deafness (Miyamoto et al., 1995; Summerfield and Marshall, 1995;

O'Donoghue et al., 1998). Specific aetiologies of deafness may, however, influence auditory performance with an implant. Aetiology affects spiral ganglion cell survival (Nadol et al., 1989) and larger dynamic ranges for electrical stimulation are related to better spiral ganglion cell survival and hence better auditory performance with an implant (Kawano et al., 1998). Cochlear implantation following temporal bone fracture can result in poorer outcomes and more frequent facial nerve stimulation (Camilleri et al., 1999). Disappointing results from cochlear implantation have been reported in a child with auditory neuropathy (Miyamoto et al., 1999b) and in a child with cochlear nerve aplasia (Maxwell, Mason and O'Donoghue, 1999). Children with enlarged vestibular aqueducts have, however been successfully implanted and show improvements in speech recognition (Bent, Chute and Parisier, 1999). Deaf children with other disabilities can achieve good outcomes from implantation providing that tuning of the device and rehabilitation can be adapted to suit any child's particular needs, such as test materials for the visually or physically impaired.

Type of device

As cochlear implant technology has evolved, children's auditory performance with implants has improved although there continues to be wide variation between the performance of different individuals with the same device. Multichannel implants have been shown to give better results than single channel implants (Gantz et al., 1988; Cohen, Waltzman and Fisher, 1993; Weston and Waltzman, 1995; Eyles, Aleksy and Boyle, 1995). Changes in speech processing strategy have also led to better outcomes from implantation for most children. Many patients originally programmed with older Nucleus strategies in the Nucleus 22 implant successfully changed to using SPEAK when the Spectra speech processor became available. Their speech perception abilities generally improved after a period of adjustment to the new strategy (Shallop and McGiun-Brunelli, 1995; Cowan et al., 1995; Lenarz and Battmer, 1995; Sehgal et al., 1998). It is too early to determine whether children will do even better with the latest generation of cochlear implants. Adults, however, have been shown to have better speech recognition with the Combi 40 and Clarion implants with CIS strategy than with the Nucleus 22 SPEAK strategy (Helms et al., 1997; Kiefer et al., 1996; Tyler et al., 1996;

Battmer, Reid and Lenarz, 1997). The Nucleus 24 implant, which has the choice of ACE, SPEAK and CIS strategies, has shown promising results (Arndt et al., 2000). Comparisons between different devices are not straightforward because the patient population is also changing. More children are being implanted at younger ages and will have greater neural plasticity, which should enable them to use the signal through an implant better. As patient performance with implants improves, candidates with more residual hearing and thus probably better spiral ganglion cell survival are being implanted. Both of these factors will improve group performances as well as more sophisticated implants and speech processing strategies.

Mode of communication

Better results are obtained after implantation if the primary environment is auditory rather than signing but rehabilitation does not have to be exclusively oral. Spencer et al. (1998) report on a case of an implanted child who used Signed English and auditory/oral communication and made significant gains in speech perception and production after implantation. Dominant auditory and vocal style of early communication one year after implantation is, however, associated with better speech and language outcomes two years later (Tait and Lutman, 1997). Children educated orally after implantation tend to have higher speech perception scores (Meyer et al., 1998), better expressive language (Miyamoto et al., 1999a) and make more use of sound (Quittner and Thompson, 1991) than those educated in total communication settings. Educational placement of children in mainstream unit or school for the deaf settings can be influenced by the age at which they were implanted (Archbold et al., 1998). Implantation and issues around education of the deaf have been discussed by Chute, Nevins and Parisier (1996).

Participation in the rehabilitation programme

Overt benefits of cochlear implantation in young pre-lingually deafened children do not accrue until the implant has been used for two or three years. Participation in the rehabilitation programme offers support and guidance to families and local education services in building on the child's interest in sound and changes in communicative behaviour. Children using hearing aids, tactile aids and cochlear implants and participating in the same rehabilitation programme all showed improvements in speech perception but the implanted children improved at a faster rate (Geers and Moog, 1991). This clearly demonstrates the need for appropriate rehabilitation to allow children to attain their full potential with any device used to assist hearing. In a study of vowel perception in implanted children the poor performance of a child implanted at five years of age was attributed to poor social support and hence lack of participation in rehabilitation (Parkinson, El-Kholy and Tyler, 1998). Better results from individual children after four years of implant use could usually be predicted from one year performance levels suggesting that it may be possible to identify children who may benefit from extra rehabilitation (Tyler et al., 1997). Successful outcomes from implantation depend also on device use that can be encouraged within the rehabilitation programme. High levels of device use (93% full-time users) have been reported for children predominantly implanted at a young age (Archbold, O'Donoghue and Nikolopoulos, 1998). A significantly higher proportion of implanted children who are minimal or non-users of their implants has been reported by Fryuaf-Bertschy et al. (1997). The children in this study were educated in total communication settings and the minimal or non-users were primarily those aged over five years at the time of implantation. Most of the minimal or non-users became so from the beginning of stimulation so it is unlikely to be entirely because they receive a poorer signal from their implants.

Cost effectiveness of cochlear implantation in children

The precise cost of maintaining a child's cochlear implant use over their lifetime is not known and neither is it possible to truly quantify the benefit of implantation in monetary terms. There are, however, increasing demands on healthcare budgets and treatments need to be cost effective to justify funding. Deafness is not life threatening and implantation reduces disability but does not restore normal hearing and as such, may be considered a lower healthcare priority than life saving and disease preventing treatments. Cochlear implantation can, however, bring significant benefit in terms of enhanced auditory receptive skills and useful levels of ability in spoken language. Better engagement and integration in education could lead to enhanced educational qualifications, better employment opportunities and an improved quality of life in adulthood. Implanted children are likely to use their implants for many years so, although healthcare costs may seem high, savings in education and better personal income as adults could be considerable (Summerfield and Marshall, 1999; O'Neill et al., 2000).

Future developments

Cochlear implants are now widely used to give profoundly deaf and, more recently, severely deaf children access to sound. Children under the age of two years are being implanted (Lenarz, Battmer and Bertram, 2000) and older children with some residual hearing who previously used hearing aids (Kiefer et al., 1998; Rubenstein et al., 1999). With neonatal hearing screening being applied to wider populations there are likely to be more challenges in assessing and implanting suitable children at a very young age. Further advances in the use of objective methods may facilitate the tuning of implants for very young children. Bilateral implantation is currently being investigated and may result in better speech perception in certain listening conditions (Van Hoesel and Clark, 1999). Any extra benefit from bilateral implantation needs to be considered along side the loss of residual hearing in the second ear and longer or additional surgery. Further developments in implant design could lead to greater miniaturization of devices and possibly wholly implantable devices. Research into speech processing and its application to implants for children will enable device settings to be further customized for each implanted child. The possibility of repair or regeneration of inner ear tissue in the future could have implications for cochlear implantation (Staecker and van der Water, 2000). Future research with pre-lingually deaf young children may reveal how implanted children use the poor signal from the implant (compared with normal hearing) to develop a representational system for attaching meaning to sound and how the implant influences information processing (Pisoni, 2000). Cochlear implants for children have given suitable candidates significant benefit in speech perception and production. Over the next few years there are likely to be further advances in cochlear implantation that will increase the benefit that they afford to severely to profoundly deaf children.

References

Abbas PJ, Brown CJ, Shallop JK, Firszt JB, Hughes ML, Hong SH, Staller SJ (1999) Summary of results using the Nucleus CI24M implant to record the electrically evoked compound action potential. Ear and Hearing 20: 45-59.

Agelfors E (1998) A comparison of speech performance in quiet and noise between persons using cochlear implants and hearing aids. Speech, Music and Hearing Quarterly Progress and Status Report 1-2: 81-8.

Allen MC, Nikolopoulos TP, O'Donoghue GM (1998) Speech intelligibility in children after cochlear implantation. The American Journal of Otology 19: 742-6.

Allen SE, Dyar D (1997) Profiling linguistic outcomes in young children after cochlear implantation. The American Journal of Otology 18: s127-s128.

Allum DJ (ed.) (1996) Cochlear Implant Rehabilitation in Children and Adults. London: Whurr.

Archbold SM (1992) The development of a paediatric cochlear implant programme - a case study. Journal of the British Association of Teachers of the Deaf 16: 17-26.

Archbold SM, Lutman ME, Marshall DH (1995) Categories of auditory performance. Annals of Otology, Rhinology and Laryngology 104 (suppl 166): 312-14.

Archbold SM, Lutman ME, Nikolopoulos T (1998) Categories of auditory performance: inter-user reliability. British Journal of Audiology 32: 7-12.

Archbold SM, O'Donoghue G, Nikolopoulos T (1998) Cochlear implants in children: an analysis of use over a three year period. The American Journal of Otology 19: 328-31.

Archbold SM, Nikolopoulos T, O'Donoghue GM, Lutman ME (1998) Educational placement of children following cochlear implantation. British Journal of Audiology 32: 295-300.

Arndt P, Staller SJ, Beiter AL, LeMay M (2000) Initial paediatric results with the Nucleus 24 cochlear implant system. In Waltzman SB, Cohen NL (eds) Cochlear Implants. New York: Thieme, pp. 207-9.

Axon PR, Mawman DJ, Upile T, Ramsden RT (1997) Cochlear implantation in the presence of chronic suppurative otitis media. The Journal of Laryngology and Otology 111: 228-32.

Balkany TJ, Cohen NL, Gantz BJ (1999) Surgical technique for the Clarion cochlear implant. Annals of Otology, Rhinology and Laryngology 108: 27-30.

Balkany T, Gantz B, Nadol JB (1988) Multichannel cochlear implants in partially ossified cochleae. Annals of Otology, Rhinology and Laryngology 97: 3-7.

Balkany TJ, Gantz BJ, Steenerson RL, Cohen NL (1996) Systematic approach to electrode insertion in the ossified cochlea. Otolaryngology, Head and Neck Surgery 114: 4-11.

Balkany TJ, Hodges AV, Gomez-Marin O, Bird PA, Dolan-Ash S, Butts S, Telischi FF, Lee D (1999) Cochlear reimplantation. The Laryngoscope 109: 351-5.

Bath AP, O'Donoghue GM, Holland IM, Gibbin KP (1993) Paediatric cochlear implantation: how reliable is computed tomography in assessing cochlear patency? Clinical Otolaryngology 18: 475-9.

Battmer RD, Laszig R, Lehnhardt E (1990) Electrically elicited stapedius reflex in cochlear implant patients. Ear and Hearing 11: 370-4.

Battmer RD, Reid JM, Lenarz T (1997) Performance in quiet and noise with the Nucleus Spectra 22 and the Clarion CIS/CA cochlear implant devices. Scandinavian Audiology 26: 240-6.

Battmer RD, Zilberman Y, Haake P, Lenarz T (1999) Simultaneous analogue stimulation (SAS) – continuous interleaved sampler (CIS) pilot study in Europe. Annals of Otology, Rhinology and Laryngology 108: 69-73.

Bent JP, Chute P, Parisier SC (1999) Cochlear implantation in children with large vestibular aqueducts. The Laryngoscope 109: 1019-22.

Bertram B (1996) An integrated rehabilitation concept for cochlear implant children. In Allum DJ (ed.) (1996) Cochlear Implant Rehabilitation in Children and Adults. London: Whurr, pp 52-64.

Bilger RC (1977) Evaluation of subjects presently fitted with implanted auditory prostheses. Annals of Otology, Rhinology and Laryngology 86 (suppl 38): 1-140.

Boggess WJ, Baker JE, Balkany TJ (1989) Loss of residual hearing after cochlear implantation. The Laryngoscope 99: 1002-5.

Boothroyd A, Medwetsky MS (1992) Spectral distribution of /s/ and the frequency response of hearing aids. Ear and Hearing 13: 150-7.

Bredberg G, Lindstrom B, Lopponen H, Skarzynski H, Hyodo M, Sato H (1997) Electrodes for ossified cochleae. The American Journal of Otology 18 (suppl): S42-S43.

Brill SM, Gstottner W, Helms J, Ilberg C, Baumgartner W, Muller J, Kiefer J (1997) Optimisation of channel number and stimulation rate for the fast continuous interleaved sampling strategy in the Combi 40+. The American Journal of Otology 18 (suppl): S104-S106.

Brummer SB, Robblee LS, Hambrecht FT (1983) Criteria for selecting electrodes for electrical stimulation: theoretical and practical implications. Annals of the New York Academy of Sciences 405: 159-71.

Burian K, Hochmair-Desoyer IJ, Eisenwort B (1986) The Vienna cochlear implant programme. Otolaryngology Clinics of North America 19: 313-28.

Camilleri AE, Toner JG, Howarth KL, Hampton S, Ramsden RT (1999) Cochlear implantation following temporal bone fracture. The Journal of Laryngology and Otology 113: 454-7.

Chute PM, Nevins ME, Parisier SC (1996) Managing educational issues throughout the process of implantation. In Allum DJ (ed.) Cochlear Implant Rehabilitation in Children and Adults. London: Whurr, pp. 119-30.

Cinamon U, Kronenberg J, Hildesheimer M, Taitelbaum T (1997) Cochlear implantation in patients suffering from Cogan's syndrome. The Journal of Laryngology and Otology 111: 928-30.

Clark GM, Blamey PT, Brown AM, Gusby PA, Dowell RC, Franz BK-H, Pyman BC, Shepherd RK, Tong YC, Webb RL, Hirshorn MS, Kuzuma J, Mecklenberg DJ, Money DK, Patrick JF, Seligman PM (1987) The University of Melbourne – Nucleus multi-electrode cochlear implant. In Pfaltz CR (ed.) (1987) Advances in Otology, Rhinology and Laryngology, Vol. 38. Basel: Karger.

Clark G, Franz B, Pyman B, Webb R (1991) Surgery for multichannel cochlear implantation. In Cooper H. (ed.) (1991) Cochlear Implants – A Practical Guide. London: Whurr, pp. 169-200.

Cohen NL (1994) The ethics of cochlear implants in young children. The American Journal of Otology 15 (suppl): 1-2.

Cohen NL, Hoffman RA (1991) Complications of cochlear implant surgery in adults and children. Annals of Otology, Rhinology and Laryngology 100: 708-11.

Cohen NL, Waltzman SB (1995) Influence of processing strategies on cochlear implant performance. Annals of Otology, Rhinology and Laryngology 104 (suppl 165): 9-15.

Cohen NL, Waltzman SB (1996) Cochlear implants in infants and young children. Seminars in Hearing 17: 215-21.

Cohen NL, Waltzman SB, Fisher SG (1993) A prospective randomised study of cochlear implants. New England Journal of Medicine 328: 233-7.

Cohen NL, Waltzman SB, Shapiro WH (1989) Telephone speech comprehension with the use of the Nucleus cochlear implant. Annals of Otology, Rhinology and Laryngology 98: 8-11.

Colletti V, Fiorino FG, Saccetto L, Giarbini N, Carner M (1999) Improved performance of cochlear implant patients using the middle fossa approach. Audiology 38: 225-34.

Cooper HR, Carpenter L, Alesky W, Booth CL, Read TE, Graham JM, Fraser JG (1989) UCH/RNID single channel extracochlear implant: results in 30 profoundly deaf adults. The Journal of Laryngology and Otology 18 (suppl): 22-38.

Cowan RSC, Brown C, Whitford LA, Galvin KL, Sarant JZ, Barker EJ, Shaw S, King A, Skok M, Seligman PM, Dowell RC, Everingham C, Gibson WPR, Clark GM (1995) Speech perception in children using the advanced (SPEAK) speech processing strategy. Annals of Otology, Rhinology and Laryngology 104 (suppl 166): 318-21.

Daspit CP (1991) Meningitis as a result of a cochlear implant: case report. Otolaryngology, Head and Neck Surgery 105: 115-16.

Davis A, Fortnum H, O'Donoghue G (1995) Children who could benefit from a cochlear implant: a European estimate of projected numbers, cost and relevant characteristics. International Journal of Pediatric Otorhinolaryngology 31: 221-33.

Dawson PW, Blamey PJ, Rowland LC, Dettman SJ, Clark GM, Busby PA, Brown AM, Dowell RC, Rickards FW (1992) Cochlear implants in children, adolescents and prelinguistically deafened adults: speech perception. Journal of Speech and Hearing Research 35: 401-17.

Dillier N, Battmer RD, Doring WH, Muller-Deile J (1995) Multicentric field evaluation of a spectral peak (SPEAK) cochlear implant speech coding strategy. Audiology 34: 145-59.

Dobie RA, Jenkins H, Cohen NL (1995) Surgical results. Annals of Otology, Rhinology and Laryngology 104 (suppl 165): 6-8.

Dorman MF, Loizou PC (1998) The identification of consonants and vowels by cochlear implant patients using a 6 channel CIS processor and normally hearing subjects using simulations of processors with 2 to 9 channels. Ear and Hearing 19: 162-6.

Dorman M, Loizou P, Rainey D (1997) Speech intelligibility as a function of the number of channels of stimulation for signal processors using sine-wave and noise band outputs. Journal of the Acoustical Society of America 102: 2403-11.

Dorman MF, Smith L, McCandless G, Dunnavant G, Parkin J, Dankonski K (1990) Pitch scaling and speech understanding by patients who use the Ineraid cochlear implant. Ear and Hearing 11: 310-15.

Dorman MF, Dove H, Parkin J, Zacharchuk S, Danowski K (1991) Telephone use by patients fitted with the Ineraid cochlear implant. Ear and Hearing 12: 368-9.

Downs MP, Owen Black F (1985) Cochlear implants for children? Counselling the parents. Seminars in Hearing 6: 91-5.

Doyle PJ, Pijl S, Noel FJ (1991) The cochlear implant: a comparison of single and multichannel results. The Journal of Laryngology and Otology 20: 204-8.

Eddington DK, Dobelle WH, Brackmann EE, Mladejovsky MG, Parkin JL (1978) Auditory prosthesis research with multiple channel intracochlear stimulation in man. Annals of Otology, Rhinology and Laryngology 87 (suppl 53): 1–39.

Eddington DK, Noel VA, Rabinowitz WM, Svirsky MA, Tierney J, Zissman MA (1994) Speech Processors for Auditory Prostheses. Ninth quarterly progress report, NIH project NO1-DC-2-2402, Massachusetts Institute of Technology, Research Laboratory of Electronics, Cambridge MA.

Eggermont JJ, Ponton CW, Don M, Waring MD, Kwong B (1997) Maturational delays in cortical evoked potentials in cochlear implant users. Acta Otolaryngology (Stockh) 17: 161–3.

Ertmer DJ, Kirk KI, Sehgal ST, Riley AI, Osberger MJ (1997) A comparison of vowel production by children with multichannel cochlear implants or tactile aids: perceptual evidence. Ear and Hearing 18: 307–15.

Eyles JA, Aleksy WL, Boyle PJ (1995) Performance changes in University College Hospital/ Royal National Institute for the Deaf single-channel cochlear implant users upgraded to the Nucleus 22 channel cochlear implant system. Annals of Otology, Rhinology and Laryngology 104 (suppl 166): 263–5.

Eyles JA, Pringle MB, Flynn SL, French ML (2000) Implantation with a Nucleus 22, an Ineraid Mk2, and a Med-el Combi 40+: a clinical case study. Poster presentation at the 6th International Cochlear Implant Conference, CI 2000, Miami Beach, Florida, 3-5 February.

Favre E, Pelizzone M (1993) Channel interactions in patients using the Ineraid multichannel cochlear implant. Hearing Research 66: 150–6.

Fayad J, Linthicium FH, Otto SR, Galey FR, House WF (1991) Cochlear implants: histopathological findings related to performance in 16 human temporal bones. Annals of Otology, Rhinology and Laryngology 100: 807–11.

Filipo R, Barbara M, Monini S, Mancini P (1999) Clarion cochlear implants: surgical implications. The Journal of Laryngology and Otology 113: 321–5.

Fishman KE, Shannon RV, Slattery WH (1997) Speech recognition as a function of the number of electrodes used in the SPEAK cochlear implant speech processor. Journal of Speech, Language and Hearing Research 40: 1201–15.

Fraser G (1991) The cochlear implant team. In Cooper H (ed.) Cochlear Implants – A Practical Guide. London: Whurr, pp. 84–91.

French ML (1999) Electrical impedance measurements with the CI24M cochlear implant for a child with Mondini dysplasia. British Journal of Audiology 33: 61–6.

Fryauf-Bertschy H, Tyler RS, Kelsay DMR, Gantz BJ, Woodworth GG (1997) Cochlear implant use by prelingually deafened children: the influences of age at implantation and length of device use. Journal of Speech, Language and Hearing 40: 183–99.

Fu Q-J, Shannon RV (1999) Effects of electrode configuration and frequency allocation on vowel recognition with the Nucleus 22 cochlear implant. Ear and Hearing 20: 332–44.

Fujita S, Ito J (1999) Ability of Nucleus cochlear implantees to recognise music. Annals of Otology, Rhinology and Laryngology 108: 634–40.

Gantz BJ, Tyler RS, Knutson JF, Woodworth GG, Abbas P, McCabe BF, Hinrichs J, Tye-Murray N, Lansing C, Kuk F, Brown C (1988) Evaluation of 5 different cochlear implant designs: audiological assessment and predictors of performance. The Laryngoscope 98: 1100–6.

Gantz BJ, Lowder MW, McCabe BF (1989) Audiological results following reimplantation of cochlear implants. Annals of Otology, Rhinology and Laryngology 98: 12–16.

Gantz BJ, Tyler RS, Woodworth GG, Tye-Murray N, Fryauf-Bertschy H (1994) Results of multichannel cochlear implants in congenitally deaf and prelingually deafened children. The American Journal of Otology 15 (suppl 2): 1-8.

Geers AE, Moog JS (1991) Evaluating the benefit of cochlear implants in an educational setting. The American Journal of Otology 12 (suppl): 116-25.

Gersdorff M (1991) Results of cochlear implants in children. Acta Otologica-Rhinologica-Laryngologica Belgium 45: 293-5.

Gibbin KP, O'Donoghue GM, Murty GE (1993) Paediatric cochlear implantation: the Nottingham surgical experience. In Hochmair-Desoyer IJ, Hochmair ES (eds) Advances in Cochlear Implants. Austria: Manz Wein, pp. 230-2.

Giles EC (1993) An outline of telephone training procedures at the Manchester cochlear implant centre. In Hochmair-Desoyer IJ, Hochmair ES (eds) Advances in Cochlear Implants. Austria: Manz Wein, pp. 604-6.

Graham J, Lynch C, Weber L, Stollwerck L, Wei J, Brookes G (1999) The magnetless Clarion cochlear implant in a patient with neurofibromatosis 2. Journal of Laryngology and Otology 113: 458-63.

Gray R, Evans RA, Freer CEL, Szutowicz HE, Maskell GF (1991) Radiology for cochlear implants. Journal of Laryngology and Otology 105: 85-8.

Gstoettner W, Plenk H, Franz P, Hamzavi J, Baumgartner W, Czerny C, Ehrenberger K (1997) Cochlear implant deep electrode insertion: extent of insertional trauma. Acta Otolaryngology (Stockh) 117: 274-7.

Harnsberger HR, Dart DJ, Parkin JL, Smoker WRK, Osborn AG (1987) Cochlear implant candidates: assessments with CT and MR imaging. Radiology 164: 53-7.

Heller J, Brackmann D, Tucci D, Nyenhuis J, Chou C (1996) Evaluation of MRI compatibility of the modified Nucleus multichannel auditory brainstem and cochlear implants. The American Journal of Otology 17: 724-9.

Hellman SA, Chute PM, Kretschner RE, Nevins ME, Parisier SC, Thurston LC (1991) The development of a children's implant profile. AAD/Reference 136: 77-81.

Helms J, Muller J, Schon F, Moser L, Arnold W, Janssen T, Ramsden R, Schon F, Von Ilberg C, Kiefer J, Pfennigdorff T, Gstottner W, Baumgartner W, Ehrenberger K, Sharzyinski H, Ribari O, Thumfart W, Stephan K, Mann W, Heinmann M, Zorowka P, Lippert KL, Zenner HJ, Bohndorf M, Huttenbrink K, Muller-Aschoff E, Hofmann G, Fiegang B, Begall K, Ziese M, Frogbert O, Hausler R, Vischer M, Schlatter T, Schlodorff G, Korves B, Doring H, Gerhardt HJ, Wagner H, Schorn K, Schilling V, Baumann U, Kastenbauer E, Albegger K, Mair A, Gammert Ch, Mathis A, Streitberger Ch, Hochmair-Desoyer I (1997) Evaluation of performance with the Combi 40 cochlear implant in adults: a multicentric clinical study. ORL 59: 23-35.

Hochmair-Desoyer IJ (1986) Fitting of an analogue cochlear prosthesis – introduction of a new method and preliminary findings. British Journal of Audiology 20: 45-53.

Hodges AV, Balkany TJ, Ruth RA, Lambert PR, Dolan-Ash S, Schloffman JJ (1999) Electrical middle ear muscle reflex: use in cochlear implant programming. Otolaryngology, Head and Neck Surgery 117: 255-61.

Hoffman RA, Cohen NL (1993) Surgical pitfalls in cochlear implantation. Laryngoscope 103: 741-4.

Hoffman RA, Cohen N, Waltzman S, Shapiro W (1991) Delayed extrusion of the Nucleus multichannel cochlear implant. Otolaryngology, Head and Neck Surgery 105: 117-19.

Hortman G, Pulec JL, Causse JB, Causse JR, Briand C, Fontaine JP, Tetu F, Azema B (1989) Experience with the extracochlear multichannel implex system. In Fraysse B (ed.) Cochlear Implant Acquisitions and Controversies. Basel: Cochlear, pp. 307-17.

House WF, Berliner KI (1986) Safety and efficacy of the House/3M cochlear implant in profoundly deaf adults. Otolaryngology Clinics of North America 19: 275-6.

House WF, Berliner K, Crary W, Graham M, Luckey R, Norton N, Selters W, Tobin H, Urban J, Wexler M (1976) Cochlear implants. Annals of Otology, Rhinology and Laryngology 85 (suppl 27): 1-93.

Huarte AI, Molina M, Manrique M (1996) Auditory pre-training and its implications for child development: the importance of early stimulation in the deaf child. In Allum DJ (ed.) (1996) Cochlear Implant Rehabilitation in Children and Adults. London: Whurr, pp. 131-43.

Inscoe J (1999) Communication outcomes after paediatric cochlear implantation. International Journal of Pediatric Otorhinolaryngology 47: 195-200.

Jackler RK, Leake PA, McKerrow WS (1989) Cochlear implant revision: effects of reimplantation on the cochlea. Annals of Otology, Rhinology and Laryngology 98: 813-20.

Kasper A, Pelizzone M, Montandon P (1991) Intracochlear potential distribution with intracochlear and extracochlear electrical stimulation in humans. Annals of Otology, Rhinology and Laryngology 100: 812-16.

Kawano A, Seldon HL, Clark GM, Ramsden RT, Raine CH (1998) Intracochlear factors contributing to psychophysical percepts following cochlear implantation. Acta Otolaryngology (Stockh) 118: 313-26.

Kiefer J, Muller J, Pfennigdorff T, Schon F, Helms J, Von Ilberg C, Baumgartner W, Gstottner W, Ehrenberger K, Arnold W, Stephan K, Thumfart W (1996) Speech understanding in quiet and noise with the CIS speech coding strategy (Med-el Combi 40) compared to the multipeak and spectral peak strategies (Nucleus). ORL 58: 127-35.

Kiefer J, Von Ilberg C, Reimer B, Knecht R, Diller G, Sturzebecher E, Pfennigdorff T, Spelsberg A (1998) Results of cochlear implantation in patients with severe to profound hearing loss – implications for patient selection. Audiology 37: 382-95.

Kiefer J, Von Ilberg C, Rupprecht V, Huber-Egener J, Baumgartner W, Gstottner W, Forgasi K, Stephan K (2000) Optimised speech understanding with the speech coding strategy in cochlear implants: the effect of variations in stimulus rate and number of channels. In Waltzman SB, Cohen NL (eds) Cochlear Implants. New York: Thieme, pp. 339-40.

King A (1991) Audiological assessment and hearing aid trials. In Cooper H (ed.) Cochlear Implants – A Practical Guide. London: Whurr, pp. 101-8.

Kirk KI, Sehgal M, Miyamoto RT (1997) Speech perception performance of Nucleus multichannel cochlear implant users with partial electrode insertions. Ear and Hearing 18: 456-71.

Kompis M, Vischer MW, Hausler R (1999) Performance of compressed analogue (CA) and continuous interleaved sampling (CIS) coding strategies for cochlear implants in quiet and noise. Acta Otolaryngology (Stockh) 119: 659-64.

Lane H (1995) Letter to the editor. The American Journal of Otology 16: 1-6.

Lawson DT, Wilson BS, Zerbi M, Finley CC (1996) Speech processors for auditory prostheses. Third quarterly progress report, NIH project NO1-DC-5-2103, Neural Prosthesis program, National Institutes of Health, Bethesda, MD.

Leake PA, Synder RL, Rebscher SJ, Hradek GT, Moore CM, Vollmer M, Sato M (2000) Long term effects of deafness and chronic electrical stimulation of the cochlea. In Waltzman SB, Cohen NL (eds) Cochlear Implants. New York: Thieme, pp. 31–42.

Lenarz T, Battmer RD (1995) First results with the Spectra 22 speech processor at the Medizinsche Hochschule Hannover. Annals of Otology, Rhinology and Laryngology 104 (suppl 166): 285–7.

Lenarz T, Battmer RD, Bertram B (2000) Cochlear implants in children under 2 years of age. In Waltzman SB, Cohen NL (eds) Cochlear Implants. New York: Thieme, pp. 163–5.

Ling D (1988) Foundations of Spoken Language for Hearing Impaired Children. Washington DC: Alexander Graham Bell Association for the Deaf.

Linthicum FH, Fayad J, Otto S, Galey F, House W (1991) Inner ear morphological changes resulting from cochlear implantation. The American Journal of Otology 12 (suppl): 8–10.

Loizou P (1998) Mimicking the human ear. An overview of signal processing strategies for converting sound into electrical signals in cochlear implants. IEEE Signal Processing Magazine Sept 1053-5888: 101–30.

Loizou PC, Dorman M, Fitzke J (2000) The effect of reduced dynamic range on speech understanding: implications for patients with cochlear implants. Ear and Hearing 21: 25–31.

Luetje CM, Jackson K (1997) Cochlear implants in children: what constitutes a complication. Otolaryngology, Head and Neck Surgery 117: 243–7.

Luntz M, Balkany T, Hodges AV, Telischi FF (1997) Cochlear implants in children with congenital inner ear malformations. Archives of Otolaryngology, Head and Neck Surgery 123: 974–7.

Lutman ME, Archbold S, Gibbin KP, McCormick B, O'Donoghue GM (1996) Monitoring progress in young children with cochlear implants. In Allum DJ (ed.) Cochlear Implant Rehabilitation in Children and Adults. London: Whurr, pp. 31–51.

MacPhearson BJ, Elfenbein JL, Schum RL, Bentler RA (1991) Thresholds of discomfort in young children. Ear and Hearing 12: 184–90.

Manolson HA (1992) It Takes Two to Talk: A Parent's Guide to Helping Children Communicate. Toronto: The Hanen Centre.

Mason S, Sheppard S, Garnham CW, Lutman M, O'Donoghue G, Gibbin K (1993) Improving the relationship of intraoperative EABR threshold to T-level in young children receiving the Nucleus cochlear implant. In Hochmair-Desoyer IJ, Hochmair ES (eds) Advances in Cochlear Implants. Austria: Manz Wein, pp. 44–9.

Maxwell AP, Mason SM, O'Donoghue GM (1999) Cochlear nerve aplasia: its importance in cochlear implantation. The American Journal of Otology 20: 335–7.

McCormick B (1977) The toy discrimination test: an aid for screening the hearing of children above the mental age of 2 years. Public Health 91: 67–73.

McCormick B (1991) Paediatric cochlear implantation in the United Kingdom – a delayed journey on a well marked route. British Journal of Audiology 25: 145–9.

McCormick B (2001) Assessing audiological suitability. In McCormick B, Archbold SM (eds) Cochlear Implants for Young Children. London: Whurr.

McCreery DB, Agnew WF, Yuon TGH, Bullara L (1990) Charge density and charge per phase as cofactors in neural injury induced by electrical stimulation. IEEE Transactions on Biomedical Engineering BME-37: 996–1001.

McDermott HJ, McKay CM (1997) Musical pitch perception with electrical stimulation of the cochlea. Journal of the Acoustical Society of America 101: 1622-31.

Mecklenburg DJ, Blamey PJ, Busby PA, Dowell RC, Roberts S, Rickards FW (1990) Auditory (re)habilitation for deaf children and teenagers. In Clark GM, Tong YC, Patrick JF (eds) Cochlear Prostheses. London: Churchill Livingstone, pp. 207-21.

Meyer EA, Svirsky MA, Kirk KI, Miyamoto RT (1998) Improvements in speech perception by children with profound prelingual hearing loss: effects of device, communication mode and chronological age. Journal of Speech, Language and Hearing Research 41: 846-58.

Miller J (1991) Physiological measures of electrically evoked auditory system responsiveness: effects of pathology and electrical stimulation. The American Journal of Otology 12 (suppl): 28-36.

Miyamoto RT, Svirsky MA, Robbins AM (1997) Enhancement of expressive language in prelingually deaf children with cochlear implants. Acta Otolaryngology (Stockh) 117: 154-7.

Miyamoto RT, Kirk KI, Todd SL, Robbins AM, Osberger MJ (1995) Speech perception skills of children with multichannel cochlear implants or hearing aids. Annals of Otology, Rhinology and Laryngology 104 (suppl 166): 334-7.

Miyamoto RT, Young M, Myers WA, Kessler K, Wolfert K, Kirk KI (1996) Complications of pediatric cochlear implantation. European Archives of Otorhinolaryngology 253: 1-4.

Miyamoto RT, Svirsky MA, Myers WA, Kirk KI, Schutz J (1997) Cochlear implant reimplantation. The American Journal of Otology 18: 560-1.

Miyamoto RT, Kirk KI, Svirsky MA, Sehgal ST (1999a) Communication skills in pediatric cochlear implant recipients. Acta Otolaryngology (Stockh) 119: 219-24.

Miyamoto RT, Kirk KI, Renshaw J, Hussain D (1999b) Cochlear implantation in auditory neuropathy. The Laryngoscope 109: 181-5.

Nadol JB (1997) Patterns of neural degeneration in the human cochlear and auditory nerve: implications for cochlear implantation. Otolaryngology, Head and Neck Surgery 117: 220-8.

Nadol JB, Young Y-S, Glynn RJ (1989) Survival of spiral ganglion cells in profound sensorineural hearing loss: implications for cochlear implantation. Annals of Otology, Rhinology and Laryngology 98: 411-16.

Nelson DA, van Tassel DJ, Schroeder AC, Soli S, Levine S (1995) Electrode ranking of 'place pitch' and speech recognition in electrical hearing. Journal of the Acoustic Society of America 98: 1987-99.

Nikolopoulos TP, Archbold SM, O'Donoghue GM (1999) The development of auditory perception in children following implantation. International Journal of Pediatric Otorhinolarngology 49 (suppl 1): s189-s191.

Niparko JK, Oviatt DL, Coker NJ, Sutton L, Waltzman SB, Cohen NL (1991) Facial nerve stimulation with cochlear implantation. Otolaryngology, Head and Neck Surgery 104: 826-30.

O'Donoghue GM, Nikolopoulos TP, Archbold SM, Tait M (1998) Speech perception in children after cochlear implantation. The American Journal of Otology 19: 762-7.

O'Neill C, O'Donoghue GM, Archbold SM, Normand C (2000) A cost-utility analysis of pediatric cochlear implantation. The Laryngoscope 110: 156-60.

Osberger MJ, Robbins AM, Miyamoto RT, Berry SW, Myers WA, Kessler KS, Pope ML (1991a) Speech perception abilities of children with cochlear implants, tactile aids and hearing aids. The American Journal of Otology 12 (suppl): 105-15.

Osberger MJ, Robbins AM, Berry SW, Todd SL, Hesketh LJ, Sedley A (1991b) Spontaneous speech samples of children with cochlear implants or tactile aids. The American Journal of Otology 12 (suppl): 151-64.

Osberger MJ, Robbins A, Todd S, Riley A, Kirk K, Carney A (1996) Cochlear implants and tactile aids for children with profound hearing impairment. In Bess F, Gravel J, Tharpe AM (eds) Amplification for Children with Auditory Deficits. Nashville TN: Bill Wilkerson Centre Press, pp. 283-308.

Ousey J, Sheppard S, Twomey T, Palmer AR (1989) The IHR/McCormick automated toy discrimination test – description and initial evaluation. British Journal of Audiology 23: 245-50.

Parisier SC, Chute PM, Popp AL (1996) Cochlear implantation mechanical failures. American Journal of Otology 17: 730-4.

Parisier SC, Chute PM, Weiss MH, Hellman SA, Wang RC (1991) Results of cochlear implant reinsertion. The Laryngoscope 101: 1013-15.

Parkin J, Stewart BE (1988) Multichannel cochlear implantation: Utah design. The Laryngoscope 98: 262-5.

Parkinson AJ, El-Kholy W, Tyler RS (1998) Vowel perception in prelingually deafened children with multichannel cochlear implants. Journal of the American Academy of Audiology 9: 179-90.

Pelizzone M, Cosendai G, Tinembart J (1999) Within-patient longitudinal speech reception measures with continuous interleaved sampling processors for Ineraid implanted subjects. Ear and Hearing 20: 228-37.

Pfingst BE, Spelman FA, Sutton D (1980) Operating ranges for cochlear implants. Annals of Otology, Rhinology and Laryngology 89 (suppl 66): 1-4.

Pisoni DB (2000) Cognitive factors and cochlear implants: some thoughts on perception, learning and memory in speech perception. Ear and Hearing 21: 70-8.

Portnoy WM, Mattucci K (1991) Cochlear implants as a contraindication to magnetic resonance imaging. Annals of Otology, Rhinology and Laryngology 100: 195-7.

Quality Standards in Paediatric Audiology. Volume III (1999) Cochlear Implants for Children. Joint review by the National Deaf Children's Society and the British Cochlear Implant Group.

Quittner AL, Thompson J (1991) Predictors of cochlear implant use in children. The American Journal of Otology 12 (suppl): 89-94.

Quittner AL, Thompson Steck J, Rouiller R (1991) Cochlear implants in children: a study of parental stress and adjustment. The American Journal of Otology 12 (suppl): 95-104.

Ray J, Gray RF, Court I (1998) Surgical removal of 11 cochlear implants – lessons from the 11 year Cambridge programme. The Journal of Laryngology and Otology 112: 338-43.

Richardson HC, Beliaeff M, Clarke G, Hawthorne M (1999) A three array cochlear implant: a new approach for the ossified cochlea. The Journal of Laryngology and Otology 113: 811-14.

Robbins AM, Kirk KI (1996) Speech perception assessment and performance in pediatric cochlear implant users. Seminars in Hearing 17: 353-69.

Robbins AM, Renshaw JJ, Berry SW (1991) Evaluating meaningful auditory integration in profoundly hearing impaired children. The American Journal of Otology 12 (suppl): 144-50.

Ruben RJ (1997) A time frame of critical/sensitive periods of language development. Acta Otolaryngology (Stockh) 117: 202-5.

Rubenstein JT, Parkinson WS, Tyler RS, Gantz BJ (1999) Residual speech recognition and cochlear implant performance: effects of implantation criteria. The American Journal of Otology 20: 1-7.

Ryals BM, Rubel EW, Lippe W (1991) Issues in neural plasticity as related to cochlear implants in children. The American Journal of Otology 12 (suppl): 22-7.

Sehgal ST, Kirk KI, Svirsky M, Miyamoto RT (1998) The effects of speech processor strategy on the speech perception performance of pediatric Nucleus multichannel cochlear implant users. Ear and Hearing 19: 149-61.

Seidman DA, Chute PM, Parisier S (1994) Temporal bone imaging for cochlear implantation. Laryngoscope 104: 562-5.

Selmi A (1985) Monitoring and evaluating the educational effects of the cochlear implant. Ear and Hearing 6 (suppl): 52s-59s.

Shallop JK, McGiun-Brunelli T (1995) Speech recognition performance over time with the Spectra 22 speech processor. Annals of Otology, Rhinology and Laryngology 104 (suppl 166): 306-7.

Shallop JK, Facer GW, Peterson A (1999). Neural response telemetry with the Nucleus CI24M cochlear implant. The Laryngoscope 109: 1755-9.

Shallop JK, Beiter AL, Goin DW, Mischke RE (1990) Electrically evoked auditory brainstem responses (EABR) and middle latency responses (EMLR) obtained from patients with the Nucleus multichannel cochlear implant. Ear and Hearing 11: 5-15.

Shallop JK, Goin DW, van Dyke L, Mischke RE (1991) Prediction of behavioural threshold and comfort values for Nucleus 22 channel implant patients from electrical auditory brainstem response test results. Annals of Otology, Rhinology and Laryngology 100: 896-8.

Shepherd RK, Franz BK-HG, Clark G (1990) The biocompatibility and safety of cochlear prostheses. In Clark G, Tong YC, Patrick JF (eds) Cochlear Prostheses. London: Churchill Livingstone, pp. 69-98.

Shepherd RK, Hartmann R, Fleid S, Hardie N, Klinke R (1997) The central auditory system and auditory deprivation: experience with cochlear implants in the congenitally deaf. Acta Otolaryngology (Stockh) 532 (suppl): 28-33.

Shipp DB, Nedzelski JM (1991) Round window versus promontory stimulation - assessment for cochlear implant candidacy. Annals of Otology, Rhinology and Laryngology 100: 889-92.

Simmons FB (1966) Electrical stimulation of the auditory nerve in man. Archives of Otolaryngology, Chicago 84: 2-54.

Skinner MW, Holden LK, Holden TA (1995) Effect of frequency boundary assignment on speech recognition with the SPEAK speech coding strategy. Annals of Otology, Rhinology and Laryngology 104 (suppl 166): 307-9.

Skinner MW, Clark GM, Whitford LA, Seligman PM, Staller SJ, Shipp DB, Shallop JK, Everingham C, Menapace CM, Arndt PL, Antogenelli T, Brimacombe JA, Pijl S, Daniels P, George CR, McDermott HJ, Beiter AL (1994) Evaluation of the new spectral peak (SPEAK) coding strategy for the Nucleus 22 channel cochlear implant system. The American Journal of Otology 15 (suppl 2): 15-27.

Slattery WH, Luxford WM (1995) Cochlear implantation in the congenital malformed cochlea. Laryngoscope 105:1184-7.

Snik Ad FM, Vermeulen AM, Geelen CP, Brokx JPL, Van den Broek P (1997) Speech perception performance of children with a cochlear implant compared to that of children with conventional hearing aids II. Results of prelingually deaf children. Acta Otolaryngology (Stockh.) 117: 755–9.

Somers M (1991) Effects of cochlear implants in children: implications for rehabilitation. In Cooper H (ed.) (1991) Cochlear Implants – A Practical Guide. London: Whurr, pp. 322–45.

Spencer LJ, Tye-Murray N, Tomblin JB (1998) The production of English inflection morphology, speech production and listening performance in children with cochlear implants. Ear and Hearing 19: 310–18.

Spencer LJ, Tye-Murray N, Kelsay DMR, Teagle H (1998) Learning to use a cochlear implant: a child who beat the odds. American Journal of Audiology 7: 24–9.

Staecker H, Van der Water TR (2000) Regeneration, repair and protection in the inner ear: implications for cochlear implantation. In Waltzman SB, Cohen NL (eds) (2000) Cochlear Implants. New York: Thieme, pp. 17–30.

Staller S, Beiter AL, Brimacombe JA, Mecklenburg DJ, Arndt P (1991) Paediatric performance with the Nucleus 22 channel cochlear implant system. The American Journal of Otology 12 (suppl): 126–36.

Starczewski H, Lloyd H (1999) Using stories / narrative assessment procedure (SNAP) to monitor language and communication changes after a cochlear implant: a case study. Deafness and Education International 1: 137–54.

Stephan K, Welzl-Muller K, Stiglbrumer H (1991) Acoustic reflex in patients with cochlear implants (analogue stimulation). The American Journal of Otology 12 (suppl): 48–51.

Summerfield AQ, Marshall DH (1995) Cochlear implantation in the UK 1990–1994. Report by the MRC Institute of Hearing Research on the Evaluation of the National Cochlear Implant Programme. Nottingham: MRC Institute of Hearing Research.

Summerfield AQ, Marshall DH (1999) Paediatric cochlear implantation and health-technology assessment. International Journal of Pediatric Otorhinolaryngology 47: 141–51.

Szilvassy J, Czigner J, Somogyi I, Jori J, Kiss JG, Szilvassy Z (1998) Cochlear implantation in a patient with grand mal epilepsy. The Journal of Laryngology and Otology 112: 567–9.

Tait DM (1987) Making and monitoring progress in the pre-school years. Journal of the British Association of Teachers of the Deaf 11: 143–53.

Tait M, Lutman ME (1994) Comparison of early communicative behaviour in young children with cochlear implants and with hearing aids. Ear and Hearing 15: 352–61.

Tait M, Lutman ME (1997) The predictive value of measures of preverbal communicative behaviours in young deaf children with cochlear implants. Ear and Hearing 18: 472–8.

Tait DM, Wood DJ (1987) From communication to speech in deaf children. Child Language, Teaching and Therapy 3: 1–17.

Tait M, Lutman ME, Robinson K (2000) Pre-implant measures of preverbal communicative behaviour as predictors of cochlear implant outcomes in children. Ear and Hearing 21: 18–24.

Teissl C, Kremser C, Hochmair ES, Hochmair-Desoyer IJ (1998) Cochlear implants: in vitro investigation of electromagnetic interference at MR imaging – compatibility and safety aspects. Radiology 208: 700–8.

Terr LI, Sfogliano GA, Riley SL (1989) Effects of stimulation by cochlear implants on the cochlear nerve. The Laryngoscope 99: 1171-4.

Tucci DL, Lambert PR, Ruth RA (1990) Trends in rehabilitation after cochlear implantation. Archives of Otolaryngology Head and Neck Surgery 116: 571-4.

Tucci DL, Telian SA, Zimmerman-Phillips S, Zwolan TA, Kileny PR (1995) Cochlear implantation in patients with cochlear malformations. Archives of Otolaryngology Head and Neck Surgery 121: 833-8.

Twomey T, Archbold S (1997) Electrode and device problems: manifestation and management. The American Journal of Otology 18: s99-s100.

Tye-Murray N, Spencer L, Witt S, Bedia EG (1996) Parent and patient centred aural rehabilitation. In Allum DJ (ed.) Cochlear Implant Rehabilitation in Children and Adults. London: Whurr, pp. 65-82.

Tyler RS (1993) Speech perception by children. In Tyler RS (ed.) Cochlear Implants – Audiological Foundations. San Diego: Singular, pp. 191-256.

Tyler RS, Summerfield AQ (1996) Cochlear implantation: relationships with research on auditory deprivation and acclimatisation. Ear and Hearing 17: 38S-50S.

Tyler RS, Gantz BJ, Woodworth GG, Parkinson AJ, Lowder MW, Schum LK (1996) Initial independent results with the Clarion cochlear implant. Ear and Hearing 17: 528-36.

Tyler RS, Gantz BJ, Woodworth GG, Fryauf-Bertschy H, Kelsay DMR (1997) Performance of 2 and 3 year old children and prediction of 4 year from 1 year performance. The American Journal of Otology 18: s157-s159.

Van Dijk JE, Van Olphen AF, Langereis MC, Mens LHM, Brokx JPL, Smoorenburg GF (1999) Predictors of cochlear implant performance. Audiology 38: 109-16.

Van Hoesel RJM, Clark GM (1999) Speech results with a bilateral multichannel cochlear implant subject for spatially separated signal and noise. The Australian Journal of Audiology 21: 23-8.

Von Wallenberg EL, Battmer RD (1991) Comparative speech recognition results in eight subjects using two different coding strategies with the Nucleus 22 channel cochlear implant. British Journal of Audiology 25: 371-80.

Von Wallenberg EL, Brinch JM (1995) Cochlear implant reliability. Annals of Otology, Rhinology and Laryngology 104 (suppl 166): 441-3.

Von Wallenberg EL, Laszig R, Gnadeberg D, Battmer R, Desloovere C, Kiefer J, Lehnhardt E, Von Ilberg C (1993) Initial findings with the modified Nucleus implant comprised of 20 active intracochlear and 2 extracochlear reference electrodes. In Hochmair-Desoyer IJ, Hochmair ES (eds) (1993) Advances in Cochlear Implants. Austria: Manz Wein, pp. 186-92.

Waltzman SB, Cohen NL, Gromolin RH, Shapiro WH, Ozdamar SR, Hoffman RA (1994) Long term results of early cochlear implantation in congenitally and prelingually deaf children. The American Journal of Otology 15 (suppl 2): 9-13.

Webb RL, Pyman BC, Franz BK-HG, Clark GM (1990) The surgery of cochlear implantation. In Clark GM, Tong YC (eds) Cochlear Prostheses. London: Churchill Livingstone, pp. 153-80.

Weber BP, Neuburger J, Koestler H, Goldring JE, Battmer R, Santogrossi T, Lenarz T (1999) Clinical results of the Clarion magnetless cochlear implant. Annals of Otology, Rhinology and Laryngology 108: 22-6.

Weston SC, Waltzman SB (1995) Performance as a function of time: a study of three cochlear implant devices. Annals of Otology, Rhinology, Laryngology 104 (suppl 165): 19-24.

Wilson BS (1997) The future of cochlear implants. British Journal of Audiology 31: 205-25.

Wilson BS, Finley CC, Lawson DT, Wolford RD, Eddington DK, Rabinowitz WM (1991) Better speech recognition with cochlear implants. Nature 352: 236-8.

Wilson BS, Lawson DT, Zerbi M, Finley CC, Wolford RD (1995) New processing strategies in cochlear implantation. The American Journal of Otology 16: 669-75.

Wood DJ, Wood HA, Griffiths AJ, Howarth CT (1986) Teaching and Talking with Deaf Children. London and New York: John Wiley.

Wood EJ, Flynn SL, Eyles JA (2000) The benefit of using an FM radio aid system with cochlear implant users. Poster presented at the 6th International Cochlear Implant Conference, CI 2000, Miami Beach, Florida 3-5 February.

Woolley AL, Oser AB, Lusk RP, Bahadori RS (1997) Preoperative temporal bone computed tomography scan and its use in evaluating the pediatric cochlear implant candidate. Laryngoscope 107: 1100-6.

Yune HY, Miyamoto RT, Yune ME (1991) Medical imaging in cochlear implant candidates. The American Journal of Otology 12 (suppl): 11-17.

Zeng F-G, Galvin JJ (1999) Amplitude mapping and phoneme recognition in cochlear implant listeners. Ear and Hearing 20: 60-74.

Zimmerman-Phillips MS, Murad C (1999) Programming features of the Clarion multi-strategy cochlear implant. Annals of Otology, Rhinology and Laryngology 108: 17-21.

Index

3M House implant 427
3M Vienna implant 427

ABaer (Biologic Corp) 246
acoustic admittance 340
 cochlear implantation 450
 Eustachian tubes 334-5
 middle-ear function 316-22, 328-9,
   332, 339-42
 peak static 319, 320-1, 329, 335,
   342
acoustic conductance 322, 340, 342
acoustic dampers 391, 393
acoustic immittance 109, 320-1, 340,
   341-2
acoustic impedance 315, 340-1, 423
 cochlear implantation 449
 hearing aid performance 387, 395
 middle-ear function 316-17, 319,
   340-1
 pure-tone audiometry 177-8, 179,
   183
acoustic leakage 166, 167
acoustic nerve 346, 397
acoustic reactance 322, 340
acoustic reflectometry 316, 332-4, 340
acoustic reflex delay (ARD) 330, 332,
   341
acoustic reflex threshold (ART) 109,
   329-32, 341
acoustic resistance 341
acoustic stapedial reflex 67, 254, 300,
   328-32, 341, 423
 calibration 339
 cochlear implantation 253, 254,
   442, 460

pure-tone audiometry 178
TMD 336
tympanometry 320
see also electrically evoked
   stapedial reflex (ESR)
acoustic stimulation including middle
   latency response (EMLR) 254
acoustic susceptance 322, 341, 342
acquired hearing loss 45, 48, 204, 249,
   359
 aetiology 14-15, 470
 age 31
 cochlear implantation 429, 436,
   441, 467-9
 prevalence 7-9
 risk factors 12-13, 18, 21
acquired stenosis 47
active electrodes
 ABR 214, 215-16
 ACR 201
 cochlear implantation 427-8,
   432-3, 451, 454, 456-7, 459
 MLR 198
acute mastoiditis 50
acute otitis media 317
acute supporative otitis media (ASOM)
   48, 50
 infection 49, 50, 51, 56
adaptation 204
adenoidectomy 54, 55, 58
adenoiditis 51
adhesive otitis media 49, 57
advanced combination encoder (ACE)
   strategy 431, 435, 456, 458, 472
aetiology of hearing loss 2, 13-15, 22,
   42, 470-1